TELLTALE
HEARTS

TELLTALE HEARTS

A PUBLIC HEALTH DOCTOR,
HIS PATIENTS, AND
THE POWER OF STORY

Dean-David Schillinger, MD

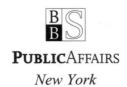

PUBLICAFFAIRS

New York

PublicAffairs
Hachette Book Group
1290 Avenue of the Americas, New York, NY 10104
www.publicaffairsbooks.com
@Public_Affairs

Printed in the United States of America

First Edition: July 2024

Published by PublicAffairs, an imprint of Hachette Book Group, Inc. The PublicAffairs name and logo is a registered trademark of the Hachette Book Group.

This book contains the opinions and ideas of its author. It is intended to provide helpful and informative material on the subject addressed. It is sold with the understanding that the author and publisher are not engaged in rendering medical, health, or any other kind of personal or professional services in the book. Readers should consult with their own medical, health, or other professional before drawing inferences from this book.

Names and identifying characteristics of all patients and most other individuals have been changed. Some dialogue has been re-created.

The Hachette Speakers Bureau provides a wide range of authors for speaking events. To find out more, go to hachettespeakersbureau.com or email HachetteSpeakers@hbgusa.com.

PublicAffairs books may be purchased in bulk for business, educational, or promotional use. For more information, please contact your local bookseller or the Hachette Book Group Special Markets Department at special.markets@hbgusa.com.

The publisher is not responsible for websites (or their content) that are not owned by the publisher.

Print book interior design by Amy Quinn.

Library of Congress Cataloging-in-Publication Data
Names: Schillinger, Dean-David, author.
Title: Telltale hearts : a public health doctor, his patients, and the
    power of story / Dean-David Schillinger.
Description: First edition. | New York : PublicAffairs, 2024. | Includes index.
Identifiers: LCCN 2023047479 | ISBN 9781541704206 (hardcover) |
    ISBN 9781541704220 (ebook)
Subjects: LCSH: Public health—United States. | Medical policy—United States. |
    Discrimination in medical care—United States. | Physician and patient—United States.
Classification: LCC RA395.A3 S3663 2024 | DDC 362.10973—dc23/eng/20240202
LC record available at https://lccn.loc.gov/2023047479

ISBNs: 9781541704206 (hardcover), 9781541704220 (ebook)

LSC

Printing 1, 2024

For my children, Micaela, Gabriel, and Eytan

Contents

viii   Contents

PART 3: STORY AS CATALYST

Chapter 18: Walking on Coals: Melanie's Story   227

Chapter 19: Melanie Goes to the State Capitol   237

Chapter 20: Melanie Goes to Court   251

Chapter 21: Melanie Goes to City Hall   259

Chapter 22: Melanie Goes Onstage   277

  Epilogue: Song for My Father: To the Dark Side and Back Again 299

             Acknowledgments   327

             Credits   331

TELLTALE
HEARTS

Prologue

AT THE PEAK OF MY CAREER AS A PHYSICIAN, MODERN MEDICINE NEARLY killed me. The year was 2010, and I was forty-five years old, happily married with three children, and had just become the chief of the Division of Internal Medicine at San Francisco General, arguably the country's finest public hospital. I had been promoted to full professor at the University of California and was a successful researcher and public health expert. I felt I had made it in medicine and, perhaps, in life.

My crisis began during a weeklong holiday on a Caribbean island where my extended family had come together to celebrate my father's eightieth birthday. I had eagerly looked forward to windsurfing, playing tennis with my brothers, and dancing at night. But I had no energy for any of it. Instead, I was overcome with a profound fatigue that forced me to sleep fourteen hours a day and made me unable to walk on the beach without getting muscular pains. I could not even write the toast I had planned to pay tribute to the longevity and success of my amazing father, who, as a Jewish teenager during World War II, had survived a year in a Nazi concentration camp and then endured solitary confinement in a Soviet prison after the war.

Back in San Francisco, my physicians carefully considered the long list of medical conditions that could be causing my symptoms. Was it hepatitis? Leptospirosis? Lyme disease, or its Caribbean cousin, babesiosis? Thyroid disease? Heart failure? Could I have acquired HIV from a needlestick at the hospital? I underwent extensive blood work and imaging studies.

But all the tests came back normal.

Over the following months, I deteriorated until I became largely confined to bed. While I managed to drag myself into work for my clinic sessions, my research and administrative work suffered. My ability to concentrate de-clined, my intellectual stamina waned, and I fell further and further behind. My day-to-day life was characterized by cycles of daytime sleep, nighttime insomnia, crying spells peppered with bouts of anxiety and panic, and an inability to interact with others in any way except to describe my physical weakness, despondency, fear, and guilt. I couldn't care for my children; my wife took on the full load. I ruminated endlessly over my sudden and seem-ingly permanent failings as a doctor, spouse, and father.

I couldn't face the possibility that I needed to request a medical leave due to what appeared to be an episode of major depression. I was afraid of being cast out by my colleagues, stripped of my titles, and told to surrender my re-search grants. Worst of all, I was convinced that being labeled mentally ill would jeopardize my hospital privileges, preventing me from working as a primary care physician for my patients, whose complex care benefited from the continuity and partnership with them that I had carefully fostered over decades.

I began to think about suicide. I hid a stash of Ativan in my sock drawer. I had nightly fantasies of sneaking out to the Golden Gate Bridge and jumping.

Eventually, I had no choice but to put a formal request in for a medical leave. A mentor—the only faculty member I discussed my illness with—advised me not to disclose the diagnosis, as doing so could jeopardize my career. While stepping away from work provided momentary relief, my depression only deepened. My doctors began talking to me about hospitalization.

Which was how I found myself in the consultation room of yet another doctor, a brawny and balding psychiatrist with a baritone voice and a South African accent. He had no medical chart by his side, not even a computer from which to review my prior history or laboratory workup.

"I'm Dr. Duncan."

We shook hands, and I took a seat.

He leaned back in his leather recliner.

"So. Tell me your story."

"It's all there in my record."

"I need to hear details from you that I can't find in the record."

His desire to hear my story made me feel hopeful for the first time in months. I had a theory that previous medical doctors—including a psychiatrist—had dismissed.

"It all started with the Thanksgiving my family spent at the rustic cottage my wife and I had just bought in Point Reyes. My twelve-year-old twin boys and I spent three days clearing the fire trail that was overrun with brush since no one had maintained the land for a long time."

Dr. Duncan did not interrupt me or hurry me along, unlike previous doctors had.

"A few days later, I was covered in red, itchy bumps that looked like a poison oak eruption but then turned into a bad case of *erythroderma*—literally, red skin syndrome. The only parts of my body that were not beet red were the whites of my eyes and the brown of my hair. Heat was discharging from my body at an astounding rate. I was shivering cold and agonizingly itchy, feeling like I needed to rip the skin off my body. The next few days were a blur of creams and prednisone pills, accompanied by tears, writhing, forbidden scratching, and uncharacteristic praying to God for relief. These symptoms progressed, forcing me to cancel my clinic sessions. A dermatologist colleague took one look at me and prescribed high-dose corticosteroids. After this monthlong course of steroids and a few-week taper, I was no longer red and itchy, and was able to return to work."

"When was that?"

"Two years ago."

"About a year later, I suddenly started feeling really fatigued, winded, and almost incapacitated. I asked my doctors if I might have Addison's disease—whether taking all those steroid pills caused my body to shut down making its own cortisol. They said that my steroid use was too distant to make it a credible diagnosis. But since Addison's can be fatal, they humored me by sending off the tests. The results proved me wrong."

"You *were* right, in a sense," the psychiatrist said.

His response surprised me.

"How so?"

"There certainly was a lot in your life that might have caused this and was perpetuating it. But you're right: it *was* the damn steroids."

"But that's not possible; I took them two years ago."

"Look, I spent twenty years working as a consulting psychiatrist on the cancer ward at MD Anderson in Texas. We learned early on that the psychiatric effects of steroids—*especially* depression—can manifest two years out or longer. Steroids get through your cell membranes and work by getting into the nucleus of the cells, into the DNA, changing the proteins produced by the neurons in your brain. With high-dose steroids, the treatment can be worse than the disease. I'm not saying you had a choice as to whether to take those steroids. I'm saying that the treatment that helped you in the short term is haunting you now."

"You think that explains all my physical symptoms?"

"Yes, and your psychiatric symptoms too. You and I both know that depression often presents with physical symptoms: pain, fatigue, you name it."

Indeed, I had known that. But experiencing an illness is entirely different from knowing its list of associated symptoms.

"Is it reversible? Or is this just the way I am going to be?"

"I'm hopeful that you'll get better if you have faith and if you work on it. You probably have some underlying vulnerability to depression, as many of us do. It just never manifested itself until you got hit with the high-dose steroids."

I nodded. *Yes, that's it*, I thought, looking down to hide my emotions.

"Does knowing this information change my treatment?"

"What strikes me about your depression is how much you've been ruminating. Running over in your mind, again and again, how stigmatizing this is, how your career is over. Depression is bad enough, but your ruminating—the catastrophizing over how your illness is ruining your life now and will do so forever—only amplifies your suffering. It adds trauma to the trauma you've already experienced from the rash and the steroids. If we can interrupt your ruminations, you will be in a place to begin to recover."

"The ruminations are like a black cloud over my head, pushing down on me. They're always there," I replied, realizing that I had just offered up the same cliché that so many of my patients with depression had said to me.

"Yes, they can be awful. So, I'm going to prescribe you something, at a very low dose, that I think will shut them down."

"*Another* medicine?" I was already on three antidepressants.

"Yes. And you'll need a special kind of therapy to help you get rid of the toxic thoughts and self-defeating actions."

I took the new medicine, no larger than the head of a pin. Four days later, at 11:05 a.m., one year after the beginning of what had become a prolonged, severe, and inexplicable depressive episode, my ruminations stopped. Entirely.

I was not happy. I was not cured. But he had elicited my story and provided me with a tailored treatment plan. And now that my mind was clear of self-defeating, noxious, and apocalyptic thoughts, I could begin to recover.

TALES FROM THE MEDICAL UNDERGROUND

This is not another book about the "doctor as patient" or a chronicle of one doctor's odyssey from illness to recovery or of the path he took from a superficial understanding of human suffering to true enlightenment. Yes, modern medicine nearly killed me. First, the literal medicine—the steroid—was a toxic exposure that damaged me. And second, my profession, which has been conditioned to devalue stories, hindered an accurate diagnosis of my illness, undermined my treatment, and delayed my recovery all because a few doctors chose not to carefully listen. And third, the stigma I experienced undermined my ability to face my diagnosis and to recover. However, the extent of the unhealthy exposures and trauma I endured was far lower than that of my public hospital patients—many of whom have had lifelong, severe exposures with more definitive health consequences. More, the hurdles I needed to overcome to tell my story pale in comparison to those that many low-income patients in hospitals across America face.

Rather, this book reveals what my patients have taught me: that the combination of stories and science holds the key to recovery. For the last thirty years, I have served as a primary care doctor in one of our country's flagship public hospitals, the institutions that disproportionately serve our nation's poor and marginalized. Here, the burden of disease is most concentrated, and our nation's stark health inequities are on display. Here, health care meets social reality. This book is about my connections with my patients, revealing how these longitudinal relationships enable the discovery of their stories and showing how these stories then uncover the hidden exposures at the root of their illnesses. Over time, such stories also weave a larger narrative about public health. Listening to public hospital patients' stories can change the approach we take to improving our entire nation's public health. When we listen to patients' stories, and when we subject these stories to scientific inquiry, our understanding shifts: we discover that most illness occurs as a result of an excess of toxic exposures and a deficit of health-promoting resources. That the state of the social and environmental conditions in which we live largely determines the state of our health. The deeper understanding that emerges after hearing story after story—what I call *narrative epidemiology*—not only can transform health care but also provides a blueprint for dismantling the structural drivers of disease in America.

Yet public hospitals, as critical as they are to the lives of those who inhabit the margins and as informative as they can be to the health of all Americans, remain secreted away. No other book has focused on the inner workings of the public hospital, accompanying the reader into what functionally is a sort of "medical underground," where the realities and inequities that society keeps closeted away—and their consequences—are exposed. What has been missing in the national discourse around health has been the experiences of patients who come from populations most affected by illness: patients in public hospitals. Bringing the voices of these telltale hearts to the table makes a narrative epidemiology possible, allowing a melding of people's stories with our best science in the hopes of shaping a more humane health care system and more effective public health policy.

FROM ONE TO MANY

Can individual stories really hold the key to unlocking the mysteries of human disease and provide answers as to how to reduce suffering on a large scale?

In 1854, John Snow, a doctor working in the midst of an epidemic decimating London, made a scientific discovery that would save tens of thousands of lives in the short term, one with the potential to change the world forever.

But his discovery didn't happen in the way that most people think it did. The simple version of Snow's breakthrough is known to many. Few people know the deeper truths behind how he arrived at his discovery and how his method of narrative inquiry both inspired and enabled him to convince those in power to act on it. This deeper story holds lessons as profound and relevant today as they were two centuries ago.

At that time, the growing populations of European cities were plagued by recurrent outbreaks of cholera, a horrific diarrheal disease that spread with brutal pace. Marked dehydration drained the life out of those afflicted within a day or two. In 1854, about thirty thousand people, or roughly 1 percent of London's residents, died of cholera in short order.

The popular version of Dr. Snow's transformative discovery is the source of his posthumous reputation as the founder of epidemiology and public health. Snow practiced medicine at a time when microbes had not yet been identified as causes of illness, and deaths due to epidemic disease were believed to be a result of immoral behavior, especially among the poor. But Snow suspected that London's water supply might be the source of the epidemic. To test this theory, the simple story goes, he applied an unprecedented degree of abstract scientific thinking and employed a systematic geocoding method that was entirely novel. First, he obtained the exact addresses of case fatalities

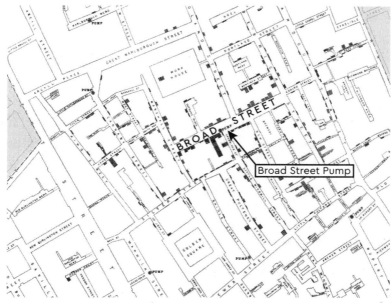

Dr. John Snow's 1854 map of London's Soho neighborhood. Stacked black lines along Broad Street and near its water pump signify the number of cholera-related deaths. C. F. Cheffins, lithograph, "Southampton Buildings, London, England, 1854," in John Snow, *On the Mode of Communication of Cholera*, 2nd ed. (London, England: John Churchill, 1855).

from municipal registries. Second, he carefully charted each case onto street maps of London. Third, he overlaid these maps with markings displaying the course of London's underground water pipe system and the positions of their associated wells and pumps. And finally, focusing in on the hard-hit district of Soho, he was able to discern a visually compelling pattern that pointed to a single communal pump on Broad Street as the likely source of the cholera epidemic. Nearly forty years later, Snow's theory was confirmed when German microbiologist Robert Koch detected that the intestines of cholera victims were infected by a waterborne bacterium, which he named *Vibrio cholerae*.

How did John Snow come to discover something so insightful and profound? Unbeknownst to many today, Snow was an avid collector of people's stories—namely, his patients'—and it was these stories that both led him to his discovery and drove his commitment to see it translated into public policy action.

This deeper story began in his childhood. Snow had drunk from the wells of the poor, both literally and figuratively. He was raised in relative poverty, one of nine children born to a working-class family in Yorkshire. His father was a laborer in a coal mine, a job with abysmal working conditions. When Snow apprenticed as a surgeon-apothecary, he witnessed firsthand some of his patients succumb to the cholera epidemic of 1831. A majority of those afflicted were coal mine workers like his father. Snow worked long and hard hours to treat the sick, and the experience had a profound impact on him. The discordance he felt between the prevailing theories of the day regarding immorality and disease causation, and his relationships with poor people of good character who were dying from cholera, undoubtedly shaped his critical thinking about the nature of disease. These early experiences also endowed him with a degree of authenticity and empathy that would engender the trust of his patients, enabling them to willingly share the details of their lives with him regardless of their station in society.

In his subsequent years as a general practitioner in London, Snow chose to work at Westminster Hospital, whose mission was to care for the sick and poor. There, he burnished a reputation among his colleagues as a fine physician and surgeon. Reports of Snow's doctoring describe him as an attentive and active listener, a sort of curious detective, an acute diagnostician, and an enlightened practitioner. In September 1838, Snow moved to 54 Frith Street,

Soho, setting up in private practice while also working in the outpatient department of Charing Cross Hospital, established as "a healing place for the poor." This work was poorly paid but gave Snow valuable experience, offering him ongoing relationships with countless patients and deep connections to the local community—assets that would serve him well in the future.

Snow continued to engage in this trench-level work even as his fame—acquired by virtue of being one of the only doctors who could safely administer anesthesia—skyrocketed. Despite being in high demand, Snow held a radically egalitarian view of his patients, viewing each as an individual no more or less worthy of his attention than the next. Within a short while of famously giving anesthesia to Queen Victoria to ease the birthing process of the future Prince Leopold, Snow could be found working with some of the poorest patients living in the most deprived areas of London. Individual stories of the poor would eventually lead to his cholera discovery.

Snow, with the help of the Reverend Henry Whitehead—a local deacon who also had his ear to the ground—elicited four stories that stand out as being instrumental. First, he learned that a subset of Soho's most destitute residents of the St James Parish workhouse, located just across the street from the Broad Street pump, were somehow spared from cholera. Such Dickensian workhouses, frequently subject to closure by the authorities for poor hygiene and mistreatment of their residents, were unfriendly to unannounced visits from outsiders, especially health authorities. This was particularly true of the guardian of St James, who wanted nothing to do with cholera talk. Snow managed to talk his way in to meet with the man. There, he learned that the workhouse had its own well and a separate piped supply from a company that drew water from the Thames at a different location.

Second, he noticed that there was not a single cholera death among the seventy workers in the Lion Brewery, located right on Broad Street. After sharing a drink with Mr. Huggins, the proprietor of the brewery, Snow learned that the workers mainly drank malt liquor and that the brewery had its own well.

Third, he was surprised to hear that a widow living far from Soho, in Hampstead, and her niece had succumbed to cholera within days of the Soho outbreak. In discussing their deaths with her family, he confirmed that neither had gone anywhere near Broad Street. It looked as though this interview was a dead end as far as his theory went. But Snow, having learned from thousands of medical encounters that truth was rarely uncovered by direct questioning and often was revealed in conversation as an afterthought, patiently gave the family time to muse further. In this way, he discovered that the widow used to live in the affected area; and that while living there, she had developed a taste for the Broad Street well water and frequently secured a supply of this water. When her niece visited on August 31, both drank from the same deadly bottle of Broad Street well water. The pieces of the puzzle were beginning to come together.

But a central piece was still missing. Believing that something critical must have happened just before August 30 to ignite the epidemic in Soho, Snow learned from Henry Whitehead of Sarah Lewis, the mother of a five-month-old infant who, on August 28, was the first to come down with diarrhea; she died on September 2. After her death, a distraught Mrs. Lewis told him that during that interval, her baby, Frances, passed copious quantities of "rice-water" stools, repeatedly soaking her cloth diapers. The mother revealed that she had rinsed the diapers in cold water and then poured that water into the cesspool located in front of their dwelling.

Snow had the final story he needed. The cesspool in front of Mrs. Lewis's building was quickly excavated. It was found to have a leak that dripped its contents into the nearest well—the well that sourced the Broad Street pump.

Impelled by this eureka moment and desperate for rapid action, Snow presented the compelling mapping data and associated elegant statistics to the civic authorities. Leaders from the church and the scientific community were unimpressed and fervently argued against his claims. As the outcome of the meeting teetered toward utter failure, Snow wondered whether he should risk his reputation as an objective scientist informed solely by quantitative data and add more personal, anecdotal evidence to the anonymity of his statistics.

As the meeting drew to its end, Snow requested one last word. He pushed his maps aside and told the real stories behind the epidemic. He told them about the St James Parish workhouse and its separate water supply, about the widow and her bottled water, and about Mr. Huggins and the malt liquor. While the authorities were still not convinced of his overarching theory that cholera was caused by some sort of exposure transmitted via London's unmonitored and poorly designed water system, they *were* moved enough to take one simple step: they ordered the removal of the handle from the Broad Street pump, temporarily disabling it.

Cases of cholera plummeted. And London was changed forever.

WHERE THE REAL STORIES CAN BE FOUND

Were John Snow alive today, where would he go to find the stories to help him understand the heavy burden of disease in America, collect the data to explain the escalating costs of US health care, and chart the maps that display the underlying structures that unequally distribute disease across our nation like cholera in London's waterways? In nineteenth-century London, he would go to his patients from the public clinics and charity hospitals, and the neighborhoods they served. In twenty-first-century America, when it comes to understanding health, the invaluable stories are still to be found in the public hospital.

I have committed my career to service as a primary care physician in a public hospital. Often called "safety net hospitals," the one hundred or so remaining American public hospitals provide care for people with limited or no access to health care due to their financial circumstances, insurance barriers, social circumstances, or stigmatizing health conditions. These hospitals exist in urban and rural areas; they are financially dependent on public subsidies like Medicaid and Medicare, as well as state and local tax appropriations. While they are money-losing institutions by design, offsetting much of the charity care provided by private and nonprofit hospitals, they are frequently on the chopping block for the fiscal insolvency they are subject to.

I grew up in a public housing project in Buffalo, New York, the son of immigrant parents: my father from Hungary and my mother from Chile. Their only wish for me—the wish of so many immigrant parents at the time—was that I would go to medical school. Many of my family, friends, and acquaintances still wonder why I work in a public hospital; why, despite my Ivy League schooling and limitless opportunities, I chose San Francisco General Hospital. Everyone understands that there are private and public schools, and that there are private sector jobs and public sector jobs. But few people appreciate all that a public hospital is and does.

My elderly parents repeatedly ask me, "What do you actually *do* there? When will you open a private practice?"

"Why would you work at a place where homeless and crazy people go?" shamelessly asks an acquaintance.

"That's where *I'd* want to be taken if I got shot or had a bad car accident," a friend says, trying to defend and justify my choice.

"That's where all the cool diseases show up, the rare stuff you'd only see if you were doing global health, right?" another asks.

"When it comes to treating poor people, we need someone who knows what he's doing," says another in solidarity.

"Thank you for all you do," says a friend. "Your hospital was the only place I could send my nanny when she had a urinary infection."

The public hospital has historically played a critical role in America. The design of my hospital, San Francisco General Hospital, tells a living history of public health in America. Our long record of public health battles has resulted in a hybrid campus with an architectural blueprint that could be entitled "Epidemics R Us." The old redbrick building that contains my research office once housed doctors and nurses who confronted smallpox, plague, cholera, influenza, tuberculosis, and polio. The aging brutalist, gray, concrete massif where I trained—and where my clinic is still located—was built to tackle illnesses related to the tobacco epidemic, such as lung cancer, emphysema, heart attack, and stroke. This building ended up serving triple duty, simultaneously battling newer scourges, such as the medical complications of IV drug use and the ravages of AIDS. And the newest cylindrical, nine-story structure built with whitened steel, green-tinted glass, and topped with a rooftop wraparound garden serves as the front line against type 2 diabetes—the terrible but unglamorous epidemic of the twenty-first century—and, most recently, COVID-19.

Public hospitals are much more than just places where poor people who are sick go to receive care. They are where health care meets social reality and where a reckoning with our nation's legacy of racism and inequality cannot be avoided. The story of our society and its impact on health is fully exposed on the wards and in the clinics of the public hospital. And while the public hospital is not the place where most Americans get their care, what this book's telltale hearts reveal here is everyone's story to one degree or another.

The stories that emerge from the public hospital force us to ask difficult questions:

Whose stories do we listen to?

What do these stories tell us about what causes disease?

What do they tell us about unhealthy exposures, about who gets over-exposed, and why?

Whom do we marginalize?

Whose lives do we value and whose health do we support?

Can we use social investment to promote health, rescue our health care system, improve our quality of life, and save lives?

Will we do so?

The answers to these questions will make the difference between life and death for millions of Americans now and many more in the future. My purpose in writing this book is to enable a broader understanding of public health in modern America by illustrating how unhealthy exposures can explain the high burden of disease in our nation, how degrees of marginalization and systemic oppression determine the risk of exposure and disease, and how stories and storytelling can provide a path to our finding a way through.

PART 1

When There Is No Story

CHAPTER 1

The Magic Bus

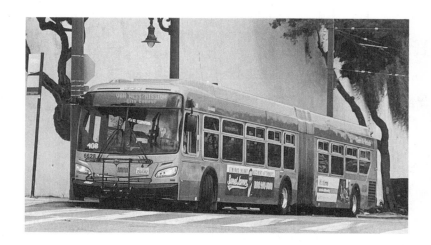

I WAS WEIGHED DOWN BY SIX WALLET-SIZE, OLD-SCHOOL PAGERS, EACH ONE with a different buzz tone alerting me to problems in a different hospital service. Five of the pagers were black, and they pulled down the belt on my waistline. The sixth pager was red and stood out from the others. The red one was known as the *Code Beeper*. It went off when someone in the hospital (or en route to the hospital) had *coded*, a term we use for an unexpected sudden death—usually from cardiac arrest. The physician of the day for the cardiac care unit (CCU) is charged to carry the Code Beeper, and it's a heavy load, filled with a strange anticipation as one waits for its alarm to sound.

The physician of the day is the leading actor in a play whose script has only a few possible outcomes, featuring fierce and frantic activity followed by the empty silence of the patient's death being the most common. The rare resurrection of this body and soul emerges as the focus of all efforts in a code, a ritual of violent intimacy.

It is the role of the code leader to make the clinical assessments, select the appropriate code algorithm, bark out the orders, respond to the evolving clinical picture, and repeat as necessary. The supporting actors are the other members of the code team, whose roles are to swiftly execute the orders of the leader, deliver the necessary supplies, carry out well-rehearsed procedures and interventions, and provide backup if things go awry. It is the code leader with the red beeper who decides if a resuscitation attempt has succeeded and whether the patient can be moved to the CCU. And it is the code leader who decides when to "call the code"—when to instruct the team that their well-orchestrated labors should stop, that their labors are now futile. All that is true, except for cases in which the code has been called in the emergency room (ER), where the ER attending physician has the final say.

ACT 1: THE ALARM

Being the CCU physician of the day for the first time was to walk in fear, in sheer terror, praying that the red pager wouldn't go off. On my first twenty-four-hour shift, my heart pounded with no visible cause, the incessant beating echoing in my ears. I had no appetite. Every beep of a black pager made me jump. My anxiety got so bad that I shifted from feeling a deep sense of dread to hoping desperately to see some real action, if only to relieve this sense of terror, to get past it. The hours passed slowly, each beat of my heart counting down the time when my shift would end. It was nearly midnight. Perhaps, this first time, I would be spared?

As my team and I were walking back from the cafeteria and our midnight meal, my pager went off again. This time, it was the Code Beeper. The vibration sent shock waves up and down my body. This pager had special radio functionality, and it roared at me with garbled words:

"CCU—TO TRAUMA ROOM 1. . . . CCU—TO TRAUMA ROOM 1!"

I felt a blast of adrenaline rush through my guts. We had to descend five floors to the Mission emergency room. I turned to my teammate Craig, whose face belied the fear that was like a mirror to mine, and we dashed to the elevators, red code backpack bouncing between his shoulders.

"Trauma Room 1," I proclaimed with a booming voice and a false light-heartedness. "Right into the belly of the beast. Couldn't ask for a better start to the night, could we?"

I forced a laugh and pressed the Down button.

Trauma Room 1. Just saying those words was enough to flood any physician at San Francisco General with a range of emotions and images. Chest x-rays that look like whiteouts, blue faces gasping for air, hands gripping bedrails, bodies bolt upright. The smell of vomit, of charcoal, of saline, of metal and flesh, of poverty, of homelessness. An entry point to healing and recovery for the lucky ones, a point of final departure for others.

The ceiling of Trauma Room 1 boasts a large bullet hole, a 1980s relic from a time when a loaded gun somehow went off during a code being run on a gunshot victim. Around that bullet hole, the doctors and nurses drew concentric circles, making it appear that the patient had hit the target in the bull's-eye, a portal to the firmament above. A twist of irony meant to highlight to subsequent generations the ambiguities and uncertainties inherent to time spent in Trauma Room 1—its futility and its godliness.

As the elevator doors on the fifth floor opened, I reached into the breast pocket of my scrubs to grab the laminated card we all carried, the one that had the treatment algorithm for cardiac arrest, the same one I had been reviewing throughout the day. I mistakenly pulled out its neighbor instead, a laminated card given to me by a rabbi—the wife of one of my colleagues—trying to bring the traditions of Jewish healing to the health professions. The card contained a Hebrew prayer—El Maleh Rachamim—the Prayer for the Soul of the Departed. I stared at it, reflexively mouthing the Hebrew words, cast a sideways glance at my teammate to make sure he hadn't caught me, and then quickly placed the prayer card back in my breast pocket. The elevator doors opened on the ground floor.

"CCU—TO TRAUMA ROOM 1.... CCU—COME TO TRAUMA ROOM 1!"

We burst into Trauma Room 1. Laid out on the gurney was a tall, olive-skinned man, possibly African American, his brown municipal bus driver shirt partially ripped off his muscular chest, his arms akimbo. Two nurses were working feverishly to place IVs in his forearms. At his head stood the respiratory therapist, repetitively hand-bagging oxygen through a tube that probably was placed into the man's trachea by the paramedics. The man's large brown eyes were wide open, fixed and dilated. They stared straight up to the ceiling.

"Muni bus driver," my ER colleague breathlessly reported, in between chest compressions. "Young guy, maybe forty.... Collapsed while on his route.... Not sure if he caused an MVA.... So, maybe some trauma.... Can't tell.... Was unresponsive for the paramedics.... Not breathing, no pulse, no blood pressure.... CPR initiated.... Intubated in the field.... Brought in by ambulance.... We called you.... My guess is a massive heart attack.... Arrhythmia, maybe.... Probably cocaine related.... Wanna take over?"

We were all too familiar with the crack epidemic in the city. So many of the city's bus drivers were heavy cocaine users that the city had begun routinely drug testing them. As the hospital contracted to provide health care to city workers, we saw our fair share of young and middle-aged Muni drivers with a cocaine habit, from those trying to quit to those suffering the addiction's consequences, such as stroke or heart attack.

I switched places with my colleague and stood on the footstool at the bedside, placed my crossed hands on the man's chest, straightened up my elbows, and started my rhythmic compressions. As I'd been taught, I used my body weight to create the most effective compressions, bending fifteen degrees or so, with my waist as the fulcrum, straightening up again, and then starting over. The repetitive movements reminded me of davening, the rhythmic swaying forward and back from the waist that religious Jews do when worshipping a God I didn't understand and couldn't decide if I believed in.

I saw that one of the nurses had successfully struck red and had gotten an IV line in. I dove in.

"Okay!... Gimme a milligram of epi push.... Let's get a monitor on him.... See if he has a rhythm.... And get the defibrillator paddles ready!"

The team snapped into action. I continued to perform chest compressions, getting a much-needed midnight workout that released all the tension and anxiety I had felt throughout the day as I dreaded this very moment. I was giving it all I had, and I was sweating, my sweat dripping onto the man's bare chest, his neck, his face. I saw his eyes again, beautiful eyes. They were still wide open, his large black pupils like big bullet holes. Brown irises surrounded his pupils, looking straight at the bull's-eye in the target above him.

Just then, the supervising ER physician, Bill W., walked in. Responsible for the care of sixty or so acutely ill patients, these are the most senior physicians in the ER, there to support and advise the medical teams. A patient cannot be discharged from the ER without first presenting the case to the senior attending. Most ER attending physicians are a fountain of knowledge and are remarkably helpful. Bill was not one of those; he was notoriously unimpressive, burned-out, and sardonically opinionated.

"Another Muni driver found down?" he inquired, feigning interest. "Gee, I wonder what it could mean? Let's see what that monitor shows us."

To my surprise, the heart monitor revealed a slow, junctional rhythm, one arising from the backup system of the heart's circuitry, beating at a rate of forty-two beats per minute. Most cardiac arrests come in either flatlining or with a very rapid and disorderly rhythm known as *ventricular fibrillation*. For V-fib, we shock the patient with a defibrillator in the hopes of resetting his native rhythm, so that the heart can go back to squeezing with its full and highly coordinated force. But this—a slow rhythm originating in the gray zone between the upper and lower chambers of the heart—triggers a different response.

"He's got a regular rhythm!" I shouted. "Weird. . . . Okay, looks junctional. . . . Let's get pacemaker gel pads on him and bring out the Zoll. . . . Give him a milligram of atropine."

I switched spots with my teammate Craig, abandoning my footstool and my chest compressions to get closer to the monitor and think. My team gently rolled him to one side and affixed a large pacemaker pad onto his back.

"Now let's start the EMD protocol."

Electromechanical dissociation (EMD) describes any situation in which heart rhythm is present (that's the electrical part) but a detectable pumping heart is absent (no pulse, no blood pressure; that's the mechanical part). So, a heart that appears to be beating on the monitor but does not generate sufficient blood flow to keep the patient alive. There are very few medical conditions that cause EMD, and we have an EMD protocol to address them all.

"Get that second IV in and push fluids. Wide open. And get me two large-bore IVs and hook them up to two 60 cc syringes. Fast. I'm gonna check for a tension pneumothorax."

I wiped his upper chest with alcohol. I was standing at the crook of his neck, between his head and his right shoulder. I was so close I could rub my cheek against his. His eyes remained locked into the target on the ceiling. I told Craig to hold the chest compressions. I then gently inserted one fourteen-gauge IV needle into the second rib space at a ninety-degree angle. I withdrew some air into the syringe and knew I was in. I then pulled out the needle and syringe, leaving behind the cannula, a thin plastic tube. Nothing. No rush that would indicate trapped air in the chest constricting the heart. I pulled out, switched sides, and tried it again. Nothing. This was not a case of pneumothorax.

I looked back at the monitor. Still slow and junctional.

"Still no pulse? Okay, restart compressions. . . . Push another milligram of epi and a milligram of atropine. . . . You're pushing fluids, right? . . . Okay, now get me the pericardiocentesis tray and wipe his chest down with Betadine. I gotta go in blind."

The hovering attending ER physician chimed in with a sarcastic, falling whistle tone, signifying how he was duly impressed with my aggressive but textbook approach.

Armed with another 60 cc syringe attached to a large and very long needle, I positioned myself so as to face the man, and I leaned in. I was now nearly on top of him, my chest touching his, our faces inches from each other, my heat on top of his unresponsive body like a brutally passionate lover facing a frigid counterpart. I placed the needle at the point where his sternum ended, just above his stomach, and, directing it at a forty-five-degree angle up toward his head and up to the heart, I slowly inserted and advanced it into his heart until blood appeared in the syringe. I withdrew 60 cc of blood and then another 60 cc. My hope was that I had just removed blood that had wedged itself in between the lining of the heart and the muscle of the heart—a fatal situation if uncorrected.

"Any pulse? No?"

I turned to Bill and pointed to the spot where I had inserted the needle.

"I'm done here, right?" I asked.

Arms folded in a smug attitude, Bill nodded.

I felt a lump in my throat and a pang of loss.

"Okay, let's give him another milligram of epi. And two amps of bicarb. Craig—let's get those compressions going again. Don't give up!"

The rhythm stubbornly remained at thirty to forty beats per minute. We were running out of what little time we had. I looked up, racking my brain in desperation. I saw the target again, the large bullet hole at its center.

"Okay. Let's try this. Maybe his rate's just too slow. Let's pace him. Set the Zoll at 80. Start at 10 mA"—milliamps—"and go up by 10 until it captures."

The team put the second pacemaker gel pad onto his chest and connected it to the pulse generator. We stepped away and the nurse turned it to 10 mA. Nothing. Still thirty-six beats per minute. 20 mA. Still nothing. 30 mA. We saw on the monitor that the heart had finally sensed the pacemaker, and the rate now was 80. This would definitely do it. My pulse quickened as I rushed to feel his. But still, stubbornly, no pulse. Not at his wrists, not at his femoral arteries, not at his carotids.

"He's still got no pulse. Keep pushing fluids, please. Damn it! Craig, start the compressions again. Gimme another milligram of epi and two amps of bicarb. And keep looking for a pulse after every five compressions."

As we repeated this cycle over the next five minutes, the monitor tracing deteriorated before my eyes, first showing pacing spikes not picked up by the heart and then, a minute later, no heart rhythm at all, only pacemaker spikes. I felt as if the floor beneath me had given way.

"We have no rhythm! Please tell me a monitor lead has fallen off."

It hadn't. So, I switched gears again.

"Okay, hold the compressions and turn off the pacer. Let's switch to de-fibrillation mode. Gimme the paddles. Set it to 200 joules. . . . Everyone—step away! Three, two, one . . ."

I pressed the paddles on his heart with all my force, stole a look at the man's face and his wide-open eyes, and delivered the shock. I leaned over to see the monitor.

"Right. Let's do it again."

I looked at the man, grabbed his hand, and gave it a squeeze.

"C'mon, man, you can do this."

My sweat dripped on his chest and neck again. I grabbed the paddles and delivered the second shock. It too yielded no rhythm.

Pointing to the flat line, Bill interjected, "You *do* know that asystole is not a shockable rhythm, don't you?"

"I know. . . . I was just hoping that . . ."

"His urine came back flagrantly positive for cocaine. I'll give you five more minutes to flail on this dead man and practice your CPR skills. And then I'm calling it. The Big Bus Driver in the Sky has called this his final stop. We need this room for the barely alive."

He turned on his heels and walked out of Trauma Room 1. He'd just pulled rank on me, the son of a bitch. We got back to work, bagging oxygen and banging on the man's chest.

INTERLUDE: THE MAGIC TRAIN

Who decides when it is that we will die?

Who gets to declare us dead or alive?

Can a soul be alive if the body is dead?

Can a soul revive a body?

How do you thank the person who has saved your life?

How do you thank the person whose life you have saved?

It is Friday, April 13, 1945. The sun is setting. My father has just turned fifteen. He lies naked on his side in the train's half-open boxcar, shivering in the same position he has been in for hours. He is one of millions of victims of a specious medical belief system promoted by the greatest physicians and scientists of the day—that eugenics and "racial hygiene" could improve human health. But when this was maliciously translated into national policy, it became the way to eliminate an entire people deemed to be the source of all problems in society. On April 10, the Nazis had packed up the few remaining survivors of the Bergen-Belsen concentration camp and stuffed them onto the train, heading east to the Elbe River. Twenty-five hundred Jews stuffed in like sardines, eighty to a boxcar. Three days later, the Nazis inexplicably turned the train back again, and a few hours later, they brought it to a halt. They then deserted the train and its prisoners for the forest, but only after stealing their striped clothes so they could pretend to be Jews on the run.*

The Americans are coming. With the British, they've been dropping leaflets for three days, promising liberation. As the sun sets, my father sees a small group of emaciated, half-naked men: prisoners, rhythmically and rapidly bending at the waist and back again, davening, rapidly chanting the prayers to welcome in the Sabbath. He looks at them with his large blue eyes. He is down to under sixty pounds, and the only part of him that appears alive are his eyes. His wasted body curled up on the floor of a train car has been consumed by bilateral tuberculosis and hepatitis. He closes his eyes. He is drifting away. How can he survive?

He first hears the sounds, and then the sounds turn into a roar. A mechanical roaring and a squeaking. He opens his eyes. Three US tanks, flanked by two dozen American infantrymen, advance from over the crest of the hill, silhouetted by the waning sun. One soldier, chewing gum, approaches him, shooing away the flies, and looks in his eyes. The eighteen-year-old soldier, burly and tough, feels for a pulse. He reaches into the boxcar and lifts my father up, gently cradling him in his arms as if the boy were made of glass. He walks with him gingerly but briskly. He looks down into my father's eyes.

"You okay?" he asks.

My father can only blink in response.

Sixty years later, on April 13, 2005, my father writes a letter to the *Sarasota Herald-Tribune*. In it, he tells the story of his liberation, of his gradual recovery from death's door, and of his immigration to the US. He writes that he wants to take this opportunity to thank the soldiers of the US Army Thirtieth Infantry, the 743rd Tank Battalion, and the 105th Medical Battalion for saving his life. His piece is published on April 14.

That afternoon, my father's phone rings.

"Hello, is this George?" the husky voice asks. "Hey, my name is Jerry Snow. I'm just an old soldier from the Thirtieth Infantry. I just read your letter in the paper, and it really choked me up. Thank you for writing that. It means a lot. So, anyway, I looked you up in the phone book. Turns out, we're neighbors. Yup. Go figure. I live only five blocks away. What do you say we get together over a beer?"

This call led to a series of annual reunions of all the survivors of that train ride and their liberators. Reunions in New York, Florida, and Israel. A few years ago, the sole surviving liberator died, and the reunions ended.

ACT 2: THE MAGIC BUS

I took over the chest compressions. The respiratory therapist at the head of the bed was still patiently bagging, and I noticed for the first time that he'd been chewing gum.

I felt Bill W. enter behind me, judging.

"Okay, people. I'm calling it. This code is officially *over*. Let's clean up, get him out of here, clear the room, and get back to work."

The first to break was the respiratory therapist. He disconnected the oxygen and the Ambu bag and casually walked out. I again looked at the man, now lying still with a tube sticking out of his mouth like a giant bent straw. I lifted my crossed palms off his chest, now adorned with monitor pads and three holes from where I had punctured his body, trying to suck the impending death out of him.

The room rapidly emptied. How could everyone have disappeared so quickly? I stepped away from the footstool, now alone with the dead man. The intensity and calamity of noise had given way to absolute silence. I looked at the young bus driver we had violently dedicated the last forty minutes to, approached him, and started to sob.

I looked at those eyes and followed their empty gaze staring at the hole in the firmament. I am not a spiritual man, but I imagined his soul floating up like smoke off dying embers, slowly getting sucked into that hole, the portal to the hereafter.

I pulled out the rabbi's laminated card and, between sobs, quietly addressed the bullet hole. I read aloud:

אֵל מָלֵא רַחֲמִים שׁוֹכֵן
בַּמְּרוֹמִים הַמְצֵא מְנוּחָה
נְכוֹנָה עַל כַּנְפֵי הַשְּׁכִינָה
בְּמַעֲלוֹת קְדוֹשִׁים וּטְהוֹרִים
כְּזֹהַר הָרָקִיעַ מַזְהִירִים, אֶת
נִשְׁמַת (פלוני בן פלוני)
שֶׁהָלַךְ לְעוֹלָמוֹ,
בַּעֲבוּר שֶׁנָּדְבוּ צְדָקָה
בְּעַד הַזְכָּרַת נִשְׁמָתוֹ, בְּגַן
עֵדֶן תְּהֵא מְנוּחָתוֹ, לָכֵן
בַּעַל הָרַחֲמִים יַסְתִּירֵהוּ
בְּסֵתֶר כְּנָפָיו לְעוֹלָמִים, וְיִצְרֹר
בִּצְרוֹר הַחַיִּים אֶת נִשְׁמָתוֹ,
יְיָ הוּא נַחֲלָתוֹ, וְיָנוּחַ
עַל מִשְׁכָּבוֹ בְּשָׁלוֹם,
וְנֹאמַר אָמֵן:

O God, full of compassion, Who dwells on high, grant true rest upon the wings of the Divine Presence, in the exalted spheres of the holy and pure, that shine as the resplendence of the firmament, to the soul of (this Muni driver) who has gone to his celestial world, for charity has been donated in remembrance of his soul; may his place of rest be in the Garden of Eden. Therefore, may the All-Merciful One shelter him with the cover of His wings forever, and bind his soul in the bond of life. The Divine was his birthright; may he rest in his resting-place in peace; and let us say: Amen.

I placed the card back into my breast pocket and took a deep breath and blew it all out, spent. As I turned to leave Trauma Room 1, I cast one last look at the dead man, my first failed code.

I imagined I saw a twitching at his neck, in the jugular area. I froze and focused my eyes. No, it was a definite twitching. I ran around to the bed-side monitor. He was back in a junctional rhythm at forty-eight. I felt a weak pulse in his carotid.

"Hey, *people!*" I yelled. "Get back in here! This guy's not dead!"

The first one in was Bill, followed by my teammate Craig.

"Start bagging this guy again," I ordered. "We got a live one!"

I looked back at Bill and flashed him a teary-eyed smile.

"Get him outta here," he said, stone-faced. "Bring him up to the CCU. And *vaya con Dios*."

We wheeled him up to the CCU and tried to convince the Cardiology attending physician to perform a cardiac catheterization to determine if our driver had had an acute heart attack—one that could be reversed by dissolving a clot or placing a stent to open up a blocked coronary artery. He was unmoved. After I told him the story of the biblical code, he begrudgingly said, "I hate cathing a dead man. It's a waste of time. But I'll do it for you because you tell a good story."

Craig jumped at the opportunity to assist on the cardiac cath. Forty-five minutes later, he ran out of the cath lab and into our CCU, breathless.

"Completely *clean* coronaries. Nothing to stent. But he's got no squeeze. His ejection fraction was only 9 percent. His heart's squeezing out only a trickle of what it should."

So, the man had not actually coded. This patient's condition was a result of very severe heart failure, a cocaine-damaged or stunned heart that was beating but just timidly pumping. He was indeed alive, but only barely so.

Over the next six hours, we lined him up and treated his heart failure with dobutamine and diuretics. As we prepared to end what would no doubt be one of our most memorable shifts, his blood pressure was 88 over 45. A very respectable blood pressure for a former dead man. Enough to go home with just a scrap of hope.

The next morning, his pressure was up to 95 over 60. His rhythm was now in normal sinus at a rate of 110. By noon, he started to move all fours and blinked in response to our questions. He was bucking the ventilator, trying to pull out the tube in his throat. That afternoon, because he was oxygenating so well, we pulled out the tube, and he breathed supplemental oxygen on his own. He passed a quiet night.

The third day, we talked. He was completely cogent. I told him about his near-death experience. He thanked me. He told me about his cocaine habit and about his three daughters, whom he wanted to see. He told me he was starving.

By day four, he was sitting up and eating and had begun to walk. We had changed all his IV medications over to oral medications. He was looking like a peach. On the morning of day five, I found him sitting up by his bed, wearing street clothes.

"Doc, I'm ready. Let's get me outta here."

He was, indeed, incredibly, ready for discharge.

"All right. I'll get the paperwork going, but you have to promise me two things."

"What's that, Doc?"

"First, promise me you'll get help for your cocaine problem. Second, let's swing by the ER on your way out, so they can meet Lazarus returned from the dead. We all have something to learn from you. They need to see you standing tall, walking out of our ER in one piece."

We took the elevator down five floors to the Mission ER. I showed him Trauma Room 1 and pointed to the bull's-eye through which I had thought his soul was ascending. Then I shepherded him around the entire ER, telling and retelling the story to anyone who would listen. I told them about the resilience of youth, the need to always remember that we can never know anything for sure, that hubris was our enemy. He had opened his button-down shirt and proudly showed the three stigmata on his chest as visible proof of his survival skills. He shook hands with everyone, like a smiling politician at a rally. We too were all smiles, and we wished him luck.

We told him we never wanted to see him again, here in the Mission.

* Information on the Bergen-Belsen death train and the liberation can be found at www.jewishgen.org/databases/holocaust/0175_Farsleben.html.

CHAPTER 2

Medical School Dropout

A QUESTION OF MEANING

I was a medical school dropout. In the 1980s, after having spent the prior four years in a liberal arts college immersed in the interior worlds of Russian language and literature, having taken only the minimum number of science courses required to enter medical school, I moved to Philadelphia. A city boiling over in the summer heat and humidity, a sort of reverse Potemkin village in which the façades of its stately colonial buildings and historic homes were fouled by bags stacked upon bags of garbage that had been uncollected for months due to a prolonged garbage collector strike. Blocks whose oppressive stench obscured the foundational breath of liberation and freedom. A city riven by distinct, block-by-block demarcations that determine where the white people should live and where the Black slums begin and end. A city reeling from the recent municipal conflagration caused by its mayor's helicopter-bombing of his own people, one that wiped out an entire block of Osage Avenue in West Philadelphia. In what was widely acknowledged to have been a disproportionate response to the rebellious lifestyles and unlawful actions of a communally living Black liberation group called MOVE, the mayor's attack on one house killed eleven MOVE members, including five children, destroying more than sixty homes in the process. Competing for a decent place to live, I settled for a sizable apartment near Osage Avenue, a dozen blocks east of that infamous urban war zone and a dozen blocks west of what was to become my medical school. Situated in a mystical gateway between the purported Hell and the supposed Sanctuary for Healing.

I suffered through the first two years in this nation's first and very prestigious medical school feeling disengaged, alienated, and lost. What did these (mostly) white men in long white coats, in these pristine and air-conditioned chambers, have to teach me about doctoring? What did the knowledge I was being fed and all the facts I was forced to memorize add up to? Where was I to find meaning and purpose? As I tried to muscle through, I shared with my closest colleagues my fantasies of dropping out, of pursuing a career as a professional musician instead. They encouraged me to repress these thoughts, feelings, and intentions, to avoid squandering the academic success I enjoyed in these first two classroom years. To just wait it out and push through until the clinical years, a time when I would begin to see how all the dots connect, a time when I would discover what medicine could do for *me*, a time when I would shift from the rote learning of facts to their application and translation into real practice.

So, I chose to suspend disbelief and hold out hope, looking to my first two-month clinical rotation in Internal Medicine: home to medicine's greatest minds, its master diagnosticians, its clinical magicians. Home to medicine's cognitively and interpersonally gifted superstars.

My supervising physician was an acclaimed kidney specialist in the university's renowned and sparkling private hospital. I was one of three junior apprentices assigned to his team. The month was deeply disheartening. I learned even more about the nephron (the basic functional unit of the kidney, responsible for filtering out toxins from the blood and producing urine) than I had during my first two years but observed nothing about how that knowledge could be applied to enhance the health of the patients I was charged with following. I learned that the forty-five-year-old Black auto mechanic we admitted to the small public ward, who was suffering from new-onset diabetes and a hypertensive emergency that threatened both his kidneys and his heart, could not be monitored or cared for in the university hospital's outpatient clinic after his discharge. He was uninsured, leaving him destined to suffer the likely complications of uncontrolled hypertension.

I learned that the City of Philadelphia had, just five years prior, torn down Philadelphia General Hospital, then the largest public charity hospital in the nation, at 1,200 beds. Situated in the university's backyard a few hundred feet from its private hospital, it had been losing too much money. I witnessed how the abandoned, gaping lot that remained was gradually being filled by newly constructed research buildings, structures that in the future would enable the university's physician-scientists to better compete for NIH funding. All in the hopes of discovering *more* treatments and more cures that, in a perfect world, would prevent suffering for all those afflicted but, in the real world, would do so for only a privileged fraction of them. I learned that the city had made an attempt to fill the void in care left by the vacant lot by creating a program it called HealthPass, providing ID cards to publicly insured and uninsured residents that would, in theory, enable access to health care. I heard that the city was never able to pay the bills submitted to HealthPass, and so clinics routinely turned such folks away. And that the only recourse for a patient would be to receive episodic care at one of the gateways to the medical underworld: the emergency department.

But I also learned from my attending's review of my month's academic and clinical performance under his watch that I was unlikely to become a successful internist. My levity with patients and colleagues he deemed to be inappropriate for the gravity of their circumstances. That this incongruous sense of humor compounded by frequent digressions in my daily work—my recurrent tendency to engage in chitchat with my patients and share what I had discovered about them and their lives with our team on daily rounds—diverted attention from the "real work" of medicine.

My second month on the Internal Medicine service, now down the street at the nation's oldest hospital, spiraled me further away. My supervising senior resident, the real team leader at any academic medical center, was a sleep-deprived Ichabod Crane, straining from the toil and burden of being an overtrained scholar subjected to the life of an indentured servant and middleman. His bald pate perpetually coated with the sweat of powerlessness, frustration, and anger, his trembling hands both suppressing yet also revealing his desire to strangle whomever crossed his path, Dr. Crane taught me that medicine was just a glorified human conveyor belt. An institutionalized assembly line whose design and ever-accelerating pace served simply as a vehicle to victimize and torture its attendant laborers while producing nothing of real value to its purported beneficiaries, who in and of themselves were utterly inconsequential. In referring to patients as GOMERs (**G**et **O**ut of **M**y **E**mergency **R**oom), he revealed to me another feature of the gateway to the medical underworld, one characterized by cynicism in the midst of the invisibility, the irrelevance, and even the *worthlessness* of the subjects of us torturing middlemen: the patients.

This was my first window into a physician attribute known as *toxicity*, a common phenomenon in which the poison of burnout slowly seeps into the soul of the physician, converting every patient from a suffering individual in the fellowship of our common humanity into an enemy to disparage, avoid, and even defend oneself from. I found it was easy to become imprinted onto Dr. Crane's behavior, to acquire his way of thinking, responding to and coping with the challenges he faced in a similar fashion. To find myself glibly referring to a mostly unresponsive, elderly male with advanced Alzheimer's dementia—whom we were admitting to the hospital with sepsis from a urinary tract infection—as a GOMER. It took me decades to clearly understand the complexities that drove Crane to this final common pathway for so many physicians during their formative years. To recognize that toxicity results from a perfect storm created by technologies in search of constructive application, misaligned fiscal incentives, destructive institutional practices, unjust social structures, and the resultant preventable and at times unbearable human suffering of patients—all projected onto entitled young clinicians who find themselves cogs in a wheel, devoid of personal agency, lacking the interpersonal skills, life experiences, moral preparation, and mindsets needed to find meaning and purpose in their work. And, above all else, lacking a basic requirement for summoning equipoise and compassion: adequate sleep.

The afternoon my Internal Medicine rotation ended, I returned to my apartment near Osage Avenue to find, as usual, two of our little neighbors hanging out on our veranda with my roommate, another medical student. We had first befriended these magnetic kids' single mother, Amelia, a Jamaican in-home support caregiver and Seventh-Day Adventist who had found a way to insinuate her beautiful children—Caleb, age seven, and Briana, age fourteen—into our lives. Sharing with us how she feared for her children's futures in this city, she had hoped that we might be positive male role models for them, perhaps helping them avoid the patterns of drug dealing or addiction, incarceration, and teen pregnancy that she had witnessed her friends' promising children succumb to by simple virtue of living in this neighborhood. Caleb was a stunning boy who, while always unwashed and in ragged clothes, boasted a shining personality but, according to his mother, could never sit still at school and was struggling with reading. He was always pleading with us to give him rides on our bicycles, begging us to buy him his own. Briana was a budding beauty, her hair always in cornrows, her skin exuding coconut fragrance. She also was smart and curious, often looking over our shoulders as we studied anatomy, sitting on our couch listening to us spout the Latin names of nematodes that invade the human GI tract, or eavesdropping as we reviewed the mechanisms of action of oral contraceptives versus IUDs. We may even have purposely reviewed and re-reviewed this particular subject, expanding the scope of the curriculum in the hopes that what reached her ears might influence her future decisions and her life. We had all become a sort of family. My roommate and I were motivated to spend our precious free time with these youths not only for the refreshing relief from the grind that their presence provided us but by an unspoken belief that our presence in their lives would bear fruit, that our attachments would somehow buffer them from the unhealthy environment in which they were growing up.

The discordance between my connection to and impact on these children, and my disassociation from the patients I was charged to care for on the medical wards, was not lost on me. My dissatisfaction with medical school had only grown and had now become unbearable. The next day, I entered the office of the dean of students, requested a brief meeting, and announced to her my decision to drop out of medical school. She respectfully listened to my explanations and then, without attempting to either validate my experience or provide counterarguments, stated that she indeed would honor my request, at least in spirit. But rather than accepting my request to drop out, she informed me that she would instead grant me a one-year leave of absence, a no-strings offer that would allow me time and space to reflect and perhaps engage in some meaningful work during that year. If I were to change my mind, she said with her stone face, I would be welcomed back to complete my medical school training. Or were I to find myself resolute in my decision, I could decide to drop out then. While at the time I begrudgingly accepted her counteroffer, now I am forever grateful to her for this wise response to my request.

Over that next year, I did indeed reflect, and I did indeed engage in meaningful work. I spent the year working at the International Physicians for the Prevention of Nuclear War (IPPNW), forging medical school exchange programs between the US and the Soviet Union in support of mutual nuclear disarmament to avoid thermonuclear holocaust, what then was called the "final epidemic." This organization, led by two courageous cardiologists who received the 1985 Nobel Peace Prize on behalf of IPPNW for this work, began to connect me to the source of my interests in medicine and started to open my eyes to public health.

And so, duly inspired yet still ambivalent, I returned to medical school one year later. At a welcome-back dinner with our Jamaican family, I discovered that Briana, now fifteen, was four months pregnant. She ignored my request to talk to her about her plans for the pregnancy and, already a very different girl from the one I had left a year prior, she excused herself from the dinner table. We never spoke about it again.

I told myself to move on, that I had other work to do. I managed to do well in, and even enjoy, many of my remaining clinical rotations. Then, in 1991, as a late senior medical student, I learned that I could participate in away rotations, opportunities to work in other institutions. I jumped at the chance and applied for a rotation at the San Francisco General Hospital (SFGH) Mission Emergency Room. Known as *the Mish*, the SFGH ER represented the quintessential down-and-dirty public hospital experience, an infamous place rumored to be run by fourth-year medical students, a place where we got to do "real stuff" on our own, and lots of it: lumbar punctures, arterial lines, nasogastric tubes, IVs galore, even minor surgery. I told myself this was a chance to really dive in and see what medicine could do for me.

FINDING THE MISSION

Nothing could have been more different from the rarefied medical school experience I had been exposed to up to that point. In the Mish, I worked harder than I ever had, serving on the front line for thirteen-hour shifts six days a week for a month. This was my first real view into the medical underworld, basement doors now cast wide open. I was exposed to—and deeply immersed in—stressful and traumatic circumstances. A violent patient striking me. A patient with an alcohol-related, potentially fatal stomach hemorrhage vomiting liters of blood on me. Diagnosing a young heroin addict with a life-threatening bacterial heart valve infection and trying to convince her to undergo cardiothoracic surgery that could save her life. Caring for a middle-aged woman with uncontrolled diabetes and no primary care who had woken up with a cold leg and in whom I could detect no pulse below her groin, but who had been waiting to be seen for fourteen hours. Figuring out that an undocumented migrant with a fever of 104 degrees was suffering from malaria. And admitting patient after patient of young men my age in various stages of dying from AIDS.

The month was a whirlwind of sensory and emotional overload—from the sense of unending trauma and death to the joy of an impossible job well done. But most often, it was the confusion I felt by the dichotomous manner in which patients and colleagues treated me: at times with spite and disrespect, at other times with gratitude and dignity. And—as I exited the double doors after each shift—a feeling of being utterly exhausted and drained, yet somehow inspired and energized. I proudly wore the institution's cheeky and informal uniform—a T-shirt on which it was written SAN FRANCISCO GENERAL HOSPITAL: IT'S AS REAL AS IT GETS. This moniker couldn't have been more different from descriptions of my experiences at the private hospitals in Philadelphia.

Like all medical students who worked at the Mish, at the end of this rotation, as I was heading out of the ER for what I thought would be the last time, I was handed a signed letter on letterhead from then mayor Art Agnos, himself a prior beneficiary of the Mish's efforts to save his life after twice being shot in the chest. The letter thanked me—yes, it thanked *me*—for "serving the people of the City & County of San Francisco in their time of need." Standing in the ER parking lot in the dawn light, I read and reread that letter. As I looked back at the sealed double doors of the ER, it was as if this letter had created an opening in those doors, revealing to my mind and my heart the idea of the practice of medicine as a form of public service, as something that I could engage in explicitly to serve others. It provided me with the tangible seed for my continuing growth toward finding meaning in medicine.

Recently, my medical school roommate from the house near Osage Avenue, with whom I speak about twice a year, texted to say he really needed to talk to me. He said he was reaching out to tell me that Amelia, the Jamaican mother from West Philadelphia—"Do you remember her?"—had found him on Facebook and had contacted him, after nearly thirty years, because she wanted to thank the two of us for always being there for her two children. She then caught him up on her life and her kids. He was calling me because he thought I'd want to know that her kids were doing well and hear what they were doing. Amelia's daughter, Briana, who'd gotten pregnant at fifteen, was a mother of three happy and healthy and now grown children of her own, and—"Can you believe it?"—she worked as a clinical pharmacist in Philadelphia. And her brother, Caleb, also was thriving as a social worker for children with autism and intellectual and developmental disabilities.

CHAPTER 3

The Luminati

THE FACELESS ONES

August 1991. I was twenty-six years old. It was the second month of my twelve-month medical internship and my first time serving on the wards at San Francisco General Hospital. I had landed at the epicenter of the AIDS epidemic, the first of a four-year stretch of unprecedented death counts from AIDS, the overwhelming majority of which were occurring at this hospital, on Ward 5A. We had only recently discovered the causative agent for AIDS, and we still had no effective treatments for it. All we had was an old tool kit of antibiotics and antiviral and antifungal agents that we industriously put to work to try to hammer out the unusual and previously rare infections these patients were succumbing to, often repurposing the drugs in the hopes of preventing these same infections that we knew would inevitably overwhelm the next patient.

One out of every two patients I admitted was in the hospital because of an AIDS-related illness. The men came to this public hospital because we had a reputation of being more welcoming and less stigmatizing than the other hospitals, and because most young men never saw the need to carry health insurance. Most of these were men my age, young men just like me: sociable, talkative, engaging, inquisitive, and sexually active. But they were gay, and I was not. They were extremely ill, while I was not. As a newly minted, sleep-deprived doctor with no experience to draw from for how to face an epidemic of this nature, I was just trying to keep my head above water. These faceless, nameless men with nine-digit medical record numbers and an active problem list nine items long: they were dying. I was busy just trying to survive.

THE INTERROGATION ROOM

It was a little after 2:00 a.m. I was catching a bit of interrupted sleep in the on-call room I shared with an intern colleague. More like a prison cell. Every fifteen minutes or so, my pager went off. The screen lit up and read x8020. The Mish, of course. Our ER. Getting this kind of call was as if you had received two passenger tickets for the *Titanic*. My eyes still closed, I prayed it was just the nursing station calling me, perhaps to replenish some potassium for the guy we admitted with an exacerbation of heart failure. I sat up in my bed and punched the four numbers into the black phone on the side table.

"ER."

"Dr. Schillinger here. Medicine Service. I was paged," I offered up in my best monotone, careful not to reveal any emotion.

I slowly stewed for the minute I was on hold.

A booming voice came on the line. *"Dr. Schillinger!* Dr. Bailey here. I have a first-class ticket for you and a friend tonight. Or should I say, this *morning*. Someone you might recognize. You interested?"

"Do I have a choice, Bailey?"

"Actually, no. You don't. But hold on to your hat. You'll never believe this *case!*"

"Hit me, why don't you."

"Actually, why don't you hit me?"

"Okay, I'll play your little game. But it isn't gonna make me feel any better, Bailey. Here goes: twenty-eight-year-old gay man with multiple partners, previously in good health, presents with progressive shortness of breath over the course of two to three weeks. No chest pain, but a worsening, dry cough. Respiratory rate 22. All other vitals stable. Dry crackles on chest exam. Chest x-ray shows bilateral infiltrates. PO_2 78. Admitted for 'Rule out pneumonia.' Done. Am I right?"

"You're an absolute medical *wizard*, Dr. Schillinger. Future chief resident material for sure. How *do* you do it?"

"Maybe because I am working at San Francisco General during the AIDS crisis?"

"Could be, Schillinger. Could be. Simply astounding, nonetheless. But bad news is his PO_2 is 68, not 78. And he's thirty-three years old, not twenty-eight."

"Bailey. Let's cut the crap. Have you done the full workup? Or are you leaving me to clean up your mess?"

"No mess, no fuss. He's all tucked in. Blood gas done, as I believe I mentioned. First sputum already collected and cooking at the lab. On Septra already. I am leaving the *weighty* decision about steroids to you and your attending. Oh, but I just couldn't fathom the idea of doing an unsuccessful dilated retinal exam in this busy and brightly lit ER. I absolutely *hate* being anything less than 100 percent effective. This is most definitely something for you to do with him in the dark, quiet moments you will be sharing during the wee hours on 5A. Oh, and if you are interested, his name is Simpson. And he has a bed ready. What do you make of that? Oh—and you're welcome."

I wheeled Simpson, hooked to an oxygen tank, up to 5A. He was talkative in the elevator. I answered in short sentences and told him we would talk once we were in his room. I mechanically carried out what unsurprisingly was a rote history and physical exam. He seemed inappropriately glib and sociable. While his HIV test had not yet come back, I asked him if he was aware that his illness may represent AIDS. That he may have a type of pneumonia caused by *Pneumocystis*, a previously rare fungal infection—now terribly common in patients with AIDS—that could fill up his lungs unless we aggressively attacked it.

"It's called PCP," I told him. "You're gonna hear us say it a lot over the next few weeks."

He changed the subject. "You single?"

I looked at him askance.

"No, no, Doc, I'm not asking for that reason. Just trying to make some chitchat to calm my nerves. Plus, you got to ask me all those real personal questions. It's only fair." His pulse ox showed only 88 percent. I readjusted the oxygen tubing in his nostrils. He smiled.

"You're right, it isn't fair. Well, okay then, I'm actually not single. I have a girlfriend."

He was listening closely. But I pushed on with my agenda.

"Look, we're almost done here. I just need to look in your eyes. HIV can affect the retina, the back of your eye. There is a kind of infection—it's called CMV—that can make people blind if we don't catch it early. About one in four people we admit to the hospital with PCP also have CMV in their eyes but don't have visual symptoms yet. So, I need to check. I'll need to put some drops in your eyes to make your pupils open up, and then turn the lights off to see inside the back of your eyes. Is that okay?"

"Does it hurt?"

"No, not at all. It can feel bright, though. I need to use a little scope that has a light at the end of it and a lens through which I can see straight through your cornea to the retina."

He nodded. "All right, then."

I pulled out the little plastic bottle I carried in my fanny pack and placed a few drops into his eyes. I then withdrew my ophthalmoscope, shaped like an upright flashlight. I showed it to him and then turned out the lights.

"Let's give those pupils a few seconds to open up."

"Ooooh, it's dark in here," he said ghoulishly.

I pointed out the little glowing red light at the end of his bed. "Please try to just stare at this little red light while I am doing my thing. Try not to move your eyes as I look into them."

I advanced my scope until we were almost eye to eye, my right eye against his right eye. Only the thin, scalloped plastic rim of the scope's lens separated our breathing faces. I felt the cool flow from his oxygen tank tickling my face, combined with the warm flow of his exhalations. I searched for the optic nerve, the central landmark in the retina where all the blood vessels and nerves emerge from and return to. It is never easy.

"Wow, that *was* blinding," he complained. "I feel like I am in an interrogation room. What more could you possibly want to know from me?"

"Shhhh."

I'd lost my path to the optic nerve, so I backed out to reboot.

"Really, no talking."

I repositioned the light into his pupil, slowly approached his right eye again, and started my scanning all over.

Staying very still, he whispered to me, "I've heard them say that when you look into the inside of someone's eyes, it's like you're staring into that person's soul."

"Don't move, please."

I located the optic nerve again and then gradually and systematically scanned the entire retinal circumference on the back of the optic bulb, looking for the characteristic pepperoni-and-cheese-pizza pattern of CMV infection, which represents retinal hemorrhages and protein that have leaked through the thin membrane. Nothing bad there. I pulled away.

"You did great, Mr. Simpson. This retina looks totally normal. Lemme switch sides. Just keep looking at that little red light, please. And then we'll be done for the night."

Now it was left eye against left eye. He stayed very still. I spun the dial around the rim of the scope's lens with my left index finger, slowly bringing the retina into focus. Optic nerve—check. I then started to slowly scan the circumference of this retina. I stopped when I saw two small hemorrhages at 7:30, at the nasal edge of his retina. Nothing anywhere else. I backed away and turned on the soft bedside light.

"I see some red spots on this one. You're not having any problems with your eyesight, right? It looks like you have early CMV in that left eye. I'll have the eye doctors come tomorrow to take a better look with their fancier machines. We probably will have to give you a second medicine that fights CMV or put some of it into that eye. We'll see what they say, okay? I'll see you at about 7:30 tomorrow morning. That gives us both a little under three hours to get some shut-eye. Good night."

I went back to my call room in the hopes of crashing for a few hours before it all started up again. As I crawled into my twin bed, I saw a pile of papers next to the black phone. Our residents and attending physicians were always passing out the latest studies to inform how we can best care for our patients. These papers had felt so irrelevant to me, so inappropriate: *Just tell me what to do or let me quickly look it up in a textbook. I am exhausted, can't you see?* This was not the ideal learning moment. This was a moment to help me get through each day without killing anyone. *What does research have to do with anything? Don't we know pretty much everything already anyway?*

But the title of the paper on the top of the pile grabbed me, something that had never happened to me since starting residency: "A Trial of Early Corticosteroids in AIDS Patients with PCP." *New England Journal of Medicine*. I quickly read through the abstract and then scanned through the full study. They asked the question, "Do steroids improve one-month survival for AIDS patients admitted to the hospital with PCP?" Turns out—yes, they do. They reduce death by 50 percent at one month. But the benefit was seen only in patients with moderate to severe PCP, defined as having a PO_2 level less than 70. That was my patient, Mr. Simpson! A PO_2 of 68, the oxygen level of a healthy person who had been dropped onto the top of a mountain that is three kilometers high. I called 5A and asked to speak to Simpson's nurse. I ordered up oral prednisone, 40 mg twice daily, to be started immediately.

A YELLOW GENIE IN THE BOTTLE

The only thing his mother told the paramedics was that Raskin had been lying on the couch of the downstairs in-law apartment for about three months. Lying on the couch, drinking vodka straight from the bottle, and watching bad TV on KOFY—channel 38—the channel that plays reruns of old sitcoms. When she went downstairs to check on him, he didn't recognize her, and he was saying some crazy stuff. So, she called 911.

My intern Craig and I approached Patient Raskin in the male ward of the Mish. The rancid smell of metabolized alcohol mixed with sweat drifted off his jaundiced skin. An adult version of the starving, wide-eyed Bangladeshi child one saw portrayed on television in campaigns to end global hunger. His face like a luminous skull, encircled by oxygen tubing, his legs spindly. And his abdomen protuberant like a pregnant woman's. And he glowed, ever so slightly, like a dim lightbulb. But the whites of his open eyes shined fluorescent neon.

He was calm and silent, nothing like the shaking and baking man in acute alcohol withdrawal that my fellow resident in the Mish had described to me over the phone. Amazing what Valium can do for a man. We were told to bring him right upstairs for a full workup. They were too full to complete it down in the Mish.

Altered mental status, jaundice, and mild hypoxia in a young alcoholic man with a massive belly. The wheels started turning and we started in on our practiced routine. The first thing was to tap the fluid in his abdomen to assess whether this was just the leaky insides of a pressurized belly choked by a scarring, cirrhotic liver—itself a significant problem. Or whether it represented liters of fluid oozing from an abdominal tumor or—worse still—trapped cirrhotic fluid that had turned into an infected cesspool, a life-threatening condition known as *spontaneous bacterial peritonitis*, or SBP.

Because Raskin was not competent to make decisions for himself, I called his mother. She gave me blanket consent to do all we could to help her son. I poured some Betadine solution on his skin down and to the left of his protruding belly button and prepped his belly for a diagnostic tap. The cool, orange fluid and my rubbing on his belly seemed to perk him up.

"Master, I have a mother-in-law problem," he mumbled.

I shot a look over at Craig, who was setting up the paracentesis kit, along with the tubes to send to the lab. He shook his head.

"Mr. Raskin, what did you say about your mother?"

"That's like comparing oranges and lemons, Major Healey," he responded.

"Mr. Raskin, I am cleaning your belly with this orange liquid soap so we can put a small needle inside to make sure you don't have a serious infection. Is that okay with you?"

"Major, you can make a man eat shredded cardboard, if you play the right tricks."

Craig let out a laugh. "We're now in Bizarro World."

Raskin's neon eyes were wide-open as if in fear, and he raised his voice. "She *can't* turn against you. You're her master. She has to obey you!"

"It's okay, Mr. Raskin," I said. "You can relax. We will take care of her and take care of you. And as her master, I will take your response as a yes to tap your belly. Craig, pass me the goods."

"Why will you not let me turn Dr. Bellows into a frog? Dr. Bellows was only doing his job."

Over the next few hours, we confirmed that Raskin had SBP and that he was in liver failure, on top of acute alcoholic hepatitis. We initiated IV antibiotics and decided we should carry out a full belly tap later to relieve his discomfort and give his lungs more room to breathe. His altered mental status was likely a manifestation of alcoholic hallucinosis, an early sign of serious alcohol withdrawal syndrome, combined with the effects of a bad intra-abdominal infection. We carried out a lumbar puncture and ruled out meningitis as an additional cause. We got a portable chest x-ray to evaluate his low oxygen level. Returning from the Radiology reading room, Craig caught up with me while I was checking lab results in the resident room.

"The new guy's got bilateral interstitial infiltrates. He's probably got PCP."

"Are you kidding me? Like we don't have enough to deal with on him?"

I called the floor nurse and ordered an HIV test on him. "And please get some Septra in him ASAP. And if he hasn't eaten today, get an induced sputum. Looks like he has PCP. And let's transfer him to 5A. Craig will come and write the orders now."

Late in the afternoon of our post-call day, we entered Raskin's room in the hopes of withdrawing the free fluid from his abdomen, armed with three single-liter vacuum bottles and several feet of clear tubing with a large-bore needle at each end. Sort of like illicitly tapping a gas tank by sucking on a hose. He was even more fluorescent, like a human glowworm. And he was more animated, mumbling to himself. The nurses had to put him in soft restraints, one for each limb, as he kept pulling off his oxygen tubing and trying to get out of bed. He was more hypoxic, so we increased the flow of his oxygen to four liters per minute.

"Mr. Raskin, we're back again. Here to get all that fluid out of your belly and lighten your load, okay? It should make you breathe easier as well."

His neon eyes stared at the ceiling as he said, emotionless, "Some men dedicate their lives to science, and some men dedicate their lives to politics. I'm dedicating my life to understanding you, Nelson."

Craig and I looked at each other.

"What the hell?" I asked him in a whisper. He shrugged and returned to setting up the IV albumin he would simultaneously infuse into Raskin's vein in an attempt to prevent his kidneys from shutting down due to the rapid fluid shifts I was about to incite.

Raskin was quite the sight. Deeply jaundiced, he had a large-bore needle sticking out from his lower belly, with a long tube snaking down to a bottle on the floor, amber fluid slowly collecting in it.

We spent the next forty-five minutes drawing out three liters of fluid, with Raskin droning on in a monotone voice all the while, as if reading from a script. Midway through, he suddenly lifted his head and locked eyes with mine.

"How are things going, Jeannie? Terrible, Master. I have to make dinner. I mean actually make it without magic. We are liable to die."

I ignored his nonsense, concentrating on ensuring that the flow of fluid continued, safe and uninterrupted.

I pulled out the needle.

"Raskin—we're done here. You can rest easy now."

"How dost thou wish to die, Master? Of old age. I'm only trying to safeguard the welfare of my astronauts, Major Nelson!"

"Okay, Raskin. We're trying to look out for your welfare too."

I gave one of the bottles to Craig and bent down to pick up the other two into one arm.

Raskin turned his head toward me as I was exiting his room and complained, "A million bottles on the beach, and I had to pick hers."

"Maybe we need to give him more lactulose, or even neomycin," I said to Craig in the hallway, implying that Raskin's increasing verbal ejaculations might be a manifestation of liver failure's toxic effects on the brain.

"I don't think this is hepatic encephalopathy," he said to me. "The things he's saying . . . they're too cogent. It's like there's some story inside his head that he's trying to get out. But I can't figure it out."

The next morning, Craig didn't show for 7:30 a.m. rounds. I paged him to find out why he was late.

"Meet me in 5R," he said, bubbling with enthusiasm, even joy. "I'm with Raskin. And I figured it out!"

Raskin, in the ICU? I trotted to 5R and saw Raskin aglow in an ICU bed, still in four-point restraints, but now wearing a full face mask with high-flow oxygen.

Craig got up from behind the nurses' station and approached me.

"Hey. So, last night—no, early this morning—he went into acute kidney failure and his O_2 sat dropped to the 80s. His repeat chest x-ray showed progression of the PCP. The night float moved him here, which made sense because, well . . . he's kinda crashing."

"Did you start steroids on him?"

"Yeah, I started them a few minutes ago, and I called Renal to see if they'll be willing to dialyze him. Doubtful, don't you think?"

"Yeah, doubtful."

"But whatever. That's not the thing. The *real* thing is that I figured it out. I figured *him* out."

"What do you mean?"

"Okay. Think about it. All this talk about 'Master this' and 'Master that.' And Major Nelson. And Roger Healey. And astronauts and bottles? And Jeannie?"

"Yeah, what about it?"

"They're all characters in the show *I Dream of Jeannie*. Which means he's been replaying episodes of *I Dream of Jeannie*. Feeding us lines—word for word—from the show. Remember, he lay on his couch for three months, maybe longer, just watching reruns on KOFY 38? While getting smashed?"

He tapped his forefinger to his temple and said, "All that's left up there is a set of scripted reactions that come from those episodes. Think about it. It's incredible. Admit it: I'm a genius."

"Okay, okay," I replied, unable to hold back my chuckling. "So, either you just figured out how the subconscious and toxified mind of a man dying of liver failure and AIDS works, or you just proved to me that you watched way too much bad TV as a kid."

"How about we say yes and yes to that?"

THE SHRILL OF THE WHISTLE

I was the intern on call at San Francisco General again, a lowly infantryman in the trenches on the front. We were making our morning rounds on my current load of patients, whistle-free for now. My attending physician was a gentle man, about forty-five years old, an infectious disease doctor whom I presumed had no choice but to become an expert in HIV. He was a fountain of knowledge. I attempted to push away the anxiety that I was feeling, the sense of impending doom, so I could try to soak up as much knowledge as I could. I looked at him closely as he spoke. He was a feeble man. He walked slowly, his hair looked like it had fallen out in clumps, and his skin was mottled. While his mini-lecturing was comprehensive and insightful, his memory for the details of our specific patients seemed paradoxically spotty. As if he were more interested in the diseases than the people. He carried a clipboard with him wherever he went, writing down every detail as we moved through our patient panel.

As rounds ended, I pulled aside my resident, Frank Massey.

"Frank, what's up with Dr. Edmunds? I mean, he's super chill and knowledgeable, but he doesn't seem to have a grasp on the details of each patient. And he carries that clipboard around, always writing stuff down. Is he just a hands-off attending? A big-picture guy, leaving the details to us? Plus, I don't know about you but, to me, he doesn't look good. Every step, every word, seems to take an effort."

"Yup. You got a good eye for an intern. You want the truth? You and I are running this service, my friend. Edmunds is sick. I heard a rumor—I can't confirm it, but I think it's true—that he's got AIDS. And now lymphoma, status post-chemo. And that he refuses to go on medical leave. He sees this as his mission in life, at least what is left of it."

"Holy shit. That both freaks me out and at the same time is super inspiring. Do you think he's competent to do this? I mean, his memory seems questionable."

"Let us be his working memory. I'll make the call if I see anything going awry. And let's keep this on the down-low, okay?"

My resident, Massey, was gay. Openly so, and in moments of levity, almost flamboyantly so. On our call night, in between hospital admissions, while eating "midnight meal" with my co-intern and two medical students, he would tell us about the experience of being gay in Indianapolis, where he was from, versus being gay in San Francisco. This gave me an opening to ask him a question I'd always wondered about.

"Frank, I've always wanted to ask: How do you guys know if someone else is gay? I mean, let's say you want to come on to someone. But you have *zero* idea if they're gay. So, it could either end up in a romantic night or a punch in the face. How do you guys navigate that? Do you have some inside signals?"

Massey burst out laughing, his cereal exploding out of his mouth.

"Dean, Dean, Dean. Are you *serious*? Yes, we all pull out little red bandannas from our back right pockets and flutter our asses like peacocks. Others have a quiet little dog whistle they blow that only we can hear. Those are our subtle signals."

"No, seriously, I'm just curious. Because not every gay man looks and acts like the stereotype," I say, trying to recover some face.

"Really? Okay then." He turned to our group of four that he supervises. "You people wanna know too, I presume? Well, here's the million-dollar answer: We're just like everyone else. We're no different."

He turned back to me and asked with a smile, "How do *you* know if someone is interested in you? How do you even know whether you should come on to them? In your case, I presume, we're talking about a woman. Fine. So how do you know?"

"Well, I just assume, you know, playing the numbers, that she's into men."

"But that's not how it works, is it? It's not whether she's into men. It's whether you think she might be into *you* and whether you have a shot, right? And then, after you make your move, you reassess, no? Based on her body language, based on what she says in response to what you've said and *how* she says it. And based on the *light* in her eyes, the sparkle. Sometimes you guess wrong, but other times you guess right. Which means that sometimes you score and sometimes you get a slap in the face—real or metaphorical. So, in answer to your very sweet and incredibly naïve question, it's like I said: we're no different from you."

I was about to ask a more important follow-up question to learn how he assessed the potential HIV status of any potential sexual partner, but our escapade into the mysteries of gay romance in the early 1990s was interrupted by the simultaneous whistles of his pager and mine. x8020. The Mish.

BRIGHT LIGHTS, BAD CT SCAN

The next morning, we were making our post-call morning rounds with Dr. Edmunds. We admitted nine new folks on top of the twelve we already had, and with Edmunds at the helm, our progress was painfully slow. Edmunds was rightly most concerned about a middle-aged HIV-positive woman—reported to be a prostitute—who presented with altered mental status. She was somnolent and only sporadically responded to sternal rubs or other forms of physical stimulation. The rest of her neurological exam was normal, and her lumbar puncture had some protein and a few white cells but otherwise was not diagnostic. The syphilis test from her cerebrospinal fluid was pending. We had her on meningitis-dose antibiotics and antifungal medications just in case. The rest of her lab evaluation had been pretty much normal, and her urine tox screen for illicit substances was positive only for cocaine.

"I'm worried about her. This is going to turn out to be something weird," said Edmunds at her bedside. "In HIV, it's often either a common problem presenting in an uncommon fashion, or an uncommon problem presenting commonly."

He paused to let us ponder that statement.

"If her kidney function's good, I would add in high-dose acyclovir to cover for herpes encephalitis," Edmunds said. "Continue all the meningitis meds. And call Neuro again to see if they can do an EEG. Herpes in the brain can give you stereotypical waveforms in a temporal lobe or two."

He then turned to me. "And what does the CT scan show?"

I looked at Massey, and he discreetly nodded.

"I think you just wrote it down, Dr. Edmunds," I reminded him as gently as I could. "She got her CT scan at 5:00 a.m., and we're waiting for the formal read. They said the attending radiologist would get in about now, so I can run down now and see what they found, or we can finish rounds if you prefer and then I can go."

"Right. I'll let you decide since you know your other patients better than I do."

This dying man had grace.

Massey confirmed it was up to me and said he could cover me for a few minutes on rounds if I wanted to check the CT scan. I decided to feed my curiosity and Edmunds's concern and break from rounds.

The CT neuroradiology room was the opposite of the patient-facing areas of the hospital. Here, everything was dark, cool, and quiet. Organized, peaceful. A backlit x-ray display panel was the only source of light. Three doctors in pristine white coats sat in a row in reclining office chairs, facing the panel. It was covered with black sheets of developed film placed into a vertically rotating carousel that rolled through the series of images at the press of a foot pedal. One of the radiologists—presumably the attending—held a small hand recorder into which she was dictating her current interpretation. She was killer smart, sarcastic, and more than a bit intimidating. I had heard she was the best neuroradiologist in the country and that she had written the textbook on HIV-related radiology of the central nervous system.

"What can we do for you?" her resident asked.

"Yeah, thanks. Medicine Service 3. Ward 5A, Bed 13. Medical record number 01077633. Forty-five-year-old lady with HIV, low-grade fever, altered mental status, nonfocal neuro exam. CD4 count 41, lumbar puncture with just a little bit of nonspecific action. Awaiting final word regarding microorganisms, so I doubt *Cryptococcus*. Still waiting for Neuro consult. So— no diagnosis yet. We're looking for *Toxo*, lymphoma, HSV encephalitis, or other, weirder stuff."

The attending wheeled her chair forward and pressed the foot pedal to reverse the carousel, the motor loudly reverberating as it flipped backward through the images.

"Right. We just looked at her scans. This is gonna be one of the weirder things. Take a look."

The nine images in front of me showed cross-sectional slices of her brain starting from the top of her scalp down to the top of her neck. The brain tissue appeared swollen, the grooves and folds less pronounced. I recognized the black fluid-filled ventricles of her brain. They were a bit larger than what I was used to. I saw the clear delineation between the gray matter and the white matter. I didn't see the grayish, ring-enhanced golf balls scattered throughout the brain that could mean toxoplasmosis, nor did I see the more geographic shape of a lymphoma. I kept scanning as I descended down her brain. Then I was hit with a bright light, a linear strip of white located above her olfactory nerves, with a contiguous white oval mass extending into her right frontal lobe. The temporal lobes looked normal to me. Feeling the powerlessness of my ignorance, I simply pointed to the blinding white region.

"Here?"

"Nicely done, Doctor," the attending quipped.

"Okay, so I can find the bright white abnormality. Hurray for me. But what is it?"

"Some sort of meningoencephalitis affecting the lining of the brain and then extending into it. The location suggests basilar meningitis. We often see that with TB and syphilis. I'd start there with your treatment, and see what the spinal fluid shows and what it grows. Then you can whittle it down. You might want to throw in some high-dose dexamethasone to get that brain swelling to go down. If you get in a bind, I'd suggest you ask the neurosurgeons to biopsy that frontal lobe. It seems accessible. And lemme know what you find out. I don't care if it's on autopsy. I *need* to know. Don't forget."

I rushed back up to 5A to tell Massey and Edmunds that we needed to get TB meds on board, but they were not there. I asked one of the nurses where they were, and he told me that they had to transfer my patient to the ICU because it looked like her brain might be herniating, a neurosurgical emergency.

As I ran over to the ICU, my pager went off: x8172, the micro lab. These guys were good. It was the Filipina lab tech, the woman whom I had gotten to know well in only two weeks on the wards here.

"Hi again, Doctor. Sorry for the delay. We think we have an answer. We needed to run it by our lab director. I first thought it was *Cryptococcus*, but I wasn't quite sure. It turns out it's an amoeba. *Naegleria. Naegleria fowleri.*"

Naegleria, Naegleria. I knew that name. I reached back to my medical school microbiology class. Yes. That strange amoeba that can crawl up your nose and through your olfactory nerves to infect the base of the front of your brain. You get it from diving into or swimming in contaminated fresh water, usually in warm countries with warm water sources. Super rare, super fatal. Not something I would ever imagine seeing in temperate San Francisco.

"You sure?"

"One hundred percent, Doctor."

I found Massey in 5R. He was at the nurses' station writing orders in her chart.

"It's *Naegleria* meningoencephalitis," I told him. He looked up at me, puzzled.

"CT scan and micro lab say so, so that's what I'm telling you," I declared. "And like I always say, in HIV, it's gonna either be a common problem presenting uncommonly, or an uncommon problem presenting commonly."

Massey rolled his eyes at me.

Dr. Edmunds was helping the nurse transfer my patient from the gurney to her new bed in the ICU. The morning light from over the hills above the highway shined on him, illuminating him like a saint in an El Greco painting. What was he doing? He's an *attending* physician. He didn't even need to be here, since once a patient from the wards was transferred to the ICU, a different attending specialist should take over the care. He certainly didn't need to be moving a patient. I rushed in to help, getting on the far side of the bed to receive the sheet that the patient was swaddled in.

Massey called out to me, "I have no idea what *Naegleria* is or how to treat it!"

Dr. Edmunds looked up. "*Naegleria?* Amphotericin B, 1.5 mg/kg in two divided doses. Follow kidney function closely. Plus, rifampin 10 mg/kg once daily. Check for drug interactions."

Massey looked at me in disbelief. I ordered the medications.

Neurosurgery arrived and took her down to the OR to place a bolt in her skull and relieve the pressure causing her brain to get squeezed, with no real exit. They left in a pressure monitor to allow us to make sure it was working. Over the next few days, I religiously administered the amphotericin and rifampin. But her cognitive function never returned. She remained in a coma.

Dr. Edmunds visited her twice daily, a familiar guest in the ICU. Or maybe he was visiting me.

"How are you doing with all this?" he asked me in her room on ICU day number four. I am quite sure he had forgotten my name.

"I'm good, Dr. Edmunds, thanks."

"You're *good?*"

"Actually, no, not entirely. This is awful. I mean, we made a quick diagnosis—kind of a superhuman diagnosis—and we started her on the right meds, and she got the bolt right away, just in time. And yet, nothing. I'm not seeing an end to this. I feel pretty powerless."

I wanted to ask him how long we should continue trying, whether it was even worth it, but I thought better of it.

"I know, I know," he said quietly. He turned, looking at me with his radiant blue eyes, eyes that seemed to emanate pure light.

"Make sure her teeth get brushed twice a day. And that she gets a sponge bath every few days. And that her hair is brushed. In fact, brush her hair yourself sometimes. With care. Don't think you're too highly trained to do that. It can be part of the job. I know I'm not your attending on this case anymore, but that's my final order. It will help her. And it will make you feel better. I promise."

Dr. Edmunds never returned to work on the wards at San Francisco General. He died of complications of AIDS-related lymphoma the next month.

A BLINDING NIGHTMARE

Dr. Edmunds's moment of commitment and mentorship began to open my eyes to the dozens of alternative responses that were emerging around this epidemic—and around me. Witnessing these acts—acts of kindness, curiosity, ingenuity, industriousness, advocacy, resilience, and love—gradually began to change me, allowing me to see and to behave differently. And, in aggregate, these acts changed the culture of the institution in which I was working, slowly converting it from an epicenter of suffering, cynicism, and sorrow to a hub for compassionate models of care, innovative science, community engagement, and broader social change. Over time, I too was transformed, becoming part of this movement, taking in some of these lessons, adapting them, and then applying them to my future work.

Many years have passed since I was a young doctor in training, caring for a thousand or so patients at the peak of the AIDS epidemic. Despite the intensity of this experience, or perhaps because of its unremitting intensity, I recall only a few faces and a few stories as conveyed here. At the time, the highly regarded *Journal of the American Medical Association* would publish a special annual issue on AIDS. While the cover of the weekly *JAMA* was traditionally adorned by a beautiful work of art, for this special issue, the editors would adorn the cover with an empty void: pure and white, with no image and no art. It was largely a blank page, an overwhelmingly bright, white page. It is only now that I recognize the statement that they were making. While I have always prided myself in my ability to never forget a face and to always remember a good story, as a formerly overworked and underprepared doctor in training, I admit that my memory from that time is mostly devoid of patients' faces and patients' stories. Many of my colleagues report similar difficulties evoking specific names and faces from that time. It was as if we all were suffering from a unique form of vicarious trauma. The kind that blinds.

Looking back, I now realize that, in the face of this surge of suffering humanity, I lost a part of my own humanity. Many of these men remain faceless. Most of what I am left with is a set of archetypes that reflects my working relationships with them, what I can only describe as *industrial* relationships. They were young men with the fate of having an intern—one who was largely disinterested or more like numb—whose job was to transition them from initial diagnosis and disclosure, through their inevitable denial, through the overcoming of their resistance, and then through a series of treatments. These treatments occasionally provided them with a few months of respite, while other treatments simply lengthened their suffering or were all-out failures from the get-go. Many of these patients were just nameless men who represented bottomless pits, the depths of which we were forced to mine in, men to learn medicine from, or, as we often said, to learn medicine *on*. Sometimes these men were to be feared as potential vectors of HIV. At other times, they were to be pitied, or glossed over, or, only sporadically, to be helped. At my worst, they were a group of men so foreign to me that my role simply became to *process* them, to efficiently move them through the different levels of care offered at this institution. And then to forget them. And to get ready to do it all over again. As if I were a *kapo* transporting skeletal concentration camp victims through the machine of modern medicine.

How is it that I was unable to see these men for who they were, that I often failed to offer hope and provide alternate ways of caring, and that I would obsessively focus on my own survival amid this plague? These are questions that are hard for me to ask, much less answer. The closest I can come to conveying this is by describing a recurring dream I began to have just after I had finished my internship year.

I am camping alone at night in a forest. I know that there are animals in the forest; it has been rumored that there are bears and wolves to contend with. I sleep an unquiet sleep. I am awakened by cries for help and quickly crawl out of my tent. It is pitch-black. I can barely see my own hand in front of my face. I hear another cry. I am not sure if it is a human cry or a wolf's howl. But I try to advance toward it. As I approach the howling cries, a bright flashlight is cast right at my eyes, blinding me. I try to shield my eyes so I can see where I am going, to establish who needs help and determine what kind of help they need so I can spring into action. But the bright light only intensifies. All I can see are brief impressions of movement, glimpses of fearful people running and of creatures in pursuit. The bright light is persistent. It stings my eyes so I cannot keep them open. And it overwhelms me.

CHAPTER 4

The Culture of Blood

The brain, when seen up close, and understood thoroughly,
has a form and function of a weapon, no more than that.

—Gonçalo M. Tavares, *Learning to Pray in the*
Age of Technique

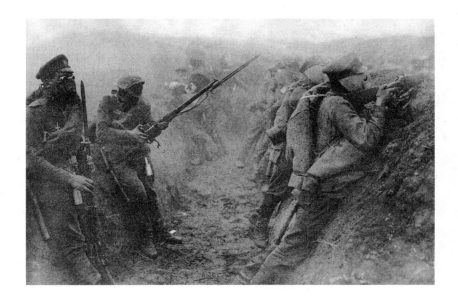

INSIDE THE TRENCHES

It was the spring of 1993. I was a twenty-seven-year-old physician, serving as a junior resident on the Medicine Service of San Francisco General Hospital (SFGH). I was like a World War I soldier serving in the medical trenches at the peak of the AIDS epidemic, another great war—but this one was being fought on the home front. I was working up to one hundred hours a week. Every fourth night, I was on call, drafted along with my two intern team members for thirty-four-hour shifts. We were tasked with admitting new patients from the emergency room (ER) while also caring for the service's one hundred or so patients during the overnight shift. Our colleagues, mummified in their scrubs and hiding under their blankets, were catching up on some sleep for a few hours, recovering from their last on-call shift and preparing for their next cycle of combat.

This was a war we were losing. My team's service had swelled to twenty-three patients. Every second patient was a young man, around my age, suffering from one or more manifestations of AIDS—so-called opportunistic infections. As their immune systems deteriorated, their bodies succumbed to organisms that usually were benign and, before the advent of AIDS, were rarely causes of illness. *Pneumocystis carinii*, a ubiquitous fungal-type microbe that infected 80 percent of AIDS patients, led to a progressive pneumonia that left these men gasping for their very lives. Or their bodies became susceptible to, then overwhelmed by, more common but normally more indolent organisms, such as *Mycobacterium tuberculosis*, the age-old infection that felled Mimi in *La Bohème*. Consumption, as TB was previously referred to, was now resurgent at SFGH. In fact, in AIDS patients, we often witnessed "galloping consumption," a phenomenon in which TB, which characteristically leads people through a slow death march, instead killed them with a racehorse pace.

Our weapons against AIDS were limited to prolonged administration of antibiotics to treat diagnosed infections, prophylactic antibiotic use to prevent imminent infections, and using a new antiviral drug—AZT—that was only slightly more effective in attacking HIV itself than spitting into the wind. One of the great medical minds of the time, our war's general, was the incomparable Dr. Merle Sande, an infectious disease specialist and chief of the Medical Service at SFGH. Dr. Sande's great passion for medicine was matched by his ego, his temper, his indiscretion, and his unparalleled ability to inspire others to fight against this great scourge of the late twentieth century. I was both fortunate and terrified to have Dr. Sande as my supervising attending physician.

It was around 2:00 a.m., and I was called to "the Mish," our nickname for the ER at SFGH (once known as *the Mission*), to admit our second "shooter with a fever." This then widely used adage referred to a patient with current IV drug use (or a history of drug use, as Merle had cynically taught us that "once a shooter, always a shooter") who was presenting with an unexplained fever. This clinical syndrome, which accounted for about 10 percent of my admissions during my service on the SFGH medicine wards, has a significant probability of declaring itself over the forty-eight hours after presentation as one of the most feared infections we know: acute bacterial endocarditis. Occurring in about 20 percent of injection drug users with a fever—often without any localizing signs, symptoms, or initial blood test abnormalities—endocarditis results when *Staph* bacteria from the skin, most commonly *Staphylococcus aureus*, enter the bloodstream at the time of injection and find their way to the valves of the heart. Once there, they adhere to the valve and set up shop. They then wreak havoc by destroying the valve and causing acute heart failure and death, or sending showers of bacteria throughout the circulation, leading to multiple abscesses (pockets of bacteria and pus) in the lungs, the brain, the kidneys, and so on, leading to sepsis and death. The only way to diagnose the infection is to obtain, at the time of presentation, two sets of blood cultures in a sterile fashion prior to any antibiotics being administered and assessing at forty-eight hours whether *both* blood cultures grow the bacterium. The admission algorithm for a shooter with a fever, therefore, is to secure two sets of blood cultures in the ER, initiate antibiotics to cover for the possibility of endocarditis, and then either continue them or peel them off once the blood cultures come back as positive or negative, respectively.

This nameless shooter with a fever was much like many others I had previously admitted and was the second such admission on this on-call shift. He was Black and, like so many users whose needle-sharing was habitual, he was HIV positive.

He was in his late fifties and was a product of his times. In the '60s and '70s in San Francisco, heroin addiction caught on like wildfire, an untoward result of the hippie movement and habits brought back by veterans returning from Vietnam. He was one of many long-term users whose body revealed the stigmata of decades of dirty injections and abscesses, with blown veins and scarred skin, and with a fully gray Afro and a deeply wrinkled face that made him look like an eighty-year-old. To treat his heroin withdrawal symptoms—which can include projectile vomiting and explosive diarrhea, not to mention pain and agony—the ER had appropriately given him a 50 mg dose of methadone. Methadone is a long-acting opiate medication related to heroin that can be used to slowly detox people, provide them with a safe alternative as a maintenance drug, or serve as a bridge during a hospitalization. As a result, he was somnolent and refused most interactions beyond the physical exam. When he did speak, he was irritable, and he answered our questions with a yes or a no or, finally, "You keep asking me the same questions over and over. I already answered them. Leave me alone!"

We were unable to obtain a detailed history. He avoided any eye contact. Further, we were unable to make a personal connection with him. My intern informed me that the patient's medical workup had already been completed by the ER physicians. We reviewed the chest x-ray and results of the blood work, all of which were unremarkable, and we admitted him to the fifth floor, with a diagnosis of "rule out endocarditis." We "tucked him in," and the forty-eight-hour blood culture vigil began.

Within hours, the calls from the nursing staff began. He was increasingly agitated, belligerent, and demanding. He had gone from being pleasantly snowed to becoming a high-maintenance patient with a history of heroin use, acting out since he couldn't get his next fix. Throughout the night, he yelled for pain medications, punctuating the monotonous beeps of the medical ward with his curses and his threats. While he demanded Dilaudid and morphine, I negotiated to provide him with another 50 mg dose of methadone, as it had become apparent that when it came to his heroin habit, he was no lightweight.

Our task for the next day was to make sure every one of our patients made it through the night and then to try to efficiently direct the human processing necessary to move as many patients as possible from presentation to diagnosis to recovery to discharge. This included ordering the CAT scans, speaking to the families, reassessing our patients, and reviewing their labs. It involved inserting the IVs, removing the catheters, reinserting the catheters, signing the death certificates, and examining biopsy results. It featured coaxing or bribing the social worker, transferring patients from the ICU to a regular room or vice versa, discussing complex cases with subspecialists, making follow-up appointments, and completing paperwork. And more paperwork.

At morning bedside rounds, I was so tired that I found myself almost envious of the emaciated AIDS patients, the shooters with fevers, the man with metastatic lung cancer, and the woman with lupus-induced kidney failure. They all had the good fortune of being in bed, of enjoying the privilege of lying down, of sleeping even. I fantasized about curling up next to them, even trading places with each of them.

As bedside rounds ended, my circadian rhythm appeared to catch up with the hectic demands of the post-call day, and we gathered in our attending physician's office to jointly establish our plan of attack. Despite having had no sleep, we provided detailed and polished presentations of our twelve new admissions to Merle. He cut through the complexities of clinical data with astounding agility, either affirming our diagnostic and treatment plans or helping us to synthesize more appropriate ones when he disagreed with ours. My intern got pulled away since his pager had been going off for the last twenty minutes. When we got to our eleventh and twelfth patients— the shooters with fevers—I stepped in and presented them with unparalleled bureaucratic efficiency, abandoning the usual protocol for presentations because we had all been through this exact case so many times before. I parroted back to Merle what he had taught us about the diagnosis and treatment of presumed endocarditis. He appeared content, and we finished rounds. We sheepishly exited his office, feeling like the walking dead, returning to the wards to execute the day's battle plans.

I caught up with my intern, who told me that all those pager calls had to do with the second shooter with a fever. He was acting out again, pulling the same stunt he had pulled the night before. I spent the next hour engaged in negotiations with the patient around pain control and opiates, all with an eye on the clock; I just needed him to stay for the forty-eight hours required to determine the blood culture results. After that, he would go back out to the street with an appointment for methadone detox that he almost certainly wouldn't keep.

While this got us through today, we learned from the on-call team the next day that the second night was much the same. Indeed, my team spent an inordinate portion of the subsequent day trying to manage his opiate withdrawal and the associated behavioral problems. All the while, we were feverishly working to care for, triage, and even discharge some of the other patients who were left on my service, each with their own sagas and their own challenges.

At the morning rounds with Merle, my interns systematically updated him on the status of our cadre of patients so the process of human processing could continue. The goals of today's rounds were again to ensure that our treatment plans were aligned with those of our attending physician while also positioning ourselves to discharge as many patients as we could to lighten our inhumane workload. When we got to our second shooter with a fever, my intern informed Merle that the patient no longer had a fever and that one of the blood cultures came back growing *Staphylococcus aureus*. I breathed a sigh of relief, for I knew Merle's teaching on the subject: if only one of two blood cultures grows *Staph*, then acute bacterial endocarditis is very unlikely; it likely represents a skin contaminant. This meant we could discharge our shooter with a fever. Predictably, Merle queried the intern as to whether only one blood culture grew *Staph*. My intern nodded, and I verbally confirmed that the second set did not grow *Staph*. I was nearly certain of this fact. I saw in my mind's eye the computer illuminating the second blood culture result: *No Growth to Date*. I told myself I would double-check that after rounds.

But I got caught up with the care of other, more acutely ill patients and never got around to it. My intern discharged the patient. This shooter with a fever was long gone and promptly forgotten.

INTERLUDE: BRIDGING THE TRENCHES

In the spring of 1916, my Hungarian great-uncle Aladar, barely a young man, was drafted to fight in the Great War. He said goodbye to his family, his girlfriend, his school, his synagogue, and his village, reassuring all that he would return soon. Since he was a subject of the Austro-Hungarian Empire, one of the great powers of Europe allied with Germany, he was immediately stationed with a battalion on the eastern front to fight the Russians in Ukraine. His battalion's mission alternated between attempting to encroach on enemy territory—one trench at a time—and defending it against the Russians, in what became known as the Brusilov Offensive.

For months, Aladar lived, slept, laughed, ate, smoked, and shat in these trenches, his rifle and bayonet his most reliable comrade. Life was characterized by stark contrasts. There were weeks of boredom, days and nights of serving as watchman to nothing, when the heat of summer, the songs of the few birds, and the blinking of the stars painted a mirage of serenity. But these long days and nights were disrupted by flurries of shelling the enemy and of being shelled, of seeking cover under any rock or ledge, of blindly shooting at the enemy from the parapet. Recurrent episodes of witnessing fellow soldiers being gunned down, and of feverishly carrying the bleeding and the wounded to the rear trenches where awaiting medics, trained in under a week, attended to them. Armin, his twenty-eight-year-old brother, one of these medics, had been killed just six weeks prior, shot in the head by a Russian sniper from a trench as he was attempting to evacuate an injured comrade to safer ground.

As this pattern repeated and repeated, with calm and grueling ennui unpredictably alternating with sheer terror, life began to take on a more monochromatic, psycho-emotional tone, one marked by hypervigilance, insomnia, and dread. Dread of the enemy—the invisible, deadly, and evil enemy. The threat of the invisible gas he was yet to be exposed to. The threat of trench fever, a sickness serious enough to knock you down for a week but not bad enough to get you sent back to a safe haven. Dread of the hand-to-hand combat that he was yet to participate in. And with this change came the change of seasons. As the days grew shorter, his hands grew colder, his feet wetter, and his spirit gloomier. How long would he live like an animal? Could he survive the coming frost? Would he ever go home?

One cold September morning in 1916, as he leaned against the trench wall in the purgatory between uneasy sleep and high alert, the gray of the predawn was set alight with a barrage of shelling that pummeled his trench. The shrill whistles of the night watch alerted his battalion to an incoming Russian infantry offensive. Chaos erupted. Before he was able to position himself at his parapet, the ursine roars of Russians advanced like a wave, extending up and down the line of his aural horizon. The roaring wave crashed down on him, and he was rolled and tossed beneath a sea of gray tunics and black boots, of fur-lined hats, bearded faces, and gap-toothed mouths. He wildly slashed his rifle and bayonet, flailing about, trying to come up for air. As he squirmed free from the morass of bodies intertwined in butchery, he tried to scramble up the wall of his trench so as to gain purchase and better defend himself. As he looked up, a massive Russian leaped down into the trench, toppling him and leaving him supine and defenseless. The bearded giant towered over him, exhaling steam like a racehorse on a cold morning. As the Russian pulled back his rifle to thrust his bayonet into the gut of his enemy, he locked his blue eyes with Aladar's. With the bayonet cocked to kill, the Russian froze for just a moment. His brows furrowed. He brought his face toward Aladar's, inspecting him closely, as would a small child who discovered what he thought was a gold coin in the black dirt.

Maintaining his intent stare, bayonet cocked, he asked, *"Tuy Zhid?"* (Are you a Jew?)

When my great-uncle didn't reply, the Russian asked in Yiddish, *"Zenen ir a Yid?"*

When Aladar vigorously nodded, the Russian quickly looked left and right, winked at my great-uncle, grabbed the lapels of his long coat, and hoisted him up and out of the trench in what felt like one fluid, superhuman motion. Now out of the trench, in no-man's-land, the Russian threw him to the ground and hugged and kissed him, telling him he would make him his prisoner and shelter him. Together, they soldier-crawled back to the Russian's trench. In this way, my great-uncle spent the next eighteen months as a Russian POW, saved by his captor—a fellow Jew.

Twenty-six years later, Aladar was murdered in Auschwitz, the end result of a pseudoscientific movement that purported that Jewish blood was not only tainted but was toxic to the health of society and therefore must be destroyed. In the midst of the bureaucratic efficiency and human processing that culminated in the gas chambers, there was not even room for one Jew to save another.

INSIDE THE TRENCHES

Seventy-seven years after my great-uncle was spared by his *landsman*, saved by the culture of blood, our team was on call again. I was called to the ER at

3:00 a.m. with the news that the shooter with a fever whom we discharged five days prior was back, now in profound heart failure, with a dangerously slow heart rate of forty-four beats per minute and a high fever. When I approached him, he was sitting on the gurney, bolt upright, breathing at thirty-two breaths per minute. His wrinkled forehead was beaded with sweat, his face exhibiting a look of desperation. I was painfully reminded of the aphorism that "when the patient is sweating, so too should the doctor." His eyes were wide-open, locked onto mine, like a suffering child looking into his parent's eyes in disbelief. But when he was unable to respond to my simple queries and could not demonstrate that he was oriented to person, place, or time, it became apparent that he was staring less at me than at the unknown world visible only to the delirious.

Working as if in a fog, I placed pacemaker pads on him, pushed more IV diuretics, and rushed him up to the cardiac care unit (CCU), transferring his care to the more senior resident in charge of that unit. At 5:00 a.m., I was called by the CCU, who informed me that my patient had expired. Racked with potential guilt, I approached the senior resident physician in the CCU—who was completing the death certificate—and advocated that an autopsy be done. He soundly squelched my request, quipping that "these guys die all the time. It's a no-brainer."

At 1:00 p.m., eight hours after the death, I got paged by the microbiology lab: a new set of blood cultures, obtained by the ER during this second admission less than twenty-four hours earlier, were both growing *Staph. aureus*.

I was shaking. Filled with dread, I found a computer and logged on. I braced myself and scrolled back through the computer record to results from eight days earlier. In disbelief, I discovered that only *one set* of blood cultures had been obtained on the first admission. The second set of blood cultures that I had reported as coming back negative had never existed. Rather, they had belonged to the first nameless shooter we had admitted that day. I ran to the on-call room and buried my head in the pillow, exhausted, moaning.

We are born into a world where differences matter. A world in which we seek the comfort of the familiar amid the danger of variance. We are a species engineered to recognize difference and to defend against it. We are hardwired to protect our tribe, to shelter and nurture those who are the "us," those from our common bloodline. But to be a civilized person engaged in service requires always being mindful of our inclination against the "other." We must be vigilant so that our breeding and our socialization to neglect or do violence against the "other" do not dictate our actions. These protective and violent inclinations—always present—become dominant during times of stress, when we are threatened, or when our basic humanity is in jeopardy. Being human means favoring the culture of blood, yet being humane requires resisting this innate tendency.

It took me many months to disentangle the complex web of personal and systems issues that led to this death—including my own complicity. It took me some years to learn about and recognize the role that implicit bias played in this fatality, to realize that my marginalization of this man due to his race, his drug habit, his HIV status, and his insufferable suffering all led me to a place where I determined that he was less than human, that he was the "other." It took me years to understand that this devaluing had dehumanized me. And that I needed to come to terms with what I had done to reconcile this act with my values and my beliefs regarding who I was and who I wanted to become.

CHAPTER 5

Man and Bird

IN 1971, A BRITISH FAMILY DOCTOR BY THE NAME OF JULIAN TUDOR HART made an observation based on his clinical experience working in the National Health Service (NHS) in Wales. He cared for a geographic swath of patients that had been assigned to him, a population that came from low-income neighborhoods. He noticed that while he worked nonstop from 7:00 a.m. to 7:00 p.m. Monday through Saturday, his colleagues assigned similar-size populations in the wealthier neighborhoods took Wednesdays off to golf, were home by 5:00 p.m. and dined with their families, and had both Saturdays and Sundays off. Cross-trained as an epidemiologist and therefore skilled in recognizing patterns related to health and disease, he carried out a formal study of the NHS in London and discovered that this pattern was replicable across all of London's municipalities and sectors. In essence, he discovered that doctors were far busier in low-income neighborhoods than in high-income neighborhoods both because of a much greater burden of illness in these neighborhoods and because of an undersupply of health care providers relative to this need. He first coined this phenomenon the *inverse care hypothesis*, and later, as the pattern was found to hold across the globe, the *inverse care law*. Tudor Hart's law states: "The availability of good medical care tends to vary inversely with the needs of the population it

53

serves. This . . . operates more completely where medical care is most exposed to market forces, and less so where such exposure is reduced."

Physicians, nurses, social workers, and pharmacists who work in safety net settings in underserved regions are familiar with the inverse care law; we feel it in our gut. Always aspiring to reverse the inverse care law, we often feel as though we struggle like Sisyphus, pushing with all our might to roll the giant boulder up the mountain, only to witness it roll back down again and having to push it up again and again.

THE MAN

One morning in 2002, I entered my outpatient clinic, twenty minutes early for my morning session. The clinic's waiting room was already filled beyond capacity: the elderly, the uninsured, and the disabled, all wedged together. The odor of unwashed clothes, soiled with layers of sweat and soured by urinary incontinence, mixed with the repugnant fragrances of cheap cologne and cheaper alcohol, came together to create a prototypical public hospital olfactory concoction. The smell of poverty, sickness, and neglect.

I carefully navigated through the already overcrowded waiting room, past the searching eyes and around the wheelchairs, and gravitated toward the back of the clinic, spotting the chin-high stack of charts that my medical assistant had obtained from the Medical Records Department and set up for my review. Volumes upon volumes of charts from the fourteen patients on my morning schedule that contained decades of visits, countless blood tests, x-ray reports, specialist consultations, vaccination records, and hospital discharge summaries.

Making the most of my prep time, I quickly leafed through any notable clinical events that had transpired in the interval between today's upcoming visit and the last. I spent most of my pre-rounding time on Mr. Garcia's chart, rereading my notes, reviewing interval data, and collecting my thoughts. A handsome and well-built, fifty-six-year-old, Spanish-speaking immigrant from Guatemala, he had spent the last twenty years working construction in San Francisco for a large, local construction company, as well as doing some side jobs as an individual contractor. Like 40 percent of our patients, he was uninsured. Because our city has a public hospital, I had had the privilege of caring for him for many years. Over this time, he had proudly shown me photos of the houses he had helped to build, the kitchen remodels he had done, and even a downtown high-rise he helped to construct.

The recent years had been less productive for him, as arthritis in his hands and knees had made it increasingly challenging for him to "keep up with the youth" and consistently put in the hours of hard labor required of the immigrant construction worker. He had to step away from some jobs, declined others, and—for his solo contractor gigs—he had been unable to deliver on time. He hadn't accrued enough income to hire help and participate in construction jobs in a more supervisory role, and his lack of English proficiency had made it impossible for him to get his contractor's license, further restricting his opportunities.

As I flipped through his chart, I recalled our prior visit. At that time, Mr. Garcia's chief complaint had been fatigue—a profound fatigue that left him unable to walk long distances, a fatigue that hit him the moment he awoke, making him feel as if he hadn't slept at all. Multiple potential medical diagnoses to explain the symptom of fatigue instantaneously peppered my mind. Yet before I fully gave in to them, I reminded myself that the most common cause of fatigue was depression. So, after eliciting more details on his fatigue and carrying out a quick review of symptoms related to organ systems whose failure could result in fatigue, I had gently queried him about his mood. He acknowledged that he was increasingly concerned about his ability to pay the rent for the two-bedroom apartment in the Mission District that housed him and his wife, their three children, and one grandchild while also needing to pay for food, clothes, and school supplies for the kids.

He then reminded me that he also had a family back in Guatemala, from a prior wife, and that he had become unable to send them the small amounts of money he had been sending them each month for two decades. He told me that things were beginning to look grim for him, that he wasn't sleeping well, and that his arthritis was bothering him more and more, making it harder and harder for him to work. He felt caught in a cycle. He began to weep silently, turning his face away to shield himself from my witnessing his suffering. I too teared up, looking away and down to my chart.

After expressing my compassion for the situation in which he had found himself, my confidence in his ability to manage this challenge, and my commitment to do my best to help him get through this, I quickly explained the common causes of fatigue, including depression and anxiety, and ordered the routine blood work to evaluate fatigue (thyroid function tests, blood count, etc.). Since he was reticent to go deep with a discussion about a diagnosis of depression and any associated treatment options, I simply asked him to take the next few weeks to consider whether he would like to receive some professional counseling, and to let me know at our upcoming visit whether he felt he wanted to talk to me more about it and get some treatment.

As I continued to leaf through his chart, I was reminded that his blood work had been notable for a fairly profound anemia, one that could very well explain his fatigue. I read my note that documented the telephone call in which I had informed him of the anemia and instructed him to obtain additional lab studies just before our upcoming visit to evaluate whether he had the type of anemia caused by iron deficiency (which prevents the adequate production of red blood cells) versus a type caused by red blood cell destruction. The day's visit would allow us to discuss the results of this second battery of tests and consider any further workup.

After we greeted each other, I asked him about his symptoms. He told me his mood and his fatigue were about the same, but his arthritis pain was worse, especially the pain in his back. I told him that I didn't recall his arthritis affecting his back.

"Well, I guess it does now," he responded.

He asked me about the most recent lab tests. Since these had not yet been filed in his paper record, I called them up on my late-twentieth-century office computer. While his anemia persisted, there was no evidence of iron deficiency. Instead, it appeared that his bone marrow was not producing new red blood cells at a pace to make up for the anemia.

As I interpreted these results for him, my brain interrupted my speech with an associative phrase: *"Anemia and new back pain. Anemia and new back pain . . . anemia and new back pain."* The connection between these two entities led my mind straight to cancer. And while many cancers can spread to the bone, there was one that originates within the very progenitor cells of the bone marrow, taking over the space where blood cells are produced, and over time seeding themselves in many parts of the skeletal system, especially the spine. Known as *multiple myeloma*, this cancer is not curable but can be treatable. Treatment can prevent suffering and prolong life. Multiple myeloma can be detected with a blood test or a urine test and is confirmed with a bone marrow biopsy, a painful but definitive procedure.

"This back pain of yours, is it *new* for you?"

"Well, you know, I always have pains, but yes, I guess it's kind of new."

I told him we needed to keep looking for the cause of his anemia, and I ordered a spinal x-ray, another set of blood tests, and a urine test. I asked him to return in one week, squeezing him onto a schedule that was already fully booked.

THE BIRD

I finished my morning clinic at 1:45 p.m. As I exited the building and took a deep recuperative breath, glad that I had that intense flurry of activity behind me, my pager went off. It was the babysitter of my four-year-old twin boys. I called back. She was hysterical. I was unable to understand what she was trying to tell me, other than something about my son Eytan. My heart was racing. She couldn't answer my simple questions. I directed her to put Eytan on the phone. A moment later:

"Hi, Daddy."

Putting on my calmest voice, I said, "Hello, Eytan. What's going on over there? Are you okay?"

"I think Dulce is sick. He just sits there on the bottom of his cage. He just stares at me. I took him out now. He's in my hand. He doesn't even fly away."

Dulce was the twin of Guapo, my other son Gabriel's parakeet. The twin boys and the two Guatemalan birds had been inseparable for over a year.

"I'm sorry, Eytan. We'll figure it out. Can you put Yasmin back on the phone?

"Yasmin, everything will be all right. Just put Dulce back in his cage. I'll call a vet and see if I can get an appointment. I'll hurry home by 4:00. For now, please read some books with the boys, but in a different room."

THE MAN

While Mr. Garcia's x-ray was normal, both the blood and urine tests were highly suggestive of multiple myeloma. As always, he arrived promptly for his visit, and I shared with him my concerns. I told him that the next step was to submit to a bone marrow biopsy, a somewhat painful procedure that was done by our blood cancer specialists, and that if the biopsy showed that he did not have bone marrow cancer, that we would have to follow him very closely to make sure it didn't develop in the future. But if it did show cancer, we would want to quickly start him on chemotherapy to prevent any progression. I acknowledged that this must be particularly tough to hear, especially since he had been grappling with his work and financial difficulties. He looked me in the eye and told me he was not scared and that he would do whatever needed to be done.

I gave him a firm squeeze on the shoulder and told him I needed to step out of the room to make a phone call to the cancer specialists to try to get him seen quickly. I looked at my watch; I was already thirty minutes behind, and he was only my second patient of the day. I paged the Oncology fellow, and a few minutes later, I got her on the phone. She told me we had to be quick because she was dealing with a very busy clinic day. After I shared with her the clinical scenario of Mr. Garcia, she informed me that their next available appointment was not for three months and offered to connect me to their clerk to get him that appointment. I calmly pressed her, as I had been through this dance before. First, they say no, then you kick and scream, and then they cry "Uncle!" and bend.

But she was different; she persisted with her hard line. Our dialogue escalated as I informed her that I was well aware that any delay could jeopardize my patient's well-being and declared that it was unacceptable that he should have to wait three months to get a bone marrow biopsy and start treatment.

She flippantly retorted that I should "just send him to California Pacific Medical Center," a chic private hospital up the road. Since we both knew that the uninsured are not welcome anywhere else in the city or Bay Area, I accused her of being stonehearted and demanded to speak to the chief of the oncology clinic. She told me she would pass my message on, that I'd get a call back at some point, and wished me and my patient good luck. I reentered Mr. Garcia's room and told him, in as soothing a voice as I could muster, that I was still working on getting him a timely appointment, that he could go home, and I would call him in a few days with the date, time, and location.

Early that afternoon, I was called by the chief of the hematology/oncology clinic. She confirmed that, indeed, she had absolutely no availability before the three-month appointment I was offered. When I forcefully pushed back, she told me about the metastatic breast cancer patients, the lung cancer patients, and the advanced colon cancer patients who were also in line, how many of their patients didn't speak English or didn't have a home, which made care even more complicated and time-intensive, how their service was swelling beyond capacity, and how one of their oncologists just quit because of the working conditions. She too was dealing with an "acute on chronic" problem of inadequate supply relative to the demand. She suggested that if I had a genuine complaint about her clinic, then I should submit it to the director of the Department of Public Health and do it on behalf of *all* the patients that are in line, because the department held the purse strings.

I thanked her for this pointless suggestion and asked her if there was a logic to her line, whether it was simply first come, first served, or a needs-based decision. She responded by asking me if my patient had visible fractures on his x-ray, any kidney failure, or a high calcium level (all complications of multiple myeloma).

I reported that, as of yet, he did not.

"Well, since you asked, that's how we make our decisions about who gets bumped up the line," she said.

I decided that, in a medical world characterized by a mismatch between high demand and low supply, her decision-making made perfect sense.

THE BIRD

I checked the internet and found the number of the Bay Area Animal Hospital just blocks from my house. I told the front desk staff that I was aware that it was already 3:00 p.m., but I was wondering whether I could get an urgent, same-day appointment. When I told them the scenario, they quickly responded that they "don't do birds." They suggested the nearby bird hospital, located about four miles southeast.

"Really? A bird hospital?"

But she had already hung up.

I phoned the bird hospital.

"Sure, we can definitely make room for Dulce. We even have evening hours if that is more convenient."

Relieved that Dulce could get seen so promptly, I set an appointment for 4:30 and called my wife so she could participate in this clinical rite of passage for our boys. I swung by my house to pick up the boys and the bird, and we all converged on the bird hospital.

As we stepped into the clinic entrance, my breath was taken away by the glimmer and shine of a pristine and empty waiting room. When I recovered my breath, I smelled an enticing trace of pine and spruce and heard the faint tweets of birdsong being piped in. We were greeted by a kind receptionist who shepherded us right into a spacious exam room.

The bird vet, donning the classic white coat but accompanied by a toylike miniature stethoscope, entered the room with a sparkling, white-toothed smile.

"So, what's going on with Dulce?" she asked my son Eytan.

"He's sick," he said, offering up the bird to her in his little cupped hands.

I took over the conversation and quickly filled her in, describing a syndrome that in allopathic medicine we term *failure to thrive*. I made sure she was aware that I was a physician.

"No problem. We can get right on this."

She carried out a cursory physical exam, including inspecting and palpating from crown to cloaca, from crest to claw. She opened the bird's beak and took a peek into his mouth, and then a quick listen with her stethoscope.

In hushed tones, she told me and my wife that she detected what might be a mass in Dulce's underbelly.

"We see this all the time in these Central American parakeets. Probably a hepatocellular carcinoma or germ cell tumor. They are prone to get these in their first few years of life."

I stole a glance at my wife and nod over to our boys, sending her a visual message that it may be time for us all to say our goodbyes to Dulce.

"But no worries. Let's perk this bird up with a quick gavage and grab an x-ray and we can take it from there."

"I've done a *lavage* before," I said. "You know, pumping someone's stomach. But what's a *gavage*?"

"It's basically the opposite. It's when we insufflate high-caloric nutrients and fluid into the bird's stomach. It really perks them up." She turned to my boys and bent down to their level. "You'll see. It's safe and easy. And your bird will be just fine in no time."

She moved toward the door to leave the room, with Dulce now cupped in her hands. As she grabbed the doorknob, dollar signs were spinning in front of my eyes like the spinning fruit in a slot machine.

I asked myself, *How much is it going to cost us for a bird that we bought for $9.99 at our local pet shop?*

I jumped in before she left: "But what is an x-ray going to show? Wouldn't you need a CT scan to find these types of tumors?"

She smiled again and gave me an empathic look. "Turns out with birds, x-rays are as good as CT scans are in humans. Sees right through them. We'll get our arms around this soon enough."

She dashed out of the room before I could stop her.

My wife and I spent the next few minutes trying to make a plan for a quick exit while trying to delicately explain to our boys that Dulce was actually *not* going to be "just fine."

THE MAN

Over the next week, I failed in my attempts to get Mr. Garcia an earlier appointment. I phoned him to let him know about the barriers I was encountering but reassured him that I would keep advocating, including reaching out to other hospitals. He told me his wife had been worried sick, but he was patient. He was gracious and grateful, and we shared a warm goodbye on the phone. I had no idea that I would never see or hear from him again.

Over the next week, I called the four other hospital systems in the city, including the university hospital and the Catholic-run hospital, but they did not offer my patient the "charity care" that they so often claim on their tax forms. I was left with only the realization that in my city, when it came to a Spanish-speaking, middle-aged, immigrant family man with an eminently treatable cancer: 1) there was a limit to charity; and 2) in a world with high demand, low supply, and even less collective responsibility, we frame needed health care as charity, not as a basic human right.

My new plan was to try to admit him to my hospital, despite his not having an urgent clinical need. While not a popular alternative with the hospital administrators, perhaps it would force the hand of my oncology colleagues and get them to do the bone marrow biopsy.

THE BIRD

The vet rushed back in. She handed the bird back to Eytan.

Again, with the smile.

"Just as I suspected!"

She tossed the x-rays onto a viewing panel, flipped on the backlighting, and pulled me over by my elbow, as one doctor revealing her clinical acumen to another, more junior doctor.

"Right . . . *here* . . . you see this bright white area? It's supposed to be translucent in a bird. This is the area of the cloaca, where they urinate and defecate. It's been obliterated by a germ cell tumor. No doubt about it."

"All right, then," I said, "so we should talk about—"

"The great news, though, is that these tumors are *super* responsive to chemotherapy. You know, a cisplatin and corticosteroid-based regimen. And more good news is we can start it today. You can bring Dulce in weekly until we begin to see a response. No cure, of course, but they definitely respond."

I stared at her in disbelief, my mouth agape. I turned my back to the boys, pulled her aside, and asked under my breath, "Can we not talk about chemotherapy, please, and maybe discuss . . . you know . . . more of a . . . palliative care kind of approach?"

"*Palliative care?*" she snarled at me, her eyes on me like daggers. "Don't you realize you could give Dulce another three to six months of quality of life?"

"Wow. Thank you, but I think we'll just take the bird home."

She looked at my wife and my boys as if searching for a sane person to rescue this clinical encounter from its deeply troubling and unethical outcome.

"Well, if you're all sure that's what you want. And to be clear, that's not what I'd do, but if you're sure, at least take home a syringe of Cipro to give Dulce twice a day for five days."

"But Cipro is an antibiotic. How is that going to help?"

"We find that it just does."

She handed me a prepackaged 3 cc syringe filled with a milky substance, holding my hand in both her hands, providing me with a degree of bedside comfort, fitting closure for a final visit with a dying parakeet's family. The syringe was already labeled *Dulce*.

THE MAN

I phoned Mr. Garcia again to give him an update, struggling with how I could encourage him to stick it out, knowing that he had a cancer that was growing while he waited. I was going to pitch the idea of trying to admit him to the hospital. As the phone rang, I imagined his family gathered around the kitchen table, anxiously asking one another when the doctor was going to call so that Papa could begin treatment. I imagined the strong face he put on for them, telling them to relax . . . that everything would be just fine.

His eldest daughter answered. When I asked for him, she told me that he wasn't in. A few days prior, he decided to return to Guatemala in the hopes of receiving care for his cancer and reconnecting with his second family. I told her how sorry I was that we couldn't start treatment as quickly as we would have liked to. She said that they are used to that in America, the fact that poor people get second-rate health care.

I winced. That stung. I had nothing to say in response other than asking her to promise to pass on my best wishes to him and requesting that they please let me know how he fared back home. Hanging up, I wondered what sort of treatments—if any—he would receive in Guatemala. I envisioned him lying in an open coffin in a mountain village church, surrounded by a tearful family, a family whose reunification was remarkable for its rapid reversal.

THE BIRD

The six of us, two of whom were now back in their cage, shuffled out of the exam room. As my family headed back to the waiting room, I edged over to the front desk clerk.

"Will this be cash or credit? Or do you have pet insurance?"

"Credit," I said gloomily.

As I was waiting, I looked at my watch. 5:15 p.m. Wow. Forty-five minutes from presentation to laboratory workup to diagnosis to treatment options to decision. This entire avian clinical cancer cascade took only forty-five minutes.

"The total comes out to . . . $437.95. Here is an itemized bill for your review."

Damn. I handed her my credit card, feeling like I'd just been conned out of a whole bunch of green. As I scanned the itemized bill—exam, gavage (procedure), gavage (contents), radiographs (2), ciprofloxacin, and 3 cc syringe—the secretary handed me a brochure with a toucan on its cover and asked with a smile:

"Would you like to purchase our health insurance for your bird?"

"*Health insurance?* We were just told that our bird has a fatal cancer. How will that help?"

"Well, our *EMBRACE* health insurance will cover all your bird's upcoming medical costs, which could be really helpful. Excluding any costs related to the cancer, of course."

I pocketed the brochure, because one day I was sure I was going to want to write a short story about this.

I approached my wife and showed her the receipt. "Let's get the hell outta here," I told her. "And quick."

Two days later, my pager went off. It was our babysitter again. I called back, and Yasmin picked up, sobbing a mixture of incomprehensible utterances and laments in what sounded like her native Arabic.

I asked her to put Eytan on the phone.

"Hey, buddy. It's Daddy. What's going on?"

"Dulce's dying. I think he's dead. I am holding him on my lap, and he's not even moving. He's kinda stiff."

"Yup, I think you're right, buddy. That's sad. I'm sorry, sweetie. Just wrap him in a nice little towel and put him on the couch or keep just holding him if you want to. I'll be home as soon as I can. It's so great that you got to hold him while he died. I'm really proud of you. When I get home, we can cry about it together, okay?"

That night, we buried Dulce under a yucca sapling in our backyard, wrapped in a Guatemalan flag I bought in the Mission District on the way home. The yucca has since turned into a healthy tree, now over thirty feet tall.

THE BIRD, ONE YEAR LATER

October 17, 2003
From: The Feathery Friends Bird Hospital

Dear Dulce:

I am writing to send you our warmest regards and to say that I hope that life is treating you well. I noticed that it's been exactly one year since I had the pleasure of meeting with you in our office. Now would be a great time to come back in for your annual checkup.

We hope you enjoy our poem of the day:

It's been a year since you were last seen,
Let's make sure your feathers maintain their sheen.
Just make a call to our waiting staff,
Whose jollity is sure to make you laugh.
Your doctor won't give you a vaccine,
But a bill of health that's squeaky clean!

Feel free to call our office at the number below, and we'll do our best to see you at a time that is convenient for you.

In good health,
Dr. Julia Freeman

THE MAN, TODAY

Mr. Garcia almost certainly passed away within months of his arrival in Guatemala. Had Mr. Garcia presented to my clinic today, fifteen years after the events of this story, things would have gone quite differently. He would have indirectly benefited from the improvements to my health system that have accrued as a result of the Affordable Care Act (ACA, a.k.a. Obamacare). Today, fewer than 10 percent of my clinic patients are uninsured, with Medicaid becoming the primary payer for those that are newly insured. Those that remain uninsured are mostly undocumented

immigrants. Because of the influx of resources that came with more Medicaid reimbursement, the San Francisco Department of Public Health has
been able to make modest investments in the city's public health care system, expanding personnel, bolstering infrastructure to improve systems,
and implementing electronic health records. In addition, some previously
uninsured patients now can access care in private settings, unburdening
our overloaded specialty clinics. Wait times for specialty clinics have fallen,
access has improved, and quality has been enhanced. While not a panacea,
the ACA has changed the story of Mr. Garcia from being the rule in my
hospital to more of the exception. As a progressive policy whose intent was
to "reverse the inverse care law," the ACA has helped bridge the obscene gap
between what was offered to the bird and what was offered to the man.

CHAPTER 6

Patagonia Pastorale

Patagonia is the farthest place to which man walked from
his place of origins . . . a symbol of his restlessness. From its
discovery it had the effect on the imagination something like
the Moon, but in my opinion more powerful.

—Bruce Chatwin, *In Patagonia*

I AM TRAVELING IN BRUCE CHATWIN'S UTTERMOST PART OF THE WORLD.
The menacing Torres del Paine erupt from the surrounding glacial planes
like a set of massive, black-stained, jagged teeth. They dwarf anyone and anything in their perimeter, including the shelters in this summer settlement on
the Rio Serrano. I walk toward the river and the great towers of stone, my legs
aching from a day of exploring, my belly full of grilled lamb. The sun wanes—
a midnight sunset—followed by a gray dusk, and then the rising full moon.

The luminous silence is interrupted by joyful yelps, distant sounds of a
pichanga, an informal, pickup football match. All the males in this impoverished, temporary outpost are playing—peasants, farmers, gauchos, migrant
handymen of all ages, sizes, and skills. Boys, their heads filled with fantasies of being the Patagonian Ronaldinho, grown men with berets and tightly

cropped beards, and nearly fossilized grandfathers with arthritic knees come together for a carefree interlude of nocturnal pleasure. The field is a transformed grazing ground for cattle and sheep, a moonlit checkerboard of windswept high grass, dirt, and mosslike turf, bordered by a wire fence. The goals are shabbily assembled wooden frames with tacked-on green plastic netting, recycled from a nearby dump.

I lean on a goalpost, watching the game. The goaltender, a hulking, hairy man with coarse features, pillar-like legs, and a booming voice, is shouting orders to his teammates. A wave of opposing players rolls toward him. A blast from the right wing careens off the far post, then off his back, and, as he watches, the ball trickles into the net. He lets out an agonized groan and slams a massive fist against the goalpost. The entire structure collapses into a tangled heap of wooden beams. A stout teammate with blackened teeth and long, bushy sideburns grabs a hammer from the sideline, pulls a few nails out of the pocket of his overalls, and, with the goalie balancing the goalposts and crossbar with his immense hands, they re-erect the goal within a few seconds.

Something about the goalie's hands—their girth, the blocky digits—captures my clinical curiosity. I then observe his thick jaw, jutting brow, and large ducklike feet—all suggestive of acromegaly. I wonder whether I should share my discovery with this man if the knowledge can't be put to use.

The golem casts a glance at me, gives me a sly wink and a half smile. "The gringo wants to play," he barks. "I'm sending him to your side."

I jump into the game. The white ball soars from one foot to another's head, arcing over the full moon. The game is filled with flashes of delight, the back-and-forth of minor disappointments, short-lived victories, and comic failures, good-natured accusations of mishandling and vocal denials, pleadings, and gentle coaxings. The local women clothed in wide-striped, woolen ponchos watch from the field's perimeter, standing in the thresholds of their shanty homes. Some stand with arms crossed, smiling while slowly shaking their heads, or covering their eyes in mock shame and giggling with their neighbors. Others gossip while only half watching the game, holding a toddler's hand or cradling a baby wrapped in blankets.

Do the inhabitants of this last place on Earth appreciate the haunting and desolate beauty of their surroundings? Do they feel as I do—small, vulnerable, yet energized in the moon shadows of the hulking towers of stone?

Our fleet-footed winger in work boots makes a rapid run down the right side and sends a lilting cross to the middle, just over the extended, shining, bald head of an aging defender. I make firm contact with the ball in midflight and redirect it to the goal, past the outstretched arm of the diving goalkeeper. I can still see that arm—thick, furry, ending in a superhuman hand with fingers of granite. The leathery arm of the *Mylodon*, the giant ground sloth, the extinct beast of Chatwin's imagination, a huge mammal that had survived the Ice Age and lingered on in the Southern Andes.

Shouts of "*Bueno*, gringo!" are interrupted by the cheering of the fallen goalkeeper, singing the praises of his eight-year-old son who, in anticipation of the cross from our winger, was hugging the far post and blocked my shot from entering. The goalie smothers the rebounding ball and then hugs his savior son. Together they roll in the grass and dirt, the giant man kissing the giggling boy to the appreciative applause of their teammates, and the begrudging smiles of mine.

I linger next to them, patting his son's matted hair so as to get a closer look at the father. As he hollers to his teammates to spread out to receive his upcoming kick, I see his irregular, widely spaced bottom teeth. Now the diagnosis is unmistakable.

His looping kick travels the distance of the field and is trapped by a teammate, his twelve-year-old son, who sidesteps a pair of cousins and places a perfect strike between the legs of our relatively diminutive goalkeeper. The smiling boy makes a wide half turn and, with his arms spread out like wings of an airplane, weaves his way back to his father. Bellowing, "GOA-OA-OA-OA-OA-OA-L-L-L-L," in honor of his sons' back-to-back accomplishments, he hoists the boys over his shoulders.

Should I tell this man—in this impoverished and virtually inaccessible place—that he has what I believe is a tumor in the base of his brain? That if it is left untreated, it will further deform him and lead to irreversible organ failure in the not-too-distant future? Do they even have access to transsphenoidal pituitary surgery? And what is best for his sons, two boys who probably have never been happier to have this man as their father?

As the game progresses, I am distracted by the vision of a man and his family, once carefree and happy, now burdened with news of a deforming and fatal disease, with no recourse for treatment or hope for cure. Visions of his head carved wide open in an operating room of a remote Andean hospital, a prehistoric cave with a team of European archeologists digging for the lost *Mylodon*. Images of two orphaned children burying their father in the permafrost, a victim of either a failed attempt at excision or a progressive cardiomyopathy.

I keep playing, but my head and heart are no longer in the game. I am frozen with indecision. Perhaps it is best not to interfere with these people's lives. They did not seek me out, and they seem happy. To disrupt this idyllic, insulated moment with such information seems as much an act of aggression as one of kindness. But not to share such knowledge seems an equally cruel and paternalistic alternative.

The game dwindles to a close. We all gather around a communal plastic well and dip ladle-like cups to drink the cool water. As the crowd thins, the man starts walking with his sons toward his well-worn motorcycle. I try to pull him aside.

"Pardon me. Do you mind if we have a few words in private?"

"Of course, compadre. You can tell me anything."

"I'm a doctor from the United States, and I am concerned that you may have a rare illness."

His sons approach us.

"You can talk freely to me, compadre, because I am as strong as an ox, and I have no fears." He slaps me on the back. "And I have no illness."

"Thank you. I believe you have a disease in which you—your brain, actually—makes a chemical that causes parts of your body to grow. Like your hands, your feet, and your jaw. It can get worse and make you very sick."

His boys' big eyes shift between their father and me, and back to their father again.

I continue, "I think you need to see a doctor."

"And how can you cure this disease?"

"Usually, you need to get a special kind of surgery, an operation where they cut into your skull and remove that portion that is making the bad chemical."

I stare at him, looking for a reaction—fear, confusion, denial, anger, confidence—anything. He smiles, revealing his widely spaced, crooked teeth, and slaps me on the back again.

"Like I said, I have no disease. I received this exact treatment over two years ago. They sent me up to Santiago from Punta Arenas. The neuro-surgeon did a fine job, and now I am strong as an ox. I had been telling my doctors here I was sick for months, but they couldn't figure it out. Then my cousin—whom I hadn't seen for nearly twenty years—came to visit, and he noticed I was a different man. A few weeks later, they figured it out. And they sent me up there. So, don't worry, compadre. I am cured."

I tell him I am very relieved, and we shake hands. He puts on his helmet, helps his boys with theirs, and they ride off. I walk back to my cabin, unable to take my eyes off the looming Torres del Paine, timeless sentinels for this uttermost part of the world.

CHAPTER 7

The Quixotic Pursuit of Quality

"Destiny guides our fortunes more favorably than we could have expected," said Quixote. "Look there, Sancho Panza, my friend, and see those thirty or so wild giants, with whom I intend to do battle and kill each and all of them, so with their stolen booty we can begin to enrich ourselves. This is noble, righteous warfare, for it is wonderfully useful to God to have such an evil race wiped from the face of the earth."

"What giants?" asked Sancho Panza.

"The ones you can see over there," answered his master, "with huge arms, some of which are very nearly two leagues long."

"Now look, your grace," said Sancho, "what you see there aren't giants, but windmills, and what seem to be arms are just their sails, that go around in the wind and turn the millstone."

"Obviously," replied Don Quixote, "you don't know much about adventures."

—Miguel de Cervantes Saavedra, *Don Quixote*

73

M R. Q. WAS ONE OF MY MOST FRUSTRATING PATIENTS, YET ONE OF MY most treasured. He had the weather-beaten face of a Greek sailor, with deep wrinkles that undulated on the high seas of his every expression. A self-described Buddhist poet of the Beat generation, he sported a Quixote-like moustache and beard. He was often clothed in tie-dye shirts, tightly pressed khaki pants, and moccasins with no socks. Too many evenings drinking in smoke-filled cafés and a constellation of medical conditions—bleeding ulcers, high blood pressure, bad diabetes, heart disease—had left him slightly dazed. A recent stroke had robbed him of his ability to speak fluently. But Mr. Q. had turned this misfortune into the sublime, developing an ornate language of the hands, a flowery display of gestures and waving aimed at replacing the subtleties once available to him through the use of words.

After experiencing a bladder infection for the fourth time in one year, he grudgingly agreed to a surgical removal of the foreskin that, in my opinion, was contributing to the problem. Getting him to agree took all the motivational interviewing skills I could muster. But then he missed the appointment three times, forgetting the date, forgetting the location, forgetting the reason. I tried to identify a family member or friend who could remind and accompany him, but it seemed that those from his cohort had faded away.

As a primary care physician, public health program director, and part-time medical administrator at a public hospital, I served on a committee whose goal was to enhance quality of care by setting benchmarks, developing recommendations and guidelines, reducing physician variation, and improving performance. In these meetings, we often grappled with quality issues in diabetes, a chronic disease that is so common, so costly, and so complex. How could we ensure that our patients receive annual eye exams? That they receive periodic measures of blood sugar control? That their blood pressure is well managed? These discussions have their roots in the quality movement, a movement with constituencies that included patients, purchasers, and providers. It is a noble cause, designed to transform each health care system into one that is accountable for the health outcomes of the population it serves. This utopian movement has become so entrenched into the millstone of health care delivery that portions of our very livelihoods can depend on the aggregate of our performance with individual patients.

On my way out of a diabetes quality-improvement meeting, I ran into Mr. Q. He placed his knobby, artist's hands together as if in prayer and stuttered, "P-p-please come. . . . I'm having . . . a . . . p-p-p-party." With a half bow and a roll of his hand, he passed me a hand-painted invitation to his circumcision party, an "intimate commemoration of this important step in my life cycle," to be celebrated at a local tavern.

How would Mr. Q. determine quality of care? What did he value in a physician and in a health care–delivery system?

Did I possess the tools to navigate the uncharted waters between his desire to adhere to a model of spiritual health and my drive to achieve more conventional goals for his physical health?

At a subsequent visit with Mr. Q., I was running very behind. I entered the room with a harried flurry of greetings, apologies, and opening questions. He responded to my pressured overtures with characteristic tranquility. His peaceful, meditative countenance belied his sky-high blood pressure and chronically elevated blood sugar. I made some simple inquiries. He couldn't remember which medicines he was taking. He hadn't brought in his pill bottles. He didn't even have the handwritten, wallet-size medication list I had prepared for him at our last visit—a list illustrated with dosing cues: a sun for morning and a moon for nighttime. I glared at him in disbelief, exasperated, my entire body tense with the memories of recurrent failures and the frustrations of future inadequacies. He calmly placed his knobby hands together, offered me a seated bow, and stammered, "I'm s-s-s-s-sorry." He then turned his hands palms up and cast his eyes to the heavens, as if to say "These things are beyond my control."

I was in a jousting mood, and I wasn't buying his story. Was it his failing memory or his Buddhist philosophy at play? I moved to the edge of my chair, closer to him, and stiffened. "Mr. Q., we have been around and around with this. What are we going to do? You have *got* to understand how important these things are. And I noticed you missed your eye clinic appointment . . . *again*. Don't you understand what diabetes can do to your vision? You could go blind! Do you *want* to go blind?" I asked that insolent, rhetorical question out of desperation. My year-to-date performance with respect to retinal exams for my panel of patients with diabetes was a pitiful 47 percent—and this while serving as chief of the Diabetes Prevention and Control Program for the state of California.

In response to my question, he slowly squinted and offered me a mischievous smile between his gray, wispy goatee, accompanied by a crooked index finger pointed skyward. "The w-world . . . m-m-may be . . . a more b-b-beau-ti-ful p-p-place . . . for those who c-c-c-c-cannot see."

"I should have known you were going to say that."

He looked down at his lap, exhaled, examined his expressive hands, and then raised them, fully clenched, observing their sheer physical power. "And I . . . I am a m-m-m-man . . . who uses his hands, n-n-n-not his eyes!"

Mr. Q. intently placed his face in front of mine, set one heavy hand on my shoulder, closed his eyes, and breathed deeply, in and out, in and out. He repositioned himself behind me. What was he doing? I could feel his rhythmic exhalations on the nape of my neck. He began firmly massaging my shoulders, worked up to my scalp with strong, warm hands, healing hands. He pounded on my vertebrae with a firmness that was almost painful. He kneaded my arms from shoulder to elbow, elbow to wrist, and shook them until they were limp as noodles. He then squeezed and pressed my hands, ministering finger by finger by finger.

"Breathe . . . in . . . and . . . out." I followed his directives and, despite my initial discomfort, accepted his remedy. These fifteen minutes would be mine.

The message of his massage—the sensual and the tangible as restorative—taught me an important lesson about the confines of the work we do, day in and day out, in our medical practices. But the underlying meaning of this role reversal still eludes me. Was Mr. Q. simply asking me to realign my values with regard to his health and well-being? Did I fail him by projecting my own needs rather than learning how best to respond to his? If so, does the predominant view of "quality" engender just such cycles of physician inadequacy—romantic and at times misdirected quests for success hampered by limited sets of tools, circumscribed behaviors, and narrowly defined goals—leaving us to attack windmills with our lances? Or was Mr. Q. simply ministering to me?

Over subsequent visits, Mr. Q. continued to provide me with massages at the end of our encounters, the first visit a ten-minute massage, the next visit five minutes, then two minutes, then one minute, and finally, wordlessly, he weaned me to none. And at each of these visits, I found myself less pressured and more present, pushing and forcing him less and less. And I found myself less attached to the belief that he must aspire to meet every metric in my book. And, in parallel, he gradually stopped resisting and feinting, and paradoxically began affirmatively responding to my gentle suggestions, first with curiosity and then with willingness. And in this way, the duel was over, and we became like Quixote and Sancho, each of us first playing one, then the other, both of us trotting off together, one on the old steed, Rocinante, and the other on the mule, el Rucio.

> When Life itself seems lunatic, who knows where madness lies? Perhaps to be too practical was madness. To surrender dreams—this may be madness. Too much sanity may be madness—and maddest of all: to see life as it was, and not as it should be!
>
> —Miguel de Cervantes Saavedra, *Don Quixote*

CHAPTER 8

The Brother

FOUND DOWN

"We have a challenging family situation that I'm hoping you can help me out with," sheepishly suggested Glen, a long-standing colleague of mine who now was working in another health system.

"Sure, of course. What is it?"

He went on, almost apologetically, "I would do it myself, but since I don't work at the General, and since it has to do with someone in my own family, and because he's not insured, I need your help."

His tone switched to one of tempered flattery. "Plus, it's kind of a strange and puzzling case—both socially and medically—that'll need some special attention. And you're the man when it comes to figuring these kinds of complicated things out and gracefully intervening. That's why I'm asking you."

I realized I was about to commit to something significant, but since it involved a colleague's family situation, I was only too willing. What goes around comes around.

"Count me in. I'm all yours."

"Thanks, buddy. So, it has to do with my father's brother, my uncle, who I haven't seen for over a decade—that was until last week. And what I just saw wasn't pretty. I think he needs to be hospitalized, get a medical workup, and may need to be placed somewhere safe."

"Okay, no problem. What's the story?"

"Like a lot of things on my dad's side of the family tree, it's kind of a weird story. And I'm not quite getting it."

His father was a well-known artist, a guy whose charm, immense talent, and tremendous and ongoing artistic output had always impressed me. He had been warm to me on the few times we had met. I recalled that his siblings, including my colleague's uncle, had not enjoyed the good fortune in life that he had and that at times he had been forced to get enmeshed in their messy lives, to try to pick up the pieces.

Of course I'd be happy to help *him* out. It would be an honor. He was a VIP in the rarefied world of art and culture. Why wouldn't I want to associate with that?

"Go on."

"So, my uncle's name is Gerry, and—like I said—I haven't been in touch with him for probably fifteen or twenty years. And I think the same goes for my father, mostly. They had a kind of falling-out back then related to Gerry's drug use and squabbles over money. I think before that, my dad had been carrying him along, you know—supporting him for quite a while, both financially and emotionally. Trying to get him to stop using and get his life back together. I think it mostly was cocaine, maybe some mental illness. A whiff of bipolar disorder? I honestly don't know. But then something must have happened in their relationship or with Gerry's behavior that turned things sour for my dad. Gerry just kinda disappeared from our lives. While I remember him from when I was a kid as the benign and goofy uncle, I figured I didn't really want that kind of influence around our kids. So, I let it go."

"I can't fault you for that," I replied with genuine understanding, having three young children of my own.

"So, anyway, maybe about a few weeks or so ago, Gerry gets back in touch with my father. And something about it gets my dad really concerned. It wasn't the first time Gerry had tried to reconnect, usually over needing money or rent or housing or something. I assume that previously my dad had either rebuffed those attempts or had gotten Gerry through whatever crunch he was in, but in a quiet way. Neither reopening the closed doors nor disrupting our familial understanding that Gerry was a persona non grata. But this time, apparently, my dad got spooked."

"Okay, you've piqued my interest."

"So, my dad calls me up a little over a week ago and asks, 'Hey, Glen, would you mind accompanying me on a little field trip?' When I was little, he used to ask me that in those same words whenever he wanted me to go with him out into the woods, on a hike or bird-watching. I'm thinking, *Okay, it's been a while, but if I can get away, why not?*"

"But this didn't turn out to be a hike in the woods, did it?"

"No. Exactly. He tells me that his brother, Gerry, has managed to get a hold of him. And that he's no longer living in Colorado or Nevada or wherever he'd been, but was now parked in the Tenderloin in San Francisco, living in an SRO. And that he sounds really bad on the phone. So, my dad begrudgingly suggests that they meet for coffee somewhere so they can check in. But Gerry tells my dad that he's got to come to his apartment. My dad tells him he'd really prefer not to hang out in the Tenderloin, so instead invites him to a nice restaurant for lunch. But Gerry declines the invitation. And when my dad pushes him on it, Gerry tells him that he can't go to lunch because he can't walk anymore. That he actually *needs* my father to come to him."

"Oh, your poor dad."

"Yeah, well, apparently he's kind of used to these sorts of calls, but this one was a bit more concerning and had a touch of the medical in it, so a field trip with me it became."

"Well, it sounds like your dad has good clinical sense," I replied.

And it was true. The hospital had just done an analysis of the common causes for hospital admissions at the General. The single most common cause? "Found down." This referred to someone who was alone in their home or apartment or street and something goes downhill—a stroke, a fall, a hip fracture, an overdose, something metabolic—that tips them over the edge. Literally and figuratively. And then they just can't and don't get up. Often for days, just lying on the floor, until someone finds them. Usually a neighbor or a friend who notices their absence. They can't get in, so they call the police, the door gets knocked down, the whole nine yards.

I pointed out to Glen, "Gerry was lucky to have someone willing to listen and to appreciate that some kind of intervention may be in order . . . before he just became another statistic."

Glen went on, "So, you understand. I head over to my dad's place, and we drive over the bridge together, and my dad gives me this whole preamble about Gerry's life that I hadn't heard before. To say that my uncle's had a colorful life was an understatement. But that's not the point. The point was we call ahead to let Gerry know we're on our way. And then we walk up four flights in this god-awful building and knock on the door. Nothing. I start pounding and yelling, 'Uncle Gerry! Uncle Gerry, can you hear us?' Still no response. But then we hear this sort of dragging, *shuffling* sound, and he's yelling back, 'Yeah, yeah. I'm coming. Hold your horses! For fuck's sake.'

"'Always the grateful brother,' my dad says to me."

I chuckled. "He sounds like a sweetheart."

"Exactly. Then more shuffling and scraping sounds from behind the door, now getting closer. The latch clicks, the doorknob turns, and the door opens a crack. Then *more* shuffling and scraping. 'Well? What are you *waiting* for? C'mon in!' I push the door forward to find a messy but otherwise empty apartment. Until I look down to the floor and see my uncle, sprawled on all fours, looking up at me like a crazy old ape. His big, white body only half-clothed, his white hair flying every which way. I mean, it was a nutty scene.

"'C'mon! In you go,' he barks, quickly spinning around 180 degrees on all fours, scrambling toward the couch. Knuckles and knees scraping on the wooden floor. Bare feet pointing inward, toes in and heels out, as he scuttles away from us. Then he drags himself onto the grungy couch. I see that his knuckles and knees are scraped and bleeding, his skin thickened and calloused at the points of contact with the ground. And his feet and ankles are sort of oddly twisted inward."

"Holy shit, Glen. That must have freaked your dad out."

"Freaked *me* out. So, he's been dragging himself around—knuckle walking—for a couple of weeks or so, and the place was an absolute disaster. The fridge is empty. His food's run out. But he's just acting normal, like everything's cool. Being kind of charming and weirdly endearing, actually. Asking us if we want a glass of water, or if there's anything else he can get us. What's he going to get us? And how?"

"Was he making sense otherwise?"

"Totally alert and oriented—cogent, actually. He starts asking me how I've been, how many kids do I have now. You know? Not appearing to have insight into the situation, the dire situation at hand. But he did call my dad for help, so that's something. I try to put together the pieces of the puzzle regarding how he's ended up on the floor—whether it's some sort of neu-rological disorder or some muscular or bony problem. He says he's had no trauma. Says he hasn't been sick recently. He turns to my dad, raises his right hand, and swears he hasn't been drinking or using for months. And he tells me his strength is fine except maybe for his lower legs, but mostly it's just that he can't straighten out his ankles and feet to walk right—sort of like he's sud-denly gotten clubfoot—and that his wrists are killing him from walking on his knuckles and palms."

"How bizarre."

"Totally bizarre. I quickly examine him, but apart from the distorted ankle and foot positions and maybe a little weakness in the calves, and apart from the calloused and bleeding knuckles and kneecaps, he checks out as normal."

"So, what do you think we should do? I mean, he can't stay there in that state. Was he willing to get medical help?"

"Right. No, he's not safe staying there, and my dad absolutely refuses to be his errand boy—bringing him food, washing his clothes, taking care of him or what have you. Which I think was what Gerry was hoping for, honestly. So, I tell him we need to get him to a hospital so someone can figure out what's going on and so we can arrange to get him help at home, assuming it's safe for him to return to his apartment. Or find him a board and care facility, or something like that, depending on what the diagnosis was. But he flat-out refuses. We try and try, going around in circles. So, I just leave my dad with him and go do a big food shopping for him and then return and do a quick cleanup—telling him I'm doing it *just this one time*."

"Okay, that makes sense."

"And after all that, he leads us to the door, crawling his way forward, and just gives us a big smile and a big thank-you. Telling me how much I've grown and how impressed he is with my doctoring, again in that endearing way. And I'm just standing at the threshold, looking down at him on all fours. My uncle Quasimodo. I tell him I'll call him every day until he agrees to my plan. Finally, yesterday, seven days after our visit, he calls me and tells me that he's really hungry. And that he's ready."

"Okay, good. I'm on service starting tomorrow. We'll figure things out, Glen. But let's get it going tonight so that by tomorrow, he's already tucked in and ready for me to take over. Do you or your dad want to drive him to the ER, or do you want me to call an ambulance to transport him? I'll make sure to call ahead to the ER and speak to the admitting resident to smooth things out and make sure Gerry comes to my team."

"I don't think my dad and I can get him down those stairs. Let me take charge of calling the paramedics. I'll make sure they bring him to the General. It'd be great if you deal with the ER and the admitting team. Knowing you'll take over as his doctor as of tomorrow will give my dad some real peace of mind. Thanks, buddy."

HOW DOCTORS THINK

The Famous Artist had chosen me to solve it all. To help extricate his brother from an untenable and chaotic social situation, to diagnose and treat a bizarre illness presenting with knuckle walking, to direct what he hoped would be his brother's related medical and (possibly) alcohol and drug-related rehabilitation, and finally to identify a place willing to accept his brother in whatever condition he found himself when all was said and done.

The next morning, on my drive to work, I began running through the list of possibilities to explain Gerry's loss of lower-leg function. I was thinking ALS, the progressive neurodegenerative illness that felled the likes of the great Yankees baseball player Lou Gehrig and the great theoretical physicist Stephen Hawking. Or maybe a reversible ascending paralysis like Guillain-Barré or a transverse myelitis? Or one of those vitamin deficiencies: the B vitamins—B1, B6, B12? Or vitamin E? Or some toxin, most likely alcohol or one of the heavy metals? Or late-stage syphilis or HIV? Or an inflammatory muscular disorder like polymyositis, or even one of those newly discovered mitochondrial defects involving the muscle cells—rare diseases that I was not up-to-date on to have any real clue about.

I rounded with my team, and we met Gerry, our VIP patient by proxy. Glen was right. He looked like a mad scientist, yet he was charming and endearing, traits that reminded me of his brother, the Famous Artist. His speech was often digressive and his thought processes at times disorganized, making it difficult to get the story straight. And there was that strange disconnect between the seriousness of the syndrome that had distorted his ankles and feet and left him unable to walk upright on the one hand, and his jovial and playful attitude on the other.

My examination left me with little to hang my hat on. The only remarkable finding—apart from the scraped and thickened skin around his knuckles and to a lesser degree his knees—was the deviation of his feet at the ankles: feet turned inward like those of a toddler who has just learned how to crawl. I was unable to straighten out his feet. It was as if he had contractures in the surrounding foot, ankle, and calf muscles, a fixed rigidity that made it impossible for me to return his feet to their normal position in the midline axis. No numbness, no loss of vibratory sense, and no abnormal reflexes. No neurologic deficits at all. And while his calf muscles did seem thinned out, there was no associated weakness. So, the atrophy was probably just a result of the underuse of his calves from his inability to walk.

I acknowledged to the team that I had no idea what could explain this presentation. I suggested we obtain x-rays of the ankles and feet to make sure the rigidity was not bony in nature and that we send off blood work to rule out the vitamin deficiencies, heavy metal poisoning, HIV, and syphilis. And most importantly—that we obtain a neurology consult. I was going to need the experts to figure this one out. The Famous Artist was relying on me.

The neurologists—specialists notoriously difficult to impress—were similarly stumped. They concurred that the only abnormalities were the unexplained contractures around his feet and ankles. They hypothesized that he may have been knuckle walking for a longer time than he had reported, and they raised the question as to whether the knuckle walking came first, which required the continual deviation of his feet at the ankles, culminating in what appeared to be resultant, fixed muscular contractures.

Turning to my team, yet still intending my words to be heeded by my specialist consultants, I replied that such a scenario could be possible were we to invoke an alcohol-related syndrome.

"I have learned over the years that when one is stumped, one has the option of switching from our usual *clinical* ways of thinking (identifying patterns of signs and symptoms that emerge *within* the patient) to, instead, relying on *epidemiologic* ways of thinking (identifying possible diagnoses based on probabilities that align with known patterns of exposures and illnesses *across* patients and populations)."

While my team looked at me as if I had conveyed something tremendously profound, their faces belied the lack of understanding that inevitably accompanied this well-worn prologue of mine.

I went on, "Another way of saying this is: a *common* illness (such as alcoholism) presenting in an uncommon fashion (such as knuckle walking) was *far* more common than an *uncommon* illness (such as a very rare neuromuscular disease that we simply cannot think of) presenting either commonly or uncommonly."

As they struggled to digest my arcane wisdom, I worked to make things more concrete.

"Let's imagine, as I think we have sufficient evidence to, that our patient has an alcohol problem. And let's further imagine that he was consistently smashed for many months before this presentation. So much so that he spent most of his time on the floor, for many days and possibly weeks or months. But this living on the floor requires, at times, that he become mobile. Say, to get that next bottle. Or to grab some slowly rotting food from the fridge before it totally turns. Or to relieve himself. So, he crawls, because he is smashed or just really hungover or weak."

They were all paying attention. Stories—real or imagined—have that effect.

"Stick with me. Each day, he drinks and then he crawls. He drinks again and he crawls again. And all over again. Someone brings him his alcohol and sometimes his food. I don't know who; it doesn't matter. But the pattern continues and gets ingrained. But his wrists start to hurt because it's hard to crawl around on your palms for weeks without hurting your wrists. So, he learns, just like our primate cousins learned, that fixing your wrists in place by walking on one's knuckles is easier on the wrists. So, he starts to do that, and in so doing, he raises up a bit, which simultaneously provides the additional opportunity to lift his butt in the air, extend his legs, and plant his feet flat on the ground. But only by turning his feet in at a fairly extreme angle. The severe angle is maintained, and over time—by virtue of needing to hyperextend his lateral peroneus muscles and abnormally contract the twenty or so muscles of his feet—this forced, unnatural angle turns into a fixed contracture."

The members of my team looked at one another, some smiling, others appearing to suppress a smile. I couldn't tell if they were impressed or thought I was pulling their leg. The neurologists were stone-faced, as always.

"Wait. I'm almost done. Now, with his feet firmly fixed in a functional-for-knuckle-walking position, but a dysfunctional-for-upright-walking position, he realizes he's stuck. That he's got himself into a bit of a clinical pickle. So, he turns to the only person who has the means and the influence to extricate him from his pickle jar: his brother, the Famous Artist. But before he can even begin to *think* of picking up that phone, he realizes he can't call on his brother if he's drunk. He's been down that road before, and he knows it's a dead end. So, he gets sober, going through alcohol withdrawal alone, at home. Which explains why we have observed no withdrawal syndromes during this hospitalization. And then, once those hellish few days are over, he pours on the charm and the neediness, and his brother—accompanied by the caring physician nephew—does the right thing and brings him to us. So, if you buy all that, then this whole presentation is just a highly unusual clinical outcome of a typical cascade of alcohol-related events. A chronic exposure and associated set of behaviors that you all must admit are extremely common—epidemiologically speaking."

I realized I might have sold them on this slightly far-fetched story. And perhaps convinced myself in the process.

The attending neurologist broke the silence.

"Your theory, my dear Watson, may have some legs, so to speak. I fully agree that some sort of prolonged immobilization or severely constrained mobility—such as what we see when people have been shackled for long periods of time—could explain this presentation. His digressive thinking and his ingratiating and endearing way of interacting with us does evoke the sense of a confabulating, alcohol-damaged brain. So, some of the pieces of this puzzle could be explained by your public exercise in imagination. And I also must admit that, in the absence of a viable competing diagnosis, we must rely on our combined knowledge of clinical medicine and epidemiology, as well as our imaginations."

To be sure they weren't missing anything, though, the neurologists recommended a spinal MRI, which, two days later, came back negative. They then carried out nerve conduction studies, poking wired needles into the legs of our patient, sending electrical impulses downstream to measure the amount of time the wave takes to evoke a muscle response. These also came back normal, making the possibility of a nerve or muscle disorder highly unlikely. They nonetheless took the final step, performing a muscle biopsy and sending it off to pathology, a sort of nowhere land when it comes to making a clinical diagnosis in a timely manner.

In the meantime, they suggested we simply treat Gerry's muscle contractures irrespective of their cause. This meant aggressive physical therapy and potent muscle relaxants, including benzodiazepines, a class of sedative-hypnotic medicines. They recommended moderate-strength diazepam. Gerry's disappointment at our not identifying a clear diagnosis appeared tempered by his discovery that diazepam simply was the generic version of Valium.

Now our job shifted to getting him to laterally rotate both feet at the ankles, to try to return the feet to a midline position, or something approximating the midline. He made very slow but gradual progress. The neurologists recommended that the doses of the muscle relaxants be increased and that we add in a low-dose opiate to help Gerry better tolerate the pain that came with the physical therapists' daily forced ankle-bending work. These additions seemed to help.

I then was contacted by the hospital's moribund utilization review nurse, who told me that while she was able to obtain Medicaid coverage for Gerry, yesterday she was informed that we would receive no further payments for this hospitalization, as he had no clear medical problems that required acute-care hospitalization. While I couldn't help but agree, I told her that he certainly was not safe to return home and that he lived on the fourth floor of a walk-up apartment building. I encouraged her to work with my team to help us identify an excellent rehabilitation facility where he could continue to receive aggressive physical therapy, with the hope that eventually he would be able to walk again and even return home.

She looked at me with a doubly doubting face: first a face that questioned the likelihood of our finding any place that would take him, let alone an *excellent* place; and a second that questioned the likelihood that he would walk on his own two feet again.

His placement was the final hurdle that I had to overcome if I were to successfully fulfill the expectations placed on me. I pulled her aside and quietly
shared with her the information about who his brother was. The Famous
Artist, the Prize-Winning Artist. I made a big deal out of it. She was duly impressed, appearing flattered and honored to have been assigned the case. She
had not been aware, she said, apologetically. I had lit a fire where previously
not even an ember had smoldered.

And miraculously, a day later, an excellent rehabilitation facility was
found. They offered up to three hours a day of physical therapy, had expertise in the rehabilitation of gait abnormalities, and owned walking treadmills
with parallel bars with which to do their good work. They had an available
bed and were waiting for him. It was nothing short of perfect.

I gave Gerry the good news. But he insisted he was going home.

I phoned the Famous Artist and let him know of the brilliant plan I was
able to finagle and of Gerry's refusal to accept that plan. The Famous Artist
said he'd visit Gerry's bedside at 5:00 that afternoon. He added that he'd
make it clear to Gerry that he had no choice but to go with the plan. He told
me not to worry, to just proceed with the plan to transfer Gerry the subsequent morning.

The rehabilitation facility called me that afternoon and told me that they
would only accept Gerry in transfer if he had a primary care physician, someone who could oversee and sign off on his treatment plans, prescribe his medications in an ongoing fashion, and provide him with follow-up after they
discharged him. I met up with the Famous Artist at Gerry's bedside that evening, and I offered to become Gerry's outpatient doctor. He seemed thrilled.
So too did the Famous Artist.

Gerry resided in the rehab facility for nearly two months. They reported
to me that he was making progress and that he had started to walk on the
treadmill with the help of the parallel bars. He still had pain and still required the muscle relaxants, but they believed that soon he would be able to
walk independently, albeit slowly and with a walker, hopefully just for the
short term. They told me they anticipated that, if all went as planned, he
would be able to navigate stairs and that they would discharge him to his
home, maybe two weeks from then. This was their signal to me that I was
about to take over his care.

A week later, I called the Famous Artist to ask if he was comfortable with Gerry being sent home or if he had come up with an alternate plan.

"I am definitely not taking him in, if that's what you're asking."

"I understand. No, I was asking if you or Glen were considering paying for him to move to a board and care facility. No medical support is provided there, but at least there are folks on-site who can check in on him every so often."

"I appreciate what you are asking. We talked about it and, given Gerry's stubbornness and, frankly, the history here—which I haven't shared with you—we decided that if Gerry says he can manage at home and if the facility thinks so too, then that's what he should do."

"Right. Okay, we can give it a shot. I expect he will be discharged on Monday. I have set up an appointment to see Gerry in my clinic on the subsequent Monday, the tenth, at 9:30 in the morning. It would really be helpful if you or Glen can make sure he gets to my appointment, even better if you can accompany him here. Whether someone makes it to their first visit to the clinic often determines their future trajectory."

"I'll be there, Gerry in tow." He paused. "And I want to thank you so much for all you've done to get him out of this mess. You've done a beautiful job. I am deeply grateful to you."

THE LIFESAVER

On the tenth, at 9:00 a.m., as I was about to enter one of my exam rooms, I saw the Famous Artist pushing Gerry, seated in a wheelchair, down my clinic hallway to get his vital signs checked. I gave them a wave and a smile.

"I'll see you guys in a few minutes, so sit tight."

Why the hell was he in a wheelchair? I expected to see Gerry hobbling down my hallway, with his brother, the Famous Artist, by his side.

Twenty minutes later, the three of us were in my exam room. Gerry was all smiles, lounging in his wheelchair, feet turned a bit inward. He had put on weight. He had a black backpack strapped to his front. The Famous Artist sat across from him, his legs crossed in an artist's pose, save for the absent cigarette.

"Hey, Gerry, great to see you. What an ordeal you've been through."

"Yeah. Man, it's good to be home again!"

"Sounds like they did a nice job with you at the rehab facility. That they got you walking again?"

"They were real nice. And great food too."

"But you *were* walking when they discharged you, right?"

"Yup. Slowly, but I was walking."

"And how's it been going since you've gotten home?"

"Not so great, actually, at least not with the walking."

I glanced over at the Famous Artist, who was looking at Gerry with a poker face.

"How so?" I asked.

"It's been hard to walk."

The Famous Artist stepped in. "I visited him two days ago, and he was back on the floor. I got him up and he was able to walk with my help, but he was in a lot of pain, and he was really hobbled."

"That's a really quick decline, don't you think? Gerry, did you expect to be able to walk when you got home?"

He looked at me, and it seemed that he was getting tearful.

The Famous Artist jumped in. "He says he was really stiff again and had a lot of pain. They only gave him three days' worth of medicine when they discharged him. That was a week ago. So, I think he ran out. I had to get to his place at 7:00 this morning just to get him here on time. And we took it one step at a time, literally. He was in agony."

"Oh, that'll do it. With no muscle relaxants and no pain medications, he'll be back at square one real quick. We've got to get him back on those meds ASAP. Since he's kind of homebound, I'll also get home PT in to see him for a few weeks to make sure he's getting help walking again. But first, Gerry, I need you to sign a medication contract with me, because these are controlled substances."

"Oh yes . . . I understand, Doc."

"Your signing this means that you cannot obtain these medications from any other doctor aside from me and that you can only refill them once per month by coming here to pick up your special prescriptions. You cannot get them refilled earlier than every thirty days. You cannot share these medications with anyone. You cannot sell these medications. And we will randomly test your urine to make sure that these medications are in your system and that no illicit drugs, like heroin or cocaine, are in your system. Any violation of these terms would represent a violation of our contract, and I would be forced to stop prescribing them for you. Which I am sure you would agree would not be a good outcome for you."

"You don't have to read me the riot act, Doc. I get it."

His brother, the Famous Artist, said impatiently, "Gerry, he is trying to help you and to be clear with you from the get-go."

"He's right, Gerry. I do these formal contracts with any patient of mine for whom I prescribe controlled substances. This has nothing to do with you personally. These medications are highly regulated by the DEA."

"The feds? We don't want trouble with the feds," he snickered.

"No, we don't. This will ensure that we have no trouble."

"I'll sign whatever you need me to sign. Thanks for being straight with me, Doc." He raised his right hand to me. "I'll be good. I promise."

After we both signed the contract, I pulled out my secure prescription pad and wrote out a thirty-day supply for diazepam, 10 mg three times a day, and Tylenol with codeine #4, two pills three times a day. I handed him the paper prescription, and he carefully placed it into the front zippered pocket of his backpack and gave it a few pats.

"Safe and sound, Doc."

I then made a few phone calls to arrange the home PT and sent them on their way.

As they got up to leave, the Famous Artist stuck his hand out to shake mine and again looked me in the eye.

"You've been really terrific, Dean. A real lifesaver. Again, I can't thank you enough."

"Not a problem," I said to him. "Listen, if anything like this comes up again, something that seems like it's not going right, don't hesitate to call me. You have my office number already, but let me give you my cell phone. It's my personal phone. Just call if problems arise, okay?"

As I gave him my number, he slowly typed it into his cell phone, with Gerry already half out the door, his back to me.

VIP CARE

Two days later, as I was leaving the hospital for the day, my cell phone rang.

"Hello, Doc, it's Gerry. Remember me?"

"Of course. Hello, Gerry. How'd you get my number?"

"You gave it to my brother, remember? I . . . uh . . . I called him, and he told me I should just call you. So, he gave me your number."

"Oh, okay. What's going on, Gerry?"

In my head, I saw the Famous Artist looking me in the eye, smiling, and shaking my hand in gratitude, thankful that I have rescued his brother yet again.

"I got jumped by two guys just outside my apartment door. They grabbed my backpack and ran. I didn't have a chance with these bum feet. The damn Tenderloin."

"Oh no. Are you all right? Are you injured?"

"Naw, I'm okay. But they stole my pill bottles. My medications were in there. I'm all out. And so, I'm having real problems walking again."

I could see it all happening, some hoodlums hanging out in hallways just waiting to prey on the older, vulnerable tenant. The ensuing scuffle. Gerry desperately trying to hang on to his backpack. Them yanking it from his grasp. The bastards. And Gerry fated to be back on all fours.

"That's horrible, Gerry. Listen. I'll do this for you, but only this once. From now on, those medications have to stay in your apartment, not in your backpack. They have to be kept under lock and key. You got that?"

"I've learned my lesson, Doc. Thank you so much. I'll call my brother and let him know you took care of it."

"Okay. I'm going to phone them in to your pharmacy right now. They should be ready in about two hours. Take care, Gerry."

"You're a lifesaver, Doc."

Two days later, again as I was leaving the hospital, my cell phone rang. Glen was the caller.

"Whassup, Glen?"

"Hey, Dean. Listen, I've got to share some bad news. We found Gerry earlier today, dead in his apartment. They're going to be sending you the death certificate soon. My guess was a heart attack."

"What? That's not possible. Oh shit."

I was shaken. A cluster of memories and images, hiding just below the surface, bubbled up and showed themselves to me. Ambivalent memories of clinical escapades involving controlled substances, mostly opioids, arise:

The greasy and stringy long hair of Dirk Ashley, a man who had been living on the streets ever since being released from state prison. He was my patient during my first decade in practice. A young guy with a history of heroin use who also had chronic pain from injuries sustained as a result of police brutality. The endless requests for ever-increasing doses of long-acting opiates, none of which appeared to quell either his pain or his addiction. The day I put my foot down and told him on the phone that enough was enough, and that he needed to enter a methadone maintenance program before we discussed any further treatment with opiates. How he threatened me on the phone that day, warning me that unless I prescribed his opiates, he would "pull another 101 California" in my clinic, a reference to a mass shooting that had recently taken place in downtown San Francisco. And my forcefully instructing him that any further references to violent behavior would be grounds to terminate his relationship with me and our clinic. Then images from his follow-up appointment in which he became increasingly agitated and threatening, one that ended in hospital security staff escorting him out of the clinic and my needing to file a restraining order to prevent him from ever setting foot on the hospital campus grounds again. And my needing to face him and to face my fear by showing up in court to make my case. A case that he fortunately failed to show for.

And then the pink and green hats, the straw and felt hats, the flowered and feathered hats of Ms. Julia Meadows. An eighty-seven-year-old woman whom I had taken care of for over twenty-five years. A woman who used to visit our ER about five times a month—always for pain control related to chronic back pain—and who would receive five or so Tylenol with codeines for the road, but nothing more. A Black woman for whom no primary care doctor would prescribe opiates for her pain because of a distant history of depression and alcohol abuse. A so-called difficult patient whose spine I discovered was so riddled with bone growths and so distorted by a condition called *diffuse idiopathic skeletal hyperostosis* that, when I met her, she was unable to stand up beyond a forty-five-degree angle. Who was barely able to make it from bed to bathroom due to her pain and rigidity. A woman with whom I was able to work over the first three years of our relationship to build mutual trust and iteratively arrive at a successful pain regimen that involved both neuropathic agents and high-dose, long-acting opiate medications—in this case 300 mcg of fentanyl in patch form—that enabled her to live a functional life over the next twenty years. A life devoid of subsequent ER visits for pain control, a life that featured no violations of our pain medication contract. A life changed by bold but careful prescribing and monitoring.

Dueling memories. I shook myself out of this reverie.

"Glen, tell me: Did you find any pill bottles in his room?"

"There was one empty bottle of diazepam. Nothing else. It's possible that he sold the codeine and the diazepam on the street. And then bought some coke with the money. And overdid it. And either stroked out or had a massive heart attack as a result. I'm not saying that's what happened, just that it's *possible*. But either way, I wanted to call you before you found out from someone else so that you wouldn't jump to conclusions and feel bad about it. Because I want you to know that you have nothing to feel bad about."

I tried to envision the chain of events.

"Wow. Thanks for being thoughtful and calling me, Glen. Of course, I *do* feel awful. I can't help but believe that I unwittingly contributed to his death. When he called, my usual defenses were down, because I made a rare exception. I somehow believed him and called in refills on both meds. In hindsight, it sounds as though he was taking me for a ride. I think I made the fatal mistake of giving him VIP care."

Glen and I both know that outcomes are rarely good when we favor a particular patient due to their VIP status. Gerry fit that definition for me by virtue of being related to Glen's father. I gave him special treatment outside the norm because of who his nephew and brother were. He was my VIP patient by proxy, and he paid the price.

"No, you're wrong," Glen continued. "This was all Gerry, classic Gerry. He always found a way to confound himself and bring others down with him in the process. Don't beat yourself up. Have some compassion for yourself. You only did what you thought was best for him."

"Maybe. But I think what's more true is that I wanted to please you guys and not run the risk of putting Gerry—and you and your dad—through three weeks of his not being able to walk just on the small but not negligible chance that he may be hoarding or selling his meds. That was an error in judgment on my part, an error that didn't necessarily come from a place of trying to do what was best for Gerry."

"I hear you. That's a subtle distinction, though. I'm calling you to say, whether or not you believe that scenario to be true, you can and should forgive yourself."

The next day, when I received the death certificate, I called the morgue and attempted to make this a coroner's case by expressing my concern that this death could have reflected an accidental overdose. They are required by law to carry out autopsies and toxicology studies on suspected overdoses. The overworked coroner's office would have none of it, claiming this to be a straightforward case of cardiovascular death in an old man. I asked to speak to the city coroner but got no further with her.

I never did get closure on what happened to Gerry. Did he overdose on the diazepam? Did he sell the drugs to get money to buy cocaine and then die of a cocaine-induced heart attack or stroke? Or was it just an everyday heart attack?

I realized that my search for the answer as to the cause of his death was just a diversionary shell game I was playing with myself, one that reflected the wrong question. The real question was how I allowed myself to be in a position where I could actually be more certain than not that the cause of his death was related to my momentary lapse in judgment. How I allowed myself to be seduced into making what likely proved to be a fatal mistake. Seduced not only by Gerry but also blinded by my own desire to fulfill some vague artistic fantasy about my special role in this VIP's family.

The experience of Gerry's case exposed a vulnerability in myself and likely in many other doctors: a tendency to unknowingly and subtly serve our own interests while purportedly serving the needs of our patients. And more, that amid the polemic of clinical versus epidemiologic reasoning resides the poorly understood and underexplored world of the physician's emotional state and its hidden influence on decision-making.

A DECADE LATER

Mr. Chambers hobbled into my office, leaning on his four-legged cane with each small step. The pain visible on his face as he slowly propelled himself toward the corner chair created the impression that his joints were audibly creaking, like those of the Tin Man before he oiled himself up and down. And while his walking was hampered by severe degenerative arthritis, his mobility problems were exacerbated when, two years prior, at the age of sixty-two, he lost his great toe to advanced diabetes.

He slowly pivoted 180 degrees and carefully backed into the corner, shuffling in reverse until he was hovering over the chair, and then collapsed onto it with a thud.

He looked up at me, big eyes poking out from beneath his jungle of long, white hair, peering out from above the forest of his thick, white mustache and beard. He was trying to catch his breath.

"Doc . . . I honestly can't . . . I can't thank you enough. For what you did . . . two weeks ago." Tears slowly began to emerge from his bulging eyes.

"It's okay, Mr. Chambers."

"No. Really, I mean it . . . I understand how . . . how you went out on a limb for me. How you went above and beyond. Especially after you shared with me what happened to you . . . er . . . I mean . . . what happened to that patient of yours the last time you did this, the last time you made an exception to the rules. It's no exaggeration when I tell you that you were a lifesaver for me."

Two weeks prior, I received a text from one of my nurses requesting that I log in to the electronic health record to see an important and time-sensitive set of messages about Mr. Chambers. I got online and read a chain of messages documented in the medical record, all dated December 23. Five sequential messages, first from Mr. Chambers to our health system's phone triage nurse; then from the pharmacy to our clinic front desk staff; from the front desk staff member to my nurse, followed by a note documenting my nurse's subsequent conversation with Mr. Chambers; and finally, a long message from my nurse to me.

The story he had told her—one that was conveyed to me in detail in my nurse's last note—was that on the previous day, his roommate had invited a friend to hang out in the apartment they shared. The friend was supposed to stay for a few hours to watch an NFL playoff game together, but midway through the first quarter, he had apologized and said he needed to run, and he took off. After the game, Mr. Chambers told her that he went to his bedroom to take his scheduled dose of the high-dose, long-acting opiate I prescribed to help him function in the context of arthritis-related pain, only to find that the entire bottle was gone. While he still had twenty-four hours' worth of pain pills that he had previously placed in his pillbox, the rest of his medication—the bottle that contained thirteen more days' worth—had been stolen from right under his nose. My nurse's note ended as I anticipated it would: "Would you be willing to refill his opiate medications early so he can get through the Christmas and New Year holiday period without having to be immobile and suffer terribly?"

Would I? I asked myself. I really didn't *know* Chambers that well. Maybe six visits over an eighteen-month period. A guy who had been transferred to me from a physician who had left our clinic and moved to another state. Chambers seemed like a good guy, seemed to always be straight up with me. I recalled he recently talked to me about whether he should try tapering his long-acting opiate regimen someday, given all he had heard about the potential dangers of opiates. He had been understandably ambivalent, since this regimen had transformed him from barely living as the Tin Man to being able to function enough to make his life worthwhile. We had decided that we would discuss giving it a try in the coming year. So that was reassuring.

On the other hand, was it a pure coincidence that he was asking me to make this exception to our pain medication contract around the Christmas holiday, during "the season of giving," the time when one was supposed to engage in acts of kindness on behalf of mankind? Could he be harnessing this holiday spirit to get me to let my guard down, pulling the wool over my eyes to get more of the good stuff?

"You know, Mr. Chambers, you're right. It was a big stretch for me to refill your medications early. At first, given what had happened to that patient I told you about on the phone, I was just going to graciously decline, as I have done many, many times both before and after that event. Because, you know, I'm not the only doctor in this clinic to whom something like that has happened, so we've talked about this exact scenario as a group. But I checked myself and decided I was going to call you with an open mind. And you told me what happened. I could hear the panic in your voice when you imagined out loud how miserable the next thirteen days would be for you if you didn't have your medications. But that didn't move me. I'd heard that all before."

"So, why'd you do it, Doc? Why'd you risk it?"

"Well, I thought I'd dig a bit further before just saying no. So, I asked if you had made a police report, and you told me you had. *Okay*, I thought, *let's play this out*. I asked you if you had a receipt from that report. You said you did. *Good*, I thought. Then I asked you to go get it, and you told me you had it in your hands. *Even better*, I said to myself. I asked you to read out the police report number, and you did. I asked you to give me the name of the officer who took the report, and you did. And finally, I asked you to give me the precinct's phone number so I could confirm your story. And you did. And I subsequently confirmed your story, one that, based on my conversation with the police officer, included a witness to the event. Mr. Chambers, you did all the right things under the circumstances. So, I made the call and made an exception for you."

I didn't like that my only means of corroborating his story was to rely on a police report. I recognized that many of my patients would not feel safe getting the police involved. Chambers, however, felt no such ambivalence.

"Doc, I'm not a hugger. But I'd give you a big hug if it didn't take so much effort just to get up and out of this damn chair."

"No need, Mr. Chambers."

"Not true, Doc. Like I said, you went out on a limb for me, and I appreciate it. How 'bout a fist bump instead?"

"You bet."

PART 2

In Story Lies the Cure

CHAPTER 9

The Disability Blues

IN 1998, I AM WORKING AT MY CLINIC, SERVING THE URBAN POOR AND THE most medically complex patients in our city. Given the undersupply of primary care physicians relative to the needs of this population and, knowing how our waiting rooms are always filled beyond capacity, I am laser focused on being efficient in order to provide care to as many patients as possible in a day.

That day, as I sit down in the empty exam room, I glance at my nurse's annotation:

NEW PATIENT—HISTORY OF SUBSTANCE ABUSE. HERE FOR DISABILITY EVAL.

Mr. E., a fifty-six-year-old man, enters my examination room. To describe him as disheveled is to oversimplify. He shuffles toward me in trash-picked sneakers whose tongues wag for want of laces. His pants bunch at his ankles like an accordion. Barely clinging to his hips, they drag down his whole being. Nose to the ground, he is forced to look straight up, past his brow and silver Afro, just to achieve eye contact. His posture suggests a question mark. He drools, unable to counter the gravitational pull on his lower lip. He is truly down and out.

I invite him to take a seat, and I wonder what will become of our inter-action. Will I diagnose ankylosing spondylitis or severe spinal degenerative joint disease? Will I obtain radiographs documenting the sorry state of his vertebral column and describe the resultant functional impairments? Will I uncover cirrhosis or HIV infection, or find no diagnosis other than "urban decay"—a diagnosis nobody wants to pay for?

I begin our interview with the standard medical questionnaire. His re-sponses are marked by an aggressive tone and frequent digressions. Our first few minutes leave me frustrated. My frustration is obvious; I can tell he is becoming equally frustrated. Our mutual agitation crescendos. I think I may be forced to end the interview and refer him elsewhere.

Changing the tone of our conversation, I ask him what type of work he used to do.

"Well, I played the trombone," he rasps. "Yeah . . . I played with the greats. . . . But no more. . . . No, sir . . . no more."

"Really?" I am stimulated, reawakened. "*I play sax.*"

He responds with an edentulous, cavernous, soaring smile. "No kid-din', Doc?"

I smile a smile of polished, ivory teeth.

"Well, I'm not so good, but it's still fun."

"That's cool, Doc. Real cool. Hey! I got a sax-playin' doc!"

He recounts the gigs with Bill Evans, Dizzy, Coltrane, and Miles—all those gigs, all the good times, all the girls, and he smiles. And as he talks, he taps his foot to a rhythm of the past.

His smile gradually gives way to a frown, surrenders to gravity's lamenting pull downward.

"But now . . . now I got no *chops*, Doc."

He tells me about the heavy drinking, the heroin, the bad times. He can't remember much after that. We talk some more—talk jazz, talk about Oak-land in the '60s and '70s. He tells me about the methadone treatment, gives me the name of his "payee" and friend at his temporary hotel.

I return to his medical history. Now he willingly shows me his abdom-inal scar from "my bleedin' ulcer," and his swollen feet. He is bad with de-tails. His short-term memory is poor. He undoubtedly has some degree of dementia. I briefly examine him, order some blood work, and ask him to return in two weeks. He takes my card with the appointment time and pockets it.

After he leaves, I wonder what would have happened had we not stumbled upon this common interest. Would we have parted angrily, each cast into a stereotyped role that neither of us was comfortable fulfilling? Are racial, social, and class differences so great that only such fortuitous connections can rescue the clinical encounter? Ours was a narrow escape from the frequent failure within the medical profession to find a way to recognize our basic shared humanity—a continual process that sustains a therapeutic relationship.

Mr. E. misses his follow-up appointment. But he returns four weeks later instead. His blood work is normal. I perform a mini mental-status exam, which contains eleven items, such as "*What is today's date?*" and "*Spell WORLD backward,*" and "*Count backward by sevens from one hundred.*" We move at a snail's pace. He is scoring miserably.

When faced with one of the final items—"*Write a sentence*"—he takes my pen and wraps himself around the paper. I tell him to take his time, and I sit down to do my charting. A few seconds later, he reaches out and passes me the paper:

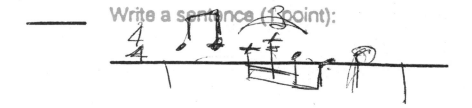

I look at his face—a smile and an unmistakable look of pride.
We've made a connection, and I know that his stories will come.
"What does it say?" I ask.
"Boom boom . . . diggiduh bmm-boom."
I decide to give him a point for this sentence.
Mr. E. remained my patient for twenty years, until the very end of his life.

CHAPTER 10

Lost in Translation

Refining the Most Common Medical Procedure

> The problem with communication is the assumption that it has occurred.
>
> —George Bernard Shaw

A THERAPEUTIC ENCOUNTER

As an experienced public hospital physician, I have witnessed how the telling—or more often the withholding—of the story governs the outcome of an individual patient's illness. How a physician's choice to elicit the narrative to inform the science or to just stick to the numbers and rely on our miraculous technology either sets the patient on the path to recovery or to premature death.

Why has the elicitation of story become a discretionary practice in medicine? We marvel at modern medicine's ever-growing ability to analyze our invisible inner chemistries, its capacity to use advanced imaging techniques with greater and greater powers of resolution to peer at the structures deep within. We have been seduced into believing that science and technology alone can divine whether each of us is destined to be sick or healthy. This has undermined our appreciation of the value of story, leaving our muscles for narrative inquiry to atrophy.

I often ask my medical students this question: *Which medical tool or procedure do you believe saves the most lives?*

Their answers range from antibiotics to cholesterol-lowering drugs, from EKGs to MRIs, from caesarian sections to IV saline, from mechanical ventilation to vaccination.

The right answer is none of those things. Rather, it is the medical interview. A procedure they perceive to have little technological flair, a communicative intervention that many—unaware of its intensely human, interactive, and revelatory features—believe to be nothing more than a mundane, standardized, and glorified questionnaire. Over a career, a primary care physician will carry out roughly one hundred thousand office-based patient interviews, making it the most common medical procedure conducted in practice. This is where communication between physician and patient takes place (or not), and lifesaving relationships can develop. Storytelling is the essential device through which the patient's experience is communicated and the physician's daily craft is realized. It is how science and narrative blend. Eliciting, listening to, and interpreting these stories: together, these narrative acts generate the most fundamental dataset from which sound clinical decisions can be made and appropriate actions taken.

Yet the interactions that comprise the medical interview have been underappreciated and undervalued in the field of medicine and largely ignored by clinical scientists. The failure to elicit the patient's story and benefit from the clinical discoveries and human connections these stories can foster results in immeasurable suffering and excess health care costs. In my own practice, I have had to learn again and again the lesson that *in the story lies the answers*. And not to make assumptions, not to impose a narrative onto my patients.

Early in my career, I worked an evening clinic that served low-income patients whose jobs as essential workers did not give them the flexibility to schedule a doctor's visit during the workday. On one of those evenings, I learned that some of the most critical stories often go untold and that the work of a primary care doctor involves the search for the hidden story.

One of my patients, John T., was a construction worker with high blood pressure that was difficult to control. He came to his appointment wearing his usual lumberjack-type flannel shirt, loose-fitting painter's pants, and work boots with the laces untied. I liked him. We got along. I respected that, at fifty-nine years old, he was able to hold his own with the younger crews doing construction.

I ripped at the Velcro and unwrapped the blood pressure cuff binding his bulky right arm. I stuffed the cuff along with its rubber tubing and rubber bulb back into the wire basket on the wall.

"Your pulse is 76, but your blood pressure is still very high: 205 over 110. It's not a safe situation, Mr. T."

Not hiding my disappointment, I extracted my stethoscope's metal tubes from my ears. More often than not, my visits with him involved blood pressure readings over 200, which led to me increasing the doses and numbers of his medications, combined with lengthy counseling sessions about the sequelae of uncontrolled blood pressure and the importance of treating this "silent killer." So named because of the lack of symptoms it causes until it's really far gone, which was something his was inching toward. I asked him:

"Are you having any headaches? Vision problems? Or chest pain?"

"No, Doc. I'm tired, for sure. But none of those other things."

I rolled my stool forward and made solid eye contact.

"Mr. T., did you take *all* your prescribed blood pressure medications today?"

"Yes, just like you told me to."

"And how about over the last two weeks? Did you miss any doses?"

"Not that I can remember, no."

I'd been treating him for escalating blood pressure for over three years, and over the last few visits, the elevated pressure had been sustained at this dangerous level. I had him taking six blood pressure medications. I had run all the usual and unusual blood and urine tests I could think of to uncover rare causes of uncontrolled high blood pressure.

I believe I have a pretty good feel for when I am being taken for a ride. I looked him in the eye again, trying to judge his sincerity. Instead, I found myself envisioning the blood vessels of his brain gradually weakening from long-standing exposure to high blood pressure, suddenly rupturing and causing a catastrophic hemorrhage and stroke. Despite my best efforts to prevent such an event, I saw the future Mr. T. paralyzed on one side, speechless, and wheelchair bound.

"Okay, Mr. T. Did you bring in your medicine bottles like I asked, so we can review them one by one?" I asked, reaching for the bag at his side.

He grabbed it first.

"Oh, no, this is just some quick food shopping I did."

"So, are you telling me you *didn't* bring your pill bottles in?"

"Well, I wanted to, but I came right from the construction site."

"But you found the time to go food shopping on your way here?" I asked in an accusatory tone.

"Yeah," he said, reaching for his back pocket. "But I brought my list of . . ."

"Mr. T., I've been trying my hardest to do right by you for over three years. I really care about you. But I need you to do your part. I have made a simple request of you on every one of the last five visits: to bring in all your medication bottles. But it's like I'm banging my head against the wall."

I felt myself escalating and saw him shrinking in parallel, slipping down in his chair and extending his legs and their untied boots farther forward.

I mercilessly pushed on.

"I simply *can't* do my job if I can't look over your pill bottles. It's not that I don't trust you. I just need to make sure there are no misunderstandings between us when it comes to your medications. And going through them one by one, together, is the best way to do that."

"Okay, Doc. I'll bring 'em with me next time."

I crossed my arms and rolled my stool away from him. "Honestly, Mr. T., that's what you've said each time before, and we're still in exactly the same place."

He looked down at his work boots. "Yeah, I know."

I surprised even myself with what I said next, because abandoning or "firing" a public hospital patient who has little recourse to alternatives was ethically troubling. But I took a calculated risk.

"So, here's what I feel forced to do. Despite your sky-high blood pressure, we're not going to change any medications this time. I will see you again in two weeks, but with your pill bottles. If you do not bring in all your medications—and I mean *all* of them, cleaning out your entire medicine cabinet—then I just don't think I can take care of you anymore. I might have to transfer your care to another physician."

He looked at me in a way that told me my threat had registered. I couldn't tell whether he had experienced my confrontation as an attempt to set limits to improve his health or to rid myself of him and his intractable hypertension. I was worried he wouldn't come back.

But two weeks later, he was back in my office. His blood pressure was 210 over 103. But this time, he had a large cardboard box at his feet. He lifted it up and dropped it on the examining table with a clatter.

"I brought 'em all in, Doc, just like you told me to."

I rolled my chair to the exam table and peered over the edge of the big box. There were dozens upon dozens of pill bottles. Transparent, orange pill bottles. Opaque, white pill bottles. Cylindrical bottles, squared-off bottles. Some small, some larger. Some labels listed a familiar medication name and had me as the prescribing doctor. But the dates seemed randomly distributed, with some going back months and others back years. Expired drugs, some with labels listing medications no longer in use: Aldomet, reserpine. Prescribed by doctors from my own clinic decades prior.

But the most striking finding was one common to all the bottles: each one was full of pills.

First, I felt anger toward him for this flagrant nonadherence. Then I felt like a fool. I swiveled my stool around and looked up at him.

"Mr. T. What's going on here? Some of these medications are really old. Others I never even prescribed for you. And all these pill bottles, even the ones I recently prescribed, look full. They don't even look like they've been opened."

He looked down at his work boots, saying nothing.

"Don't get me wrong. It is *fabulous* that you finally brought these all in for me to see. But what does it mean?"

He looked up at me like a child gingerly trying to stand up for himself after having received a scolding. "I . . . well . . . I never told you this, Doc."

I waited, but he kept looking back down at his boots. "Never told me *what*, Mr. T.?"

I waited a good three seconds.

It was then I realized I bore equal blame. And that I needed to de-escalate the tension here. That if I was ever to learn the reasons behind this boxful of pills that could have treated the high blood pressure of a small army, I had to make his nonadherence acceptable.

"Whatever it is, Mr. T., it'll be okay. And *we'll* be okay."

His gaze remained fixed at his boots. "I never told you . . . that I just . . . okay . . . that I just can't *swallow* pills. I've never been able to swallow pills, Doc. No matter how hard I try."

He looked back up at me. There was sweat visible above his brow, and I could see that he was trying to read me, awaiting my judgment.

I burst into relieved laughter, rolled my chair toward him, and placed both my hands on his shoulders.

"Oh, Mr. T.! You and me—we have both been incredibly foolish. The blind leading the mute."

He let a big breath out and started to laugh too. As our laughter mixed together and the tension drained from the room, I felt a profound sense of relief. Because we had reached a place where his willingness to share his struggle had filled the vacuum created by my blindness.

I squeezed his shoulders.

"This is no big deal, my friend. Lots of people have trouble swallowing pills."

"They do?"

"Yes, and it's my fault for not thinking that might be a problem for you."

I let go of his shoulders, rolled my stool back to my desk, and grabbed my pen and prescription pad.

"How about liquids? Would you be able to swallow medications if I gave them to you in liquid form?"

"Sure. But can they do that?"

I switched him over to liquid versions of atenolol and amlodipine, the two preparations available at our pharmacy.

A month later, Mr. T. arrived at my clinic with a toiletry bag that contained two near-empty bottles—one for atenolol and the other for amlodipine. His blood pressure was 155 over 92. I shook my head in disbelief, and we shared another laugh. I congratulated him and refilled his medications.

I have kept that box with the pill bottle collection for safekeeping. It's something I treasure, a reminder, something tangible that I show my students and residents to teach them it is dangerous to assume that the details are unimportant, and foolhardy to presume you understand the lives of your patients. To show them that, in medicine, the story holds the truth. And often you have to dig to find it.

COMMUNICATION, CAPILLARIES, AND CLINICAL CARE

Mr. T. and I had laughed over the fact that his inability to swallow pills was missed by four primary care physicians over twenty years of treating his uncontrolled hypertension. But there was a hidden tragedy in this story, both for him and for the millions of others whose clinical encounters have gone awry. While he was fortunate to have avoided a stroke or kidney failure during this time period, this decades-long disconnect may yet have untoward consequences for him, as his exposure to uncontrolled hypertension will likely find a way to take a toll on his body.

What gets in the way of open communication between patient and physician, of achieving "shared meaning"? As I have come to study and learn, very many things can and do get in the way. For Mr. T., the power imbalance he experienced and the shame he felt in disclosing his pill-swallowing "problem" presented significant barriers to open communication. Attending each visit with me must have been a painful exercise in overcoming the ambivalence he felt between the need to attend to his physical well-being and the need to protect and prioritize his pride and emotional well-being. For me, my perceived need to efficiently solve the conundrum of his intractable high blood pressure led me to prioritize direct interrogation to uncover medication nonadherence or expensive diagnostic searches for rare diseases—what we call *medical zebras*—over fostering in him a deeper sense of trust in me to enable open communication and disclosure without any associated stigma.

The profound influence of health communication with respect to the clinical trajectories of my patients gradually became apparent to me over the course of my career. This was most striking when I grappled with the challenges that I faced with my patients who had communication barriers, such as limited literacy and language skills, or when I saw my own communication failures reflected back at me. There is nothing like failure to motivate physicians to do better. Attempting to remedy such failures in communication has been my objective for much of my career, shaping my clinical work and being the subject of my research.

Despite being a procedure central to the delivery of health care, and despite its tremendous potential impact on the lives of anyone in need of health care, the medical interview does not receive as much attention as it should. There has been relatively little research conducted to understand the basic communicative processes needed to enhance this critical interaction. To this day, inexplicably, the relative investments made in health communication science remain a trickle compared to those made in the basic biologic sciences. We have discovered that cells communicate with one another; which chemical messengers they use to communicate; the complex mechanisms through which these messengers convey their messages to other cells; the ways that these messages get amplified and spread across cellular networks; and the fundamental processes by which those messages are translated into cellular expression and cellular behavior change. Yet we have focused far less on how doctors can better communicate, better elicit, better express, and better care for their patients through this communication.

At times, a single health communication event—such as the one with Mr. T.—can dramatically change a life. At other times, communication manifests its healing capacity over time and space: the hundreds of thousands of capillaries emanating from one primary care physician and her patients, when multiplied by the hundreds of millions of clinical encounters that take place across our nation every year, collectively can convey the power of a turbine.

A LESSON FROM MY FATHER: A BEDSIDE COMMUNICATION SPECTACLE

In 1980, my father, hoping that I would follow in his footsteps and become a surgeon, invited me to make hospital rounds with him on the weekends. At times, he even allowed me to gown and glove up to observe his emergency surgeries. He was an excellent surgeon who prided himself in the skills he had honed over the course of three surgical residencies: the first in Hungary, the second in Israel, and the third in the US. In the US, he was labeled a "foreign medical graduate."

My father had a heavy Hungarian accent and, because the Hungarian language lacks pronouns, he would often confuse *he* and *she*. He had set up his practice in South Buffalo, New York, a working-class neighborhood populated mostly by second-generation, hardscrabble Italian and Polish families, a place that was not exactly trusting or welcoming of new immigrants.

Despite the high stakes involved in the goings-on in the operating room, my clearest and most impactful memory of my time with him in the hospital was not of a heroic surgical procedure but of a clinical conversation that occurred at a patient's bedside.

I am sixteen years old and already stand above my father, who is only five feet, six inches tall. He is wearing a suit and tie under his newly dry-cleaned white lab coat. As we walk down the corridor of Mercy Hospital early one Sunday morning, he tells me that we are about to go into the room of a boy to obtain informed consent from the parents to take their son to the operating room. The boy is likely suffering from a torsion of the testicle, he tells me, an emergency situation in which one testicle rotates on its own axis. As a result, the spermatic cord that brings blood from the abdomen to the testicle also gets twisted, cutting off the blood supply to the testicle.

We enter the room to find the boy, maybe eight or nine years old, lying in bed. From time to time, he moans, writhing in discomfort. At the foot of his bed towers his father, a brawny man with slicked-back hair. He is wearing a T-shirt with rolled-up sleeves that reveal an impressive set of biceps, one of which is adorned with an anchor tattoo. My guess is that he works at the local Bethlehem Steel or General Motors plant. Or, perhaps more accurately, that he *had* worked at one of those plants until he got laid off, like half of South Buffalo's working-age men at the time. The muscles of his squared-off jaw are vigorously pumping as he holds back what looks like pent-up anger. To his right sits his wife, a small woman with a beehive hairdo and a worried look on her face.

Brief introductions are made, and then the boy's father takes over.

"Doc, listen. My boy's been in pain ever since the sixth inning of his ball game last night. But then he wakes up at about three in the morning in a lot more pain. I hate to admit it, but he says to me that his balls hurt. But he didn't get hit in the balls, so I'm thinking we just wait it out. And then he vomits a couple times. So, Judy here, she decides we need to bring him in. We been here since five in the morning. As far as I can tell, nothing's been done for him."

My father calmly responds, but his accent and grammar make me cringe with teenage embarrassment.

"I see your boy, he having pain. This is why they call me to come to see him. I understand dat her testicle is painful. So, I need to examine your boy now."

I watch the man exchange a long, concerned look with his wife.

"Go right ahead, then," he finally says. "I guess that's why we come here."

He squares off his jaw toward his son.

"Kevin, the doctor and his assistant are gonna take a look at you now. You just do what they say so they can figure it out."

Kevin, bedsheet pulled all the way up to his chin, shifts his eyes to his mother, who nods reassuringly.

"Hello, Kevin," my father says with a kind smile. "I need to look under your gown. Don't vorry, I going to be gently."

The boy looks up at me with fear. The mother shifts forward to the edge of her seat, but the man places a heavy hand on her shoulder so she can't move any closer.

I move to the head of the bed and tell Kevin to give me his hand, and I hold it. It is sweaty and cool.

My father pulls down the sheet and lifts the gown.

"Kevin, please open your legs for me and bend at your knee."

I squeeze Kevin's hand, and he follows my father's instructions.

"You see," my father says to me, or maybe also to Kevin's parents. "Her right scrotum is swollen and red. And watch, when I gently rub inside of the left leg, his left testicle—it move up. That is called *normal cremaster reflex*. You see dat? Now, but when I rub other side, her testicle do not move. Like it is stuck. No reflex."

"Yes, I see that," I answer and look back at Kevin.

"Also, when I feel his testicle . . ."

Kevin writhes in pain as my father, still manipulating the right testicle, looks up at him.

"Aha, it is very tender," my father says. "Especially at the tip, what we call the *pole of the testis*. This mean torsion."

I look back at the man and see that he has turned away, avoiding the scene altogether. The wife is dabbing her tears with a tissue.

I let go of Kevin's hand. My father pulls the gown down and lifts the sheet back to cover the boy and pats him on the leg.

"We fix dis for you, Kevin. It's okay. Tomorrow, you feel better."

My father steps away and vigorously washes his hands at the bedside sink, methodically dries them, and then turns to the parents, assuming his most professional tone.

"Your son, he have what we call *torsion of testicle*. It is true emergency. The testicle hangs from body by a cord, and it is become twisted and very painful in Kevin. The testicle is getting strangulation, so no blood to feed it. Without enough blood, Kevin has risk of losing testicle. This is not so common, but a serious problem in some boys."

Kevin's father looks at his wife and then asks my father in an accusatory tone, "How did this happen?"

"Maybe he move funny when he playing baseball. Maybe not. Many time it just happen for no reason. But if we go fast, we can fix it and save Kevin testicle."

"How you gonna do that?"

"I take him to operating room." My father then looks at his watch. "It's been . . . about twelve hours, so I will put him to sleep and make a small cut to look under the skin and inside at the testicle. If it is healthy, I turn it back to position, make it hang straight again. I can then tie down cord and it won't ever happen again. I sew him up, and he feel better tomorrow. If it is not healthy, I am sorry, but we have to take it out. But he still feel better tomorrow."

"Whoa, whoa there, Doc. Cool your jets. You ain't cutting into my boy's balls. No way, no how!"

The wife reaches up to place a hand on his arm. "Honey, the doctor is saying it's an emergency and—"

He yanks his arm away.

"He's gonna be just fine, Judy. There's a lot of money to be made around here, and they ain't gonna make it off my Kevin."

My father glances at me and, with a small smile, shifts to my side and places a hand on my shoulder.

"Mr. Kovalski, I understand. I vould not want my own son here to get surgery, especially in such sensitive area."

"Exactly what I'm saying, Doc. No way, no how. So, I'm glad we agree on this."

"But . . . on the other hand . . . if I *need* to do it to save my own son testicle, I do it. I agree to it. Because right now, your son is not getting blood to her testicle. If we vait any longer, it is like watching someone strangling without trying to rescue dis person. And I am sure you would agree that—"

"What about medications?" his wife meekly asks, her hands tightly clasped together before her face, her knuckles white.

"Well, we giving Kevin pain medication, but I am sorry there is no medication to fix this. Only surgery."

The man moves toward me to his son's bedside and rips back the sheet. "Kevin, let's buck up, boy. Put your clothes back on and let's get on home."

The boy looks at me in fear again, but this time, it's a different kind of fear.

"Mr. Kovalski, if I may," says my father, gently moving the man aside and stepping in between him and his boy. "So sorry. I need to get this tool."

He grabs the blood pressure cuff from its metal basket hanging on the wall at the head of the bed. "This is big decision for you and your wife. Let me demonstrate what we do in surgery."

"Like I said, Doc, I ain't agreeing to no—"

"I know, I know. But let me first show. Please. If I may?"

The man takes a step back and crosses his arms—massive biceps and thick forearms—striking an impenetrable pose.

With one raised hand, my father holds the blood pressure cuff upside down, with the large rubber bulb at the bottom. The bulb sways slowly back and forth as it hangs from the long, spiraling rubber tubing. He then reaches down with his other hand and gently grasps the rubber bulb.

"This was your son's testicle before yesterday. You see it was free and moving easy back and forth? It was happy because it was getting plenty blood through this long cord. This cord, it is also open and free. So, all is good here. Yes?"

My father gives him a smile. He pumps the bulb with his hand a few times and the air audibly flows.

"You agree all is open and flowing? All very good here, yes?"

The man is as unmoved as a statue, arms still crossed. "I see that, yes."

My father continues, now turning to the mother. "But then yesterday . . ."

My father's face slowly contorts into a grimace. I recognize this as one of his many acting faces.

The man's wife sits bolt upright, holding her breath. White hands still clasped before a face now drained of all blood.

"Yesterday, something bad happen."

He begins to deliberately turn the bulb on its axis with one hand while twisting the cord in the opposite direction with his other hand, slowly but surely shortening the distance between the bulb and the wall. With each turn, his grimace tightens and his speech becomes more pressured and strained, his voice more constricted.

"The testicle spin around and around, and the cord begin to strangle it."

I watch as the fixed, defiant features of Kevin's father's face begin to drop, and the closed look begins to soften. With each turn of the bulb, his arms slowly uncross and gradually descend.

My father pumps the bulb again, straining to do so, but now no airflow is audible.

"As the testicle strangles, it lose flow of blood and begin to die. You see?" He tries to pump again. "You see how now there is no flow? And you feel the pain?"

The man's resistance has waned, and his arms have dropped to a V shape, his hands now fully cupping the area over his own testicles, his own face contorting with each turn of the screw.

"And then," my father rasps as he twists and twists the very life out of that blood pressure bulb, "then at the very end . . ."

The man is now hunched over, his face a greenish hue, looking as if he had just gotten kicked in the groin.

He shoots one arm up, waving up at my father in surrender.

"Enough, Doc, *enough*! Please . . . please, just take my son. Take him to the operating room. Untwist that cord!"

With that, my father releases his grip on the bulb, holding the blood pressure apparatus up high. We all watch in silence as the bulb untwirls and untwirls on itself, round and round, until it swings free again.

My father stuffs the blood pressure cuff back into the metal basket at the head of Kevin's bed. He turns back to Kevin's father. "I am so glad you understand now."

The man pulls a handkerchief out of his pocket and slowly wipes his face with it. He lets out a big breath. "Yes, I understand now."

Now, four decades after that bedside spectacle, I realize that that event was what made me curious as to whether and how human interactions, whether conveyed through words, props, imagery, touch, or tone, could alter the trajectory of a medical condition with as much potency as a surgical knife.

CHAPTER 11

Detectives of Social Vulnerability

W HEN I WAS IN RESIDENCY TRAINING, MY CLINIC WAS LOCATED AT the university hospital. My patients came largely from middle-class backgrounds: many were seniors on Medicare, only a few were low-income patients on Medicaid, and none were uninsured. My patients had the usual infirmities, and in general, they did well over the course of my three years of service. In this period, only three of my patients passed away, and none of these deaths came as a surprise to me.

I was fortunate enough to be chosen to serve an extra year as chief resident, selecting to carry out this term at San Francisco General Hospital, the safety-net institution that cared for the city's most marginalized patients. Here, I cared for a panel of patients who had similar sets of diseases to those in my university clinic panel. And I worked as diligently and compulsively at the public hospital clinic located in the flats as I had "up on the Hill." But in terms of outcomes, things couldn't have been more different. By the end of my first year, six of my patients had died, half of them unexpectedly. Two more suffered big strokes, and three others were hit with end-stage kidney failure and could only survive with dialysis.

What was I doing wrong? How could the same diseases lead to such vastly different trajectories and outcomes in clinics located just four miles away from each other, staffed by a set of objectively, identically qualified physicians? Was I misdiagnosing my ailing patients?

HOW DOCTORS USUALLY THINK

Perhaps one of the most fundamental cognitive tasks that a physician must learn, practice, and master is the act of the *differential diagnosis*. Developing and refining a differential diagnosis involves the process of weighing the probability of one disease against that of many other diseases possibly accounting for a patient's symptoms and illness. This iterative method is applied from the moment the patient first presents and continues throughout her course until a definitive answer is identified. As physicians are well aware, generating a comprehensive differential diagnosis first requires possessing deep scientific knowledge and experience regarding how a wide range of diseases might present themselves. In addition, sifting through this differential diagnosis to generate a single accurate diagnosis requires an associative ability that matches a patient's symptoms or combination of symptoms to the right set of diseases, combined with the mathematical facility to apply epidemiologic principles related to disease and symptom prevalence versus rarity.

Then there are the tests we do. Much weight is now paid to the value of findings generated by the "sexier," hard-science tools in physicians' diagnostic tool kits—like results derived from blood and genetic tests, and the miraculous images produced by high-cost radiologic studies. Yet research has shown that over three-fourths of the process of "nailing the right diagnosis" (and therefore the right treatment plan) falls under the umbrella of the "soft sciences": the art of taking a good history.

DOCTORS IN PUBLIC HOSPITALS NEED
TO THINK DIFFERENTLY

San Francisco General Hospital has provided me with ample opportunities to learn and relearn the value of eliciting a comprehensive and accurate narrative from the patient. Socially marginalized patients often present with a broad range of medical conditions. These can be conditions considered to occur only in the developing world, rare conditions presenting typically, or common conditions presenting atypically. But most of all, we see illnesses that reflect the interaction between the "purely medical" and the "purely social." We need to maintain a deep sense of curiosity and relentlessly pursue lines of inquiry that are as focused on the sociologic as the biologic. We should be guided by a systematic approach to the differential diagnosis in marginalized patients that merged the rigor of the clinical sciences with a holistic worldview derived, in part, from the social sciences but, more importantly, informed by my patients' lived experiences. I learned that I could only have the luxury of applying this dualistic approach if I let myself be open to discovering my patients and their social contexts through their narratives.

A FRIDAY-NIGHT CALL

I am twelve years into my practice. I think I have seen it all, that I've heard every variation on any theme. Then I receive a call from the hospital service late one Friday night at the start of a long weekend. They inform me that my patient, Mrs. Jimenez, has been hospitalized for a severe hypoglycemic episode (low blood sugar).

"Her serum glucose was undetectable in the field," the on-call ICU resident tells me. "The paramedics treated her right away. But it was only 19 when she hit the ER door."

I hold my breath and wait to hear the rest, as I know that 19 is a blood sugar level that, if left unaddressed for too long, is not compatible with life.

"I'm sorry to bug you so late," he continues. "I'm hoping you can maybe give us some insights because her blood sugars hovered in the 30s for the last few hours despite a couple of amps of D50. She's in the ICU on a D10 drip now. It seems to be holding her blood sugar for now, like in the 80s, but whenever we dial it down, her blood sugars plummet."

I close my eyes and call up a mental image of Mrs. Jimenez. A stocky woman, sharp mind, usually lighthearted. She is an English-speaking Latina immigrant in her late fifties. She works as a housekeeper, is married, is a mother of three, and has five grandchildren. She has been under my care for nearly ten years, and I know her well. She has had diabetes for maybe fifteen years and over the last five has become insulin-dependent. She already has early kidney disease and retinal disease and also has hypertension, high cholesterol, degenerative joint disease, and a history of depression. In addition to taking long-acting insulin, she takes seven oral medications. She misses about a quarter of our scheduled visits, probably because she has a full-time job and often has to care for her grandkids on top of it all. She has a supportive family, though. She makes all her appointments when her daughter or her husband bring her to them. Her husband seems like a good guy, really dedicated.

"Wow. That's odd. I saw her maybe three, four weeks ago. Her blood pressure was excellent, her kidney function was suboptimal but unchanged, but her blood sugar control was pretty god-awful. If I recall, I increased her long-acting insulin dose a touch, you know, just hoping to delay any decline in her kidney function or her vision."

I can virtually hear our minds clicking through the differential diagnosis of hypoglycemia in a person with diabetes, a condition whose hallmark is *high* blood sugar, not low.

I continue, "I can't believe that that small of a change in insulin would be responsible for this severe an episode . . ."

"Well, I gotta think that *is* what did it," replies the ICU resident. "That's the only thing that's changed."

"Right. I hear you. But I can't see how a 5-unit change could do this. Maybe she took the wrong dose—took an overdose by accident? Or maybe her kidney function has gotten worse, and she's not clearing the insulin like she had in the past?"

"Yeah, we thought about that, but her kidney function's just the same as it was when you saw her a month ago. We can't ask her about the insulin dose she took, 'cause she's still kind of out of it. But the husband and a huge rotating set of family members have been by her side from the moment they brought her to the ER. Her daughter and husband are here with me now, and they both say she's really good about measuring out her insulin."

"Okay, yeah, I think they're right about that."

So, I go further down my virtual list, touching on the less likely possibilities.

"Liver failure, then? Gastroparesis? Or sepsis—how about sepsis?"

"Yup. We thought about those too. Liver function is rock solid. You'd know if she has bad gastroparesis because she'd have a history of vomiting or feeling full after eating only a little. Doesn't happen overnight. So that's out. And no signs of infection. Urine's clean, chest x-ray's clean, white blood count's normal. But we drew two sets of blood cultures anyway and are giving her broad-spectrum antibiotics just to cover her until we have a better handle on this."

"Got it. Well, without talking more to the family, or to her, I'm sorry—I'm at a loss and can't be that helpful. All I'd say is see if you can get into the weeds a bit more with the family. And ask them to bring in her insulin vials tomorrow. See if the pharmacist can back-calculate how much she has left versus how much she should have left. Maybe we'll find out that she actually did take too much. And hey—thanks for touching base. Gimme a call tomorrow or if anything gets worse."

Mrs. Jimenez stays in the ICU for two and a half more days, requiring continuous IV glucose. She slowly becomes more alert; her appetite returns, and she is provided meals. She gradually becomes able to maintain her blood sugar at a normal level. The inpatient team remains puzzled by the length of the hospital stay related to this episode, having carried out a thorough medical workup to determine the root cause, including ruling out the rare insulin-secreting tumor. In response to their queries about her insulin, she accurately reports to the team that she had recently changed her bedtime dose at the order of her doctor, increasing it from 45 units at bedtime to 50. Her glucose control remains stable for twenty-four hours. She is discharged on day four on 45 units of insulin, with a follow-up appointment to see me the following Monday. No clear cause for the episode is established and, despite her poor diabetes control, I am given a recommendation to avoid increasing her long-acting insulin again.

RUNNING MY LIST

At her follow-up visit, she comes alone. Equally puzzled by the episode, I share my concerns with her.

"Mrs. Jimenez, it is so good to see you up and about and back to yourself. This was your first and only attack of low blood sugar, I think. But it was a really bad one. I want to work closely with you to get to the bottom of this one so we can make sure it never happens again, okay?"

"I don't even remember it, Doctor. But don't worry—it won't happen again."

It is endearing when my patients try to take care of me this way, but this feels like a deflection. So, having ruled out the most common "medical causes" of hypoglycemia, I begin to "run my list" of the differential diagnosis of the fifteen most common *social vulnerabilities* (see table) that can generate illness or make its management more difficult.

The Differential Diagnosis of Social Vulnerability

V iolence and trauma
U ninsured
L iteracy and Language barriers*
N eglect/abuse*
E conomic hardship/food insecurity*
R acism, race/ethnic discordance
A ddiction
B rain disorders, e.g. depression,* dementia, personality disorders
I mmigrant status
L egal status
I solation/Informal caregiving burden*
T ransportation problems
I llness Model
E yes and Ears*
S helter problems

*These specific social vulnerabilities were high on my list as possible causes for her hypoglycemic episode.

T. King, M. Wheeler, A. Bindman, A. Fernandez, K. Grumbach, D. Schillinger, and T. Villela, eds., *The Medical Management of Vulnerable and Underserved Patients: Principles, Practice, and Populations*, 2nd ed. (New York: McGraw Hill Education, 2016).

My first concern is that there may be a previously undetected communication barrier—health illiteracy or vision loss—that makes it difficult for her to safely administer her insulin. My research team was the first to discover that limited health literacy and limited numeracy are not only common in people with diabetes but also are associated with worse diabetes control and higher complication rates, including poor vision. We also found higher rates of serious hypoglycemia among people with diabetes who have limited health literacy, presumably due to physician-patient miscommunication about the dose, difficulties drawing up the correct dose at home due to poor numeracy or vision problems, or lack of appreciation of the need to be well fed when taking insulin.

To explore these possibilities, I first step out of the room and bring back a vial of saline and an insulin syringe.

"Okay. Since you can't remember much from that day, the first thing I want to do is ask you to show me how you usually get your insulin into the syringe. Let's pretend that it's bedtime and you have to inject your insulin. Show me what you'd do and exactly how you'd do it. I want to make sure I've explained it well."

I hand the works over to her. She performs the task perfectly: the insulin meniscus lands exactly halfway between the 40- and 50-unit mark.

"Nicely done."

So, she's got good enough vision and math skills and has understood the dosing instructions I have given her so far. But maybe she is taking her insulin but not eating during the day or evening? I proceed with my stepwise interrogation.

"Now can you tell me what you *always* need to do during the day to safely take your bedtime dose of insulin? Again, I want to make sure I have explained things well to you in the past."

"Well, you always told me that I need to eat regular during the day. So that's what I try to do. Three meals."

That's what she *tries* to do, I say to myself. So, she knows *what* to do, but maybe she can't always *do* it. Maybe this is a case of food insecurity, another common social condition among low-income populations with diabetes? Our group has shown that food insecurity is associated with diabetes and with hypoglycemia-related hospitalizations at the end of the monthly income cycle. I pursue this line of inquiry.

"Well, Doctor, you know I have many mouths to feed and that I don't have a lot of money. It may not be the best quality of food, but I do put food on the table."

"Including for you? How do you manage to do it?"

She describes how she accesses multiple food safety net resources, including food banks, food pantries, and food stamps. She proudly reports that there is not a day in the month when her children or grandchildren go hungry. She also tells me that she never has to skip her own meals to preferentially feed her grandchildren.

Having ruled out food insecurity, I proceed to assess for depressive symptoms or caregiving burden that might have led to decreased appetite or self-neglect. She denies any current depressive symptoms and seems to be handling the childcare well, even enjoying it.

Finally, nearly at my wit's end, I turn to my trusted clinical friend: the use of unabashed praise in the form of heartfelt compliments. And I really do mean it.

"Mrs. Jimenez, I am super impressed with how on top of things you are. You have learned so many skills, and you don't give up when things are difficult. You are juggling so much, especially when it comes to taking care of your diabetes and your family. You really inspire me."

I pause and watch as the pride washes over her face.

"So, I was hoping I could count on your smarts to help me figure out what happened that day, or the night before this attack. To figure out why your blood sugar went so low. Can we walk through that day and the night before, one step at a time? Were you *asustada*?" I ask, referring to an illness-related belief common among immigrant Latinas, one that links fear or some form of a shock with subsequent sickness.

It is then that she lets down her guard and begins to tear up.

"*Susto*—yes, *susto*. I am even frightened to talk to you about this, Doctor."

I hold my breath and look her in the eye, hoping to convey a sense of nonjudgmental support, and maybe even tenderness.

"But I feel now that I can trust you."

I breathe out, relieved. "Yes. Yes, you can."

"Okay. My husband—he is a good man. I have loved him. But . . . I am scared of him. More than five years, I am very scared."

She doesn't say more, yet. She just cries, silently. I pass her a box of tissues. She quickly extracts a handful.

"I can see how hard this is for you."

She nods vigorously, hiding behind her tissues.

"And I can understand how hard it is for you to talk about it too."

Her head down, she releases an anguish-filled wail into her handful of tissues.

"No one deserves to be scared or to be hurt, Mrs. Jimenez. Tell me—has your husband ever hit you?"

She shakes her head equally vigorously, wiping the tears away. "No . . . he doesn't hit me."

She slowly lifts her tearstained, mottled face, looks straight at me, and says in an even and eerie tone:

"He uses my insulin instead."

I sit back in my chair and try to take it in.

"He uses your insulin?" I ask, not quite understanding. "Does he have di-abetes too?"

"No, that's not it, Doctor."

She then proceeds to tell me how her husband wields her insulin shots as a weapon, often withholding them from her as a means of punishment and control. But the day prior to her hospitalization, he had come home drunk. They got in a fight, and things escalated. He held her down and administered massive doses of her long-acting insulin. She attempted to eat more that day to compensate but acknowledged that she did not know how much insulin he had given her, so she was guessing. When she awoke, she was in the ICU.

"Wow, Mrs. Jimenez. I am so sorry this has happened to you. I had no idea."

Then I lean forward.

"Thank you for sharing all that. That is a horrifying story. It sounds as though you've been terrorized by him. I want to say this again: you don't de-serve this. And I'm here to help you in any way I can. I know how difficult these situations can be. But there are things you can do . . . whenever you're ready to. I will write down in your personal medical record what you have told me today in case you ever need it as evidence."

Our talk leaves her drained but visibly unburdened. She has regained her composure. I perform a lethality assessment and determine that, based on her experience, she is not in imminent danger. I also confirm that the chil-dren have never been abused, nor have they witnessed any abuse. I then review a safety plan with her, one that involves the help of her daughter, the only person in the family who knows about the abuse. She tells me she is not ready to leave him and that she is worried he will retaliate if he learns that she told me—or told anyone, for that matter.

This leaves me in a bind. She told me that she trusts me. She confided in me. Yet she has also described a serious abusive episode that likely represents a criminal act, one that may have had lethal intent and could have had a fatal outcome. Yet she has also so much as forewarned me that alerting the authorities could endanger her more, a belief that has been borne out to be valid based on prior research of intimate partner violence. The first few weeks after disclosure often represent the highest risk period for victims, as perpetrators at times do retaliate, with brutal force.

I had previously done some research in the field of domestic violence that could inform how I might be able to help her navigate this challenge. In the 1990s, as domestic violence became more widely recognized as a significant clinical and public health problem, clinicians and health systems, especially in US emergency departments, began identifying domestic violence in many women presenting with serious injuries or even nonspecific symptoms. At the same time, laws were being passed around the country intended to activate law enforcement—historically an entity that would look the other way in domestic disputes—and health care providers to proactively involve themselves in this social and legal problem, one that often had medical consequences. As such, laws mandating that physicians report cases of domestic violence to the police began to appear across different states. In 1995, recognizing the potential risks and benefits inherent in implementing such laws, and in response to a new law passed in California, our research team summarized and synthesized all relevant laws across all fifty states. Published in the *Journal of the American Medical Association*, the article was intended to clarify the legal responsibilities of the treating physician while also taking into account their primary responsibility: the patient's well-being.

In our analysis, we concluded that, while there were theoretical benefits to laws that require physicians to report injuries caused by domestic abuse, both the facts on the ground around what transpires after reports are made and the ethical implications of overriding women's autonomy could backfire. The real risk of retaliation, combined with the undermining of the physician-patient relationship, could paradoxically lead to a chilling effect on disclosure and a further disempowerment of victims.

"Mrs. Jimenez, I want to give you a number of a legal aid office, one that can help you get what's called a temporary restraining order. This is a court order that would forbid your husband from going near you for a period of time. You could get one of these court orders while you figure out what to do next. Only if you want to. Please take this number, share it with your daughter, but keep it hidden from your husband. I don't know your exact situation, of course. But my advice is that you get one of these orders. Don't wait too long."

She slips the phone number into an inside zipper of her purse and looks down into its black hole.

"Thank you, Doctor. I think about it," she whispers.

"Of course. That's exactly what you should do. And talk it over with your daughter too."

I grip myself before making my last point.

"There's one more thing before we go. I need to tell you that I am so glad you put your trust in me and that you got this off your chest. It is a really important step. I know you want and need me to keep this conversation private—just between you and me. I deeply respect and will do all I can to honor that."

"Thank you, Doctor. Yes, that is very important to me."

"I have to tell you that in California, there is a law that requires all doctors to make a report to the police whenever a patient has suffered from this kind of abuse. Because it is a crime and because you could be in danger again. I would be breaking the law if I didn't make such a report."

She looks crestfallen.

"But trust me," I reassure her. "You're not the first person to have this happen to her. We have worked closely with the police in cases like yours. I will let the police know what happened so they can document it for their records. This could be helpful to you in the future. But I will then tell them that you are really worried that your husband will get back at you for telling them, to just hold on to the report. They likely won't go to your house or try to find your husband unless you change your mind and ask them to. So, I'll do all I can to make sure that happens, okay?"

"I understand, Doctor. Thank you for explaining it to me."

PUTTING IT ALL TOGETHER

Marginalized populations are subgroups that, because of social, economic, structural, political, geographic, discriminatory, or historical forces, are exposed to a *greater risk of health risks* and are thereby subject to health disparities. The lesson from Mrs. Jimenez's experience is the importance for doctors and health professionals to expand the differential diagnosis to include social vulnerabilities, especially when caring for complex patients. We can only develop appropriate diagnostic and treatment plans if, as doctors, we use the necessary interpersonal and communication skills to understand that symptoms and potential root causes may be silent or stigmatizing. Truth is more likely to be attained if the physician is grounded in the lived experiences of her patients and cultivates a worldview that incorporates "nonmedical" (e.g., psychological, environmental, and/or social) factors into her diagnostic process. This is most successfully performed in the context of a trusting relationship.

Let me return to where I started: grappling with the question of why my clinic patients at San Francisco General Hospital fared far worse over one year than my patients at the university clinic had fared over three years. This, despite having the same diseases and being cared for by similar-caliber physicians. I have discovered that the marginalization experienced by my patients at San Francisco General Hospital leads to stark differences in their social contexts and their socio-environmental exposures. And these exposures are largely to blame.

Within the clinic walls, our research team has shown that marginalization also influences health care outcomes through three pathways, often working in concert (see figure).

In the first pathway, exposure to a social vulnerability—such as homelessness, for example—can *directly* lead to a new illness, such as pneumonia. This is fairly straightforward. In the second pathway, a marginalized patient with an established illness, such as heart failure, may have a social vulnerability such as limited literacy, making it especially challenging for her to successfully self-manage her illness, leading to poor health outcomes. In this case, the social vulnerability is a *mediator* in the pathway between the disease state and its outcome. The third pathway revolves around whether and how the physician caring for a patient with a disease—take diabetes, for example—identifies and responds to marginalization such as intimate partner violence.

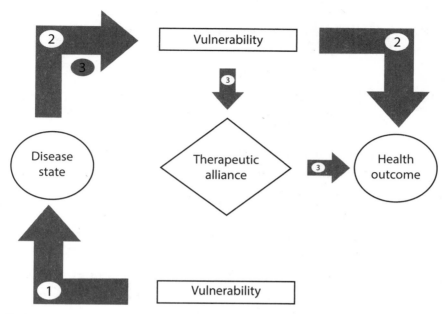

Pathways connecting social vulnerability to disease and outcomes in marginalized populations. T. King, M. Wheeler, A. Bindman, A. Fernandez, K. Grumbach, D. Schillinger, and T. Villela, eds., *The Medical Management of Vulnerable and Underserved Patients: Principles, Practice, and Populations*, 2nd ed. (New York: McGraw Hill Education, 2016).

If the patient is exposed to a physician who is able to bridge social distance, destigmatize vulnerability, harness a patient's resilience, and garner local resources, all in service of a *therapeutic alliance*, then outcomes can be optimized and health disparities mitigated. This pathway is *indirect*, one that links marginalization, vulnerability, and disease to health outcomes as a function of the physician-patient relationship.

These pathways toward better health care required me to broaden my worldview to include social causes of illness. In the case of Mrs. Jimenez, after exhausting the purely medical possibilities, I systematically tackled social vulnerabilities that the medical literature suggests might be a root cause of her severe hypoglycemia: limited health literacy, visual impairment, food insecurity, caregiver burden, and mood disorder. Having ruled these out, I focused on her resilience and her worthiness as a human being and asked open-ended questions in the spirit of partnership. Having created the context for effective intervention, I was able to create a safe space for her to newly disclose the trauma to which she had been subject for many years. While intimate partner violence has been shown to be common in patients with chronic diseases, and especially common among women seeking emergency care, few physicians—including, at the time, me—are aware that perpetrators can attempt to control a victim's medical care and medical treatments as a means to exert power.

Over the next few weeks and months after Mrs. Jimenez's disclosure, I worked together with a psychologist and a women's advocacy program to empower Mrs. Jimenez to make the kinds of difficult decisions that ultimately were in her best interests. She eventually decided to file a police report, first obtaining a temporary and then a permanent restraining order. She ended up cooperating with the district attorney in successfully pursuing criminal charges against her husband. Since then, she has had no additional hypoglycemic events, her blood sugar control has been excellent, and she and her family have felt safe in their home.

Rather than chalk health disparities up to external social forces beyond our control, physicians must actively engage in the struggle to understand how social context and structural forces shape health and illness. If we expand our roles in this way, we can attempt to foster change within our patients, in their families, and in society at large.

CHAPTER 12

Racism as a Public Health Threat: "It's About Time"

IN 2020, IN THE WAKE OF GEORGE FLOYD'S MURDER AT THE HANDS OF THE Minneapolis police, the American Medical Association's board of trustees released a statement recognizing that racism in its systemic, structural, institutional, and interpersonal forms is an urgent threat to public health. And in the spring of 2022, in the wake of the COVID-19 pandemic and in the face of overwhelming data demonstrating the disproportionate toll that the virus was taking on communities of color, the Centers for Disease Control and Prevention (CDC) also declared that racism is a serious public health threat and stated that it would be taking specific action to address the issue.

These declarations, while long overdue, were notable not only for their pointed clarity but also for what was *not* included in them. The CDC did not declare, for example, that food insecurity, housing insecurity, crowded living conditions, poor working conditions, incarceration, or mistrust in medicine—all risk factors for COVID acquisition and/or death—are serious public health threats. Rather, they recognized that communities of color are disproportionately subject to all these risk factors and to other unhealthy social and environmental exposures as a result of the racism that is baked into our society. The power of these statements rest, in part, on the fact that they acknowledge that racism is not just the driver for horrid and newsworthy events—such as the mass shootings of Black folks in supermarkets or churches by racist gunmen or the recurrent killings of innocent Black men by police officers—but that racism is also a driver—a root cause—of the ordinary medical events that play out in hospitals and emergency rooms across America every day: amputations among Black individuals suffering from type 2 diabetes, deaths from asthma among Hispanic children living in previously redlined areas of our inner cities, and excess morbidity from end-stage renal disease among Native Americans.

———— ❧ ————

As soon as the COVID-19 epidemic hit the US, my primary care clinic, like many in the country, transitioned from providing patient care via in-person visits to one that largely relied on telephone visits. The purpose of this shift was less to protect the clinicians and more to prevent viral exposure and spread between our patients, nearly all of whom are poor people of color. They often have several co-occurring chronic diseases that make them especially susceptible to death from COVID.

On one of those early days, before the COVID vaccines had been developed, a particularly endearing and challenging patient of mine, a promising young artist in the local rap scene who rarely kept his doctors' appointments, actually showed up—in person.

Marshawn entered my room with the remnants of a limp, as he was still learning to walk without the pivot point of the big toe that he'd recently lost to a type 2 diabetes–related amputation. Once a disease of the elderly, the ravaging effects of type 2 diabetes have extended into the population of lower-income, young adults of color. I was surprised to see him, as nearly all my other patients were trying to stay away from hospitals if they could.

He dropped into the chair in the corner, casually sliding down, and stretched out his long legs into the center of the room. He leaned back with the flat bill of his cap sloping over his brow, part of his face shrouded behind beaded locs, the rest of his face obscured by a poorly donned surgical mask. Out of his earbuds leaked the tinny articulations of a rapper and the staccato sounds of a backbeat.

Some would interpret his attitude as disrespectful, but I chose to take no offense. He had first presented to my hospital in diabetic ketoacidosis, a severe and potentially fatal electrolyte imbalance. But he had never connected with any doctors in follow-up. And apart from that ICU stay, he had not taken insulin since. Ten years later, in the early days of our relationship, I had attended to a then-bedridden Marshawn on a ward of San Francisco General Hospital. As I treated the bone infection in his foot in an attempt to ward off an amputation, I learned that Marshawn had grown up in abject poverty in a largely Black neighborhood. That he was forced to subsist on "syrup sandwiches" and Kool-Aid for much of his childhood. As a teenager and young adult, he had witnessed two of his closest friends get shot and killed. So, I knew that "meeting him where he was at" needed to be my go-to MO.

I motioned to pull out his earbuds, and we exchanged pleasantries. I carefully examined his stump while probing him with questions about his blood sugar levels and asking whether he had housing and adequate food right now. As I was inspecting the state of his postoperative foot, all I could think of was the fact that his poorly controlled diabetes made Marshawn particularly vulnerable to both acquiring and dying from COVID-19.

Toward the end of our visit, I reviewed the importance of his keeping an eye out for any COVID symptoms and about masking and maintaining social distance as keys to prevention.

He told me that he got it. But I had learned over my thirty years of practice that getting concrete was the only way to discover whether my patients and I were truly on the same page. So, I asked him what his plans were for the rest of the day.

He told me that right after our visit, he was going to head out to a closed studio session to record a new tune with about ten other musicians.

I knew how, for him, making music was both a source of pride and a source of strength. But given the state of COVID, I took a deep breath and firmly recommended he *not* go to the studio at this time, that it was dangerous to be exposed to others who might have the virus.

"Yeah, Doc, I appreciate what you trying to do, what you are saying. But this ain't no big thing for me."

"What do you mean, Marshawn?"

"It's like everybody's freakin' out."

"Well, I think people are freaking out for good reason."

"Nah, I mean it's like people finally got *spooked*. Like now they suddenly know what *fear* feels like, and so they just freakin' out. You know what I'm saying? I'm not freakin' out about it; I'm trying to stay chill. Because my life's been like this every day. *Every day*, Doc. This is just a blip for me. This corona thing ain't nothing compared to what I been going through every day of my life. So now, suddenly, people are freakin'?"

I let that rhetorical question sit.

Shaking his head back and forth slowly, he said, almost to himself, "Damn. So, yeah. It's about time."

"Marshawn, what do you mean, 'It's about time'?"

"I mean *it's about time* that rich white folks feel what I feel all the time. What *we* feel. The fear that anything can hit you at any time. That life ain't safe—no time, nowhere. Like something's just waiting for you around the corner. It's ugly and it's gonna take you, and make you go from bad to worse. That's what I mean."

In the face of an epidemic, it is easy for the larger story of public health to get lost in its smaller stories: the specifics related to what makes smallpox so virulent, the details about what makes a host vulnerable to HPV infection and its associated cancers, the physics around how TB transmission occurs, the mechanisms whereby hepatitis C causes liver failure, or the hope and wonder surrounding emerging discoveries that could prevent HIV infection or diabetes, or ward off death from COVID or tobacco addiction. When we think about epidemics and their public health response, we naturally think about them in this narrow way.

Yet, behind the individual stories from each of these waves of epidemics that my public hospital has been built and rebuilt to confront, there lies a unifying and much larger public health story: the story of how marginalization functions to cause disease. Marginalization, a cousin to and a consequence of racism, is a primary determinant of exposure, vulnerability, and disease, whether we consider the pathogen *M. tuberculosis*, the vectors of tobacco or sugar-sweetened beverages, or the transmission of trauma and violence. The extent to which a society marginalizes certain of its members determines who gets exposed, who succumbs and who recovers, and who lives and who dies. That is what the CDC meant when it declared that racism is a public health threat.

It's been two years since I had that visit with Marshawn. Much to my dismay, he hasn't accepted my repeated offers to provide him with a COVID vaccine. So far, he hasn't gotten COVID. Six months ago, when I tried yet again to convince him to get the vaccine, he just shook his head, telling me how he had just witnessed one of his cousins get shot and killed, and how he hasn't been able to sleep. How his son had just been expelled from high school because of drug possession, and how worried he was that his son was going to have to deal with the police as a result. I again recommended he see our clinic behaviorist to help him deal with the post-traumatic stress that continually threatens his emotional and physical well-being, and again, he declined.

One month ago, he begrudgingly agreed to blood work to assess his diabetes control. While I was drawing his blood, he told me he was sure that he was going to lose the temporary city housing I had helped him secure as part of the state's COVID-related Project Roomkey. The next day, his blood work came back, revealing that, at the age of thirty-nine, he had developed significant diabetic kidney disease.

Marshawn and I have an appointment coming up to discuss what this blood test likely will mean for his health down the line and for his medical care now. I hope he will show, but given prior patterns, there's a good chance he won't. If he does, I know I will have to work very hard to convince him to add an ACE inhibitor and an SGLT2 inhibitor—medications that can slow the inevitable progression of his kidney disease—on top of the insulin that I had finally succeeded in getting him to agree to. I also know that we will have to strategize around his unstable housing. But I predict that we will end up spending most of our time talking about the latest murder of a Black man at the hands of the state and all the ways hearing about it is impacting Marshawn's life and darkening his vision for his future. Discussing how to delay or avoid a future with kidney failure will take a backseat to grappling with his past, current, and future experiences with the public health threat of racism.

While I know that the effort needed to reach the day when racism is no longer a public health threat will be herculean and that this degree of change will take time, that day can't come too soon. For Marshawn, every day marked by another episode of police brutality or a shooting of a close friend, every day he is at risk of being forced to live on the street, and every day without taking an ACE inhibitor—together take a serious toll. For Marshawn, whose future health lies in the balance . . . it's also about time.

CHAPTER 13

The Telltale Heart

M s. L. was a sixty-eight-year-old woman and former profes-sional singer whom I had followed in primary care for over a decade. I found her to be fiercely independent and emotionally labile: at times sweet and endearing, at other times bitingly sarcastic and even downright nasty. She had difficulties from a recent stroke, with associated right-sided weak-ness and problems articulating words, speaking as if in slow motion. She also had chronic low back pain from spinal stenosis, hypertension, depression, and type 2 diabetes.

On our first visit, she was unsure of the names of her medications, know-ing only that she takes "a whole bunch of pills" for pain, blood pressure, and diabetes. She had smoked for fifty years but had quit five years prior. She did not drink alcohol or use drugs. While she had once been a jazz singer, since retiring she had enjoyed singing in her gospel choir. She was barely able to get by on her social security and disability benefits and lived with her adult son in a subsidized public housing unit.

On this first visit, she expressed to me her greatest regret: ever since the stroke, she had lost her ability to lead her choir. Her mellifluous singing voice, once the prize of her church, now generated imprecise and wavering tones or, sometimes, more like a jangle of dissonant punctuations. This loss, which she felt as absolute and final, was a major source of her depressive symptoms.

After expressing empathy for her loss, I tried a different tactic.

"Is it possible that the difficulties you experience with your singing voice are not that bad? At least, not to others? That you might just be being a perfectionist? Do you have to *lead* the choir? Can't you just *sing* in it?" I threw out these hopeful but likely unhelpful questions, based on the relatively mild articulation difficulties I had heard in her speech.

She just sneered at me and slowly said, "You shush now. I know what I'm talking about. I once sounded like a nightingale. Now I sound like a toothless hound dog who's lost his mama."

THE LUNGS VERSUS THE HEART

A few months after this first visit, she presented to clinic wearing a nightgown and slippers, an outfit that I began seeing her wear with greater frequency. As usual, she complained about her chronic back pain but also "bad asthma," with shortness of breath progressing over the last several months. While she previously had been hospitalized for the stroke, for aspirin-induced gastrointestinal bleeding, and for a burn, she had never been hospitalized for asthma and did not carry this diagnosis. She reported that she now had to walk slowly with her cane and could only walk one block, when previously she could walk five. Her back pain had been stable for years but had worsened over the last few months. Acetaminophen with codeine taken three times daily no longer soothed the pain, giving her relief for only two to three hours at a time.

I suspected either emphysema (vanishing lungs from heavy smoking) or progressive heart failure due to long-standing high blood pressure. Finding nothing remarkable during the physical exam, I pursued a number of tests of her lungs and heart. While her chest x-ray was normal, she was unable to perform formal lung function testing due to her inability to form a tight seal around the tube through which she needed to blow. An EKG showed a thickened heart, and an echocardiogram was remarkable only for difficulty in the relaxation phase of the heartbeat and a mildly leaky valve. She declined a workup to evaluate whether she might have coronary artery disease, which can produce shortness of breath on exertion and the form of cardiac dysfunction that her echocardiogram showed. Given her inability to walk for any significant duration or speed on a treadmill, this evaluation would have required that she undergo a nuclear medicine test.

"At almost seventy years old, you'd think I know what's wrong with my body," she jabbed at me. "Well, I do," she continued, jutting her jaw out at me. "And it's asthma. I'm convinced of it. It's not any heart condition, Mr. Important MD."

And then she actually rolled her eyes at me.

Duly reprimanded, I prescribed her an inhaler, not because I believed she had asthma but because I knew I needed to foster a therapeutic alliance, that invaluable and intangible bond of mutual trust and goodwill between physician and patient. I then suggested that we change her opiate regimen to a lower-dose, more long-acting preparation of morphine so as to better avoid the ups and downs of her pain. At her request, I also made arrangements for her son to formally serve as her in-home support aid, whereby he would receive some remuneration for the assistance with her activities of daily living that he was already providing. She seemed quite content with this set of recommendations.

With that door open, I gently suggested that, while asthma was a good bet, it was still *possible* that her symptoms could be a sign of heart failure and that, to be on the safe side, it would be wise for us to add a medication or two to make the work of her heart easier. She agreed.

While she didn't end up getting the full monty for her breathing symptoms, or even the standard of care, I felt that I had won a small victory and that, with time, we could make more progress—on her terms.

But Ms. L. missed several follow-up appointments. Eventually returning, she now complained of exertional chest discomfort and more shortness of breath, including at night. This was not a good sign. Her blood pressure was sky-high, and she had gained over twelve pounds. But with the exception of some swelling in her legs, her physical exam had not changed. A repeat chest x-ray revealed a mildly enlarged heart and some fluid on her lungs.

"I'm afraid that the asthma and the heart are ganging up on you," I said. "While you seem to be doing a good job handling any asthma, your heart isn't pumping blood out fast enough. And so, the blood's backing up into your lungs and your legs. The twelve pounds you gained isn't fat—it's all fluid. We've got to turn this around fast and get you feeling better. And then figure out why it's happening so we can prevent it from happening again, okay?"

Following my logic, she agreed to a short stay in the emergency room for the treatment of heart failure. There, she was treated with diuretics to quickly eliminate some of the excess fluid and was given more medications to lower her blood pressure. Tests revealed that, thankfully, she was not having a heart attack. She felt better by the next morning and, before the twenty-three hours of the short stay had passed, demanded to be sent home with her son. The ER physicians, however, were not comfortable with her going home without her first agreeing to an assessment for coronary artery disease, a frequent and treatable cause of worsening heart failure. They called me in to try to break this stalemate.

PLAYING CHESS TO WIN

When I approached her gurney, I saw by the look on her face that we were in for a standoff.

With that defiant look, she unequivocally informed me, "I am *not* getting any more tests, Mr. Important MD. Enough is enough."

I decided, rather than take her head-on, to veer right. I looked at the chessboard, took a deep breath, and went to plan B.

"Oh, Ms. L., I have been so *worried* about you since yesterday. And I was so happy to hear from the nurses that you are feeling so much better . . . and so quickly! And that you feel you're ready to go home. That's awesome."

Her arched back and jutting chin visibly relaxed.

"Listen," I whispered, furtively looking left and then right as if in cahoots with her. "This was a close call. And we need to be careful moving forward, okay? I'd like to talk the next steps over with you. I usually like to do this with a close friend or family member, because this stuff is complicated. And these decisions can be hard. Can I call your son to join us?"

She withdrew from me and shook her head, more vigorously than I had expected. "Nah . . . no way. He can't help with this."

I thought about asking her why he couldn't be helpful but felt that a different tack might be more fruitful. I took another deep breath, scanned the board, and made my next move.

"Well, who, then? Who could help? Whom are you close to? Who cares about you the most? Whose opinion do you really respect?" I asked, fearing that she'd come up with no one. Fearing that this elderly former nightingale was now largely alone with her illnesses, her pains, and her worries, locked into well-worn patterns of denial, avoidance, depression, and nihilism. And that I'd somehow be left holding the bag.

She cast her eyes past me at the drawn curtain that separated this intimate inquisition into her social support system from the jumbled and competing noises of beeping monitors, barked orders, piercing screams, and comforting words emanating from just beyond.

As I feared, she offered nothing. There was no one.

I reached, as I have gradually learned to do over many years, away from her vulnerabilities and toward her points of resilience.

"Do you still attend the church where you used to lead the choir?"

"Of course. Every Sunday. And sometimes I sit in for the rehearsals. Just talk to my pastor and my old choir friends."

"Are you close to your pastor?"

"Everyone in my church is close to Pastor Dale. He is a wise man. Sometimes I think I wouldn't know what to do if I couldn't talk to him."

"Does he know about your health problems?"

"Sure—well, he knows about the stroke."

"Does he know you've been having a hard time these last few months . . . like with your breathing?"

"Well . . . I'm sure he noticed that I haven't been coming to rehearsals regularly, but I still *have* been going to church, religiously. So, I don't know."

"Ms. L., I would really appreciate it if you could let me talk to your pastor. And just invite him to come visit you here. Or just have him talk to you on the phone so you can tell him what's been happening with your health so he can lend you a sympathetic ear. And maybe he can give you some of his wisdom and some of his prayers. It won't take long. Based on what you say about him, this is the kind of thing that he went into his line of business to do, right? To help people when they are in a difficult spot. What do you say? Can I call him and tell him what's going on with you?"

Forty-five minutes later, Pastor Dale was at the side of her gurney. We held a three-way conversation in which I summarized the situation for them and then described the why, the what, and the how of our recommendation to explore whether she had any blocked coronary arteries. After a private, closed-curtain conference with Pastor Dale, she informed me that she agreed to the nuclear medicine test.

Another small victory on the chessboard. I enthusiastically phoned the cardiology service and managed to get her squeezed in three days later.

The test indicated that it was unlikely that she had significant blockages of her coronary arteries, suggesting that it was either her high blood pressure or perhaps a worsening of that heart valve problem that had gradually affected the function of her heart. Over the next few days, I tried to reach her by phone to share the good news about the coronary arteries and make a plan about how to proceed, but she never picked up. I would just have to tell her in person at our upcoming visit.

INTO THE BIG HOUSE

Ms. L. again missed several visits and ultimately was admitted to my hospital for another episode of congestive heart failure. She brought with her many full and outdated bottles of pills. She received an aggressive diuretic regimen. Cardiac catheterization, a dye-assisted visualization of her coronary arteries, revealed a partial blockage of a branch of one of her three main arteries and mild disease in a second artery—neither of which was felt to be clinically significant enough to explain her worsening heart failure. The pictures revealed that her heart had moderate dysfunction in its ability to squeeze and pump blood, and, because of the enlarged heart, a moderate-size leak in the mitral valve, which led to some blood being pumped backward, in the direction of her lungs.

Three heart failure medications, which I had prescribed previously, were increased. Her blood pressure became well controlled, and her weight decreased by seventeen pounds. Depression and cognitive screening tests were obtained to assess why she had been nonadherent, but both were unrevealing. After she was given an updated medication list, she was able to accurately report how she would take her medication regimen at home. She also received a locally generated and highly effective, literacy-appropriate, thirty-minute patient education session on the self-management of heart failure, including instructions on how to weigh herself daily and make diuretic adjustments based on any significant weight changes. She verbally demonstrated her understanding by being able to correctly "teach back" to us how she would manage any changes in her weight and her symptoms. A visiting nurse follow-up was recommended, just to check up on her, but she declined. She agreed to home oxygen until her breathing improved to the point where it would not be necessary. I felt we had made significant progress and that we were both beginning to win in this chess game.

THE TELLTALE HEART

Ms. L. then had a series of admissions to outside hospitals for florid heart failure, as our hospital was full and "on divert." I learned little about what transpired. Then, in short order, she was readmitted to our hospital. This time, she required intubation (being placed on a breathing machine in the ICU). These hospitalizations were determined to also have been a consequence of medical nonadherence; despite her receipt of self-management education and understanding of the treatment plan, she had not followed through with the appropriate actions—again.

At the post-discharge visit, while examining her neck veins, heart, and lungs, I noticed for the first time that she was wearing a makeshift rosary around her neck, with a bottle-shaped pendant resting on her sternum. I asked her if I could look inside. When she opened it, I found that it contained her morphine tablets and a few random heart pills. And when I examined her backside, I saw that she had a small bedsore on her tailbone.

"Why are you wearing your medications on a rosary necklace, Ms. L.? Does it help you to remember to take them on time?" I asked. Commending her ingenuity, I added, "Seems like a smart idea."

She quickly brought her pill bottle closer to her chest and slowly and begrudgingly acknowledged, "I do it 'cause I gotta make sure my medications don't get stolen."

"Stolen? Who would take them from you?"

"My son and his awful crew."

Suddenly, the chessboard had taken on an entirely new appearance. Had I been playing only part of the board? Had I been playing at the wrong game this whole time?

After just a five-minute conversation, it became apparent that Ms. L. had been living in an unsafe environment, one that she was deeply ambivalent about changing. Using a communication technique known as *motivational interviewing*, I managed to get her to agree to a home visit by a public health nurse and, if indicated, to receive ongoing home care services. My additional hidden agenda was to get some trained eyes into her home to make an assessment of her living conditions.

A week later, the visiting nurse reported back to me that she had discovered that many people were living in Ms. L.'s single-bedroom, public housing unit. Unwashed clothes, dirty dishes, brimming ashtrays, drug paraphernalia, and Ms. L.'s pill bottles were scattered throughout the apartment. A pile of garbage was maggot infested. Her oxygen tank was stashed in a corner, unused. The nurse had found Ms. L. sitting on the commode, unattended, where she had been for hours, unable to move by herself. The new paid in-home support service worker, someone who the son had transferred caretaking responsibilities to, was sleeping in a drug-induced stupor in the corner. The nurse took several photos to document the state of affairs. The images revealed an apartment that looked as though it had been hit by a hurricane.

The nurse brought the patient to my clinic the next day. Ms. L. was still wearing her slippers and robe, all in tatters, and her appearance was now dirty and unkempt. I gave Ms. L. a long hug and I sat her down. *It was her turn in this new chess game*, I thought, so I waited for her to make her move. She slowly explained to me that she had not sought help to intervene with her son's substance-use problem, fearing she would risk his parole and might lose her public housing. She had felt trapped. We engaged in a long conversation about what needed to happen and why, and while never explicitly agreeing to my plan, she silently allowed things to proceed as I suggested they should.

Adult protective services (APS) were activated. The son, getting wind of what was about to happen, skipped town. Over time, APS determined that Ms. L. was unsafe to live at home alone and facilitated a move to a long-term care facility. In the year prior to this move, she had required twenty-two chest x-rays and five hospitalizations. After moving to the long-term care facility, she required no further x-rays or hospitalizations.

HEALTH AND ILLNESS ARE FAMILY AFFAIRS

After reviewing the photos the nurse had sent me, I realized that I had failed to consider how Ms. L.'s medical nonadherence, frequent hospitalizations, and general decline may have been a marker for profound family dysfunction—in her case, her son's serious substance-use disorder and the resultant abuse and neglect to which she was subjected. Considering how problems at home might explain an old woman's illness, and contemplating how a mother's love, or her fear, might contribute to her decline, was certainly the stuff of the "art of medicine." But the science of medicine also demonstrates that these vulnerabilities are predictors of suffering and death as potent as any physiologic characteristic. Ms. L., for far too long, was exposed to unhealthy social conditions and, as a result, experienced largely preventable health-related suffering. She also underwent a long and costly series of treatment episodes and diagnostic evaluations. In the end, the most important procedure that cracked the case was a disclosure based on a fortuitous physical exam finding on her chest. It was not a cardiac finding but an observation of a strange pendant on a necklace—one with a weighty backstory. It was this discovery that ultimately led her to accept what turned out to be an impactful nurse home visit. I might have prevented her decline had I taken a more family- and psychosocially oriented approach to her care from the very beginning.

In hindsight, the moves I made on the chessboard would have been different had I been more mindful of some of the clues: a son who never accompanied her to her clinic visits; a son whom she did not trust enough to share in her decision-making at a critical time in her life; and a previous hospitalization for a burn, something I had never fully investigated. Getting better at chess requires analyzing one's wins and losses, critically reviewing one's strategies and choices, and studying from the masters. And getting back to the board for another match, and then another.

I paid a social visit to Ms. L. at her long-term care facility not long ago. Wearing a brand-new nightgown and fuzzy slippers, she smiled at her "Mr. Important MD." She told me that she was content at the facility, where she had developed many friendships—and that she had started a small choir that she directed but adamantly refused to sing in.

CHAPTER 14

The Mood of the Bay

Long years of unhappiness cause a person more degradation than a fatal illness.

—Olga Tokarczuk, *Drive Your Plow over the Bones of the Dead*

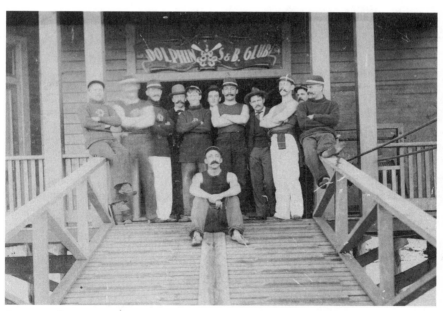

Courtesy of San Francisco Maritime National Historical Park, photo A12.07843.

SAUNA WISDOM

I exit the waters of San Francisco Bay, riding the high of my chilly, invigorating, thirty-minute early-morning swim at Aquatic Park. I ascend the stairs from the sandy little beach up to the Dolphin Club, a two-story wooden structure: San Francisco's first swimming club, built in 1877. A few swimmers—ranging in age from about twenty to ninety—guardedly make their way down to the water's edge, their golden swim caps, google-eyed goggles, and goose-pimpled bodies making them look even more bizarre than they are. No matter how many times one has swum in these frigid waters, and no matter how much pleasure one knows one will derive from each experience, a trace of the fear of entry is always present.

As the most recent one just out of the Bay, I am peppered with the usual set of friendly questions. Questions purportedly about me but whose clear intent is to reassure the questioner. These brief interchanges on the beach move people through their dread, past their indecision, and into the waters.

"Good swim?" asks one.

I smile, then spit out some salt water. "You know it was."

"Feeling alive again?" asks a second.

"It never fails," I say reassuringly.

"You warm it up for me?" asks the third.

"Can't say that I did, 'cause I know you wouldn't enjoy it as much if I had."

A ninetyish-year-old lady who, like many of us, is a regular, approaches me last.

"So, what's the mood of the Bay today?" she furtively asks.

This is my favorite question, an existential question asked only by truly experienced Bay swimmers. An endless array of fast-changing factors interact to create "the mood of the Bay": the wind conditions; the nature of, and variation in, the size, shape, and directionality of the waves; the water temperature and its microclimates; the outside weather; the placement and intensity of the sun and its frequent unwelcome companion—the fog; the presence or absence of sea mammals (seals, usually); the burden of floating obstacles, such as branches; and, of course, the tide. This assortment of external factors generates an intrinsic but ever-changing affective aquatic state. We swimmers respectfully acknowledge that this body of water—like people—has its moods, and we must contend with them.

"She looks gentle, but she's tricky today," I concede, beginning to shiver. "Almost felt like I was swimming in two different Bays. She can't decide when to be freezing cold or when to be balmy-like warm. It's all about how you respond. But I don't need to tell you that."

As the old woman self-assuredly makes her way into the deepening water, she looks back over her left shoulder. "You should hit the sauna, young man."

I walk onto the wooden deck to start toweling off behind the wood-and-glass wind barrier, entering the next stage of the Dolphin Club gauntlet. Four older men—two Italians and two Slavs—seated in a line to catch the morning sun as it peeks over the clubhouse roof, their backs to the Bay, are watching the comings and goings as they do every sunny morning. The Geriatric Swimmers' Roasting Club. Hands on canes, heads covered with berets and beanies, they look my shivering body up and down and start in on me, laughing at one another's one-liners.

"She's a real shrinker today, eh?"

"Still using a towel, eh? Don't you people have an app for that?"

"You're so blue, you look like you need a psychiatrist."

"Maybe it's time for a shot of schnapps, my boy."

"Didn't you get the memo? This ain't the Mediterranean!"

"Forget the sauna, kid. You need a good woman to warm you up!"

I smile and salute them palm up, Mussolini-style. "*Buongiornio, buoni signore! Alla doccia.*"

"Ah, *maroni . . .*"

I take a quick hot shower and make a beeline to the sauna, the Bay swimmers' mandatory transition zone prior to reentry into the real world. Our fifteen-minute dry-land sanctuary.

As usual, five or six naked guys are waxing eloquent about their lives, their interests, and the state of the world—both in and out of the water. I find a spot in the corner and quietly settle in, getting a feel for the flow of the conversation.

"Yeah, I'm still running a workshop for super-specialized tools. Fine tools. Meticulous, painstaking work. Pain-in-the-ass work, more like. Thank God I have this place to escape to. Keeps me sane. Johnny, how's your book goin'?"

"The shits. I been sitting at my desk for two straight weeks. Only five hundred words a day, average. At this rate, I'm not gonna make my deadline. And for the first time ever, I got an advance on this one. I'm screwed. But look at me: I'm laughing at it now, since I just had my daily dip."

"Got that right," says the third. "I just lost a case I've been working on for over two years. A jury trial. Depressing as all hell."

"So how come you smiling?" quips the fourth.

A wave of knowing laughter, followed by a powerful upsurge of heat as someone pours another ladle of water onto the coals.

I jump in to fill the heated silence.

"Hey, did you guys feel those drastic changes in water temperature today? I mean, one minute it felt like a five-degree drop and so I'm freezing my ass off. And then a minute later, it's ten degrees higher and it's like I'm basking in a bathtub. And then—boom!—freezing cold again. Back and forth the whole time. I couldn't acclimate. What's up with that?"

"Yeah, that happens, especially after a big rain," says the fifth man, Anson, a veteran of the Dolphin Club, kind of a well of open-ocean-swimming wisdom.

"The river runoff from the rains mixes with the snowmelt to create these deep underwater currents, flowing all the way from the Sierras through the delta and then dumping into the Bay. Does it every time."

"Really, that's the cause?"

"Yup. But you should know that the variation in water temperature is not ten degrees, or even five degrees," he says, looking at his waterproof watch. "It's about *one-quarter* of a degree, at most. It's just that with the temperature of the Bay being about fifty-eight now, it *feels* like a five- or ten-degree difference to your body."

"You're kidding me, right? There's *no way* that was a quarter-of-a-degree difference. Not what I was feeling."

"The Watch never lies," he says, pointing to his three-dialed watch. "This gives me the second-by-second water temp. It's like Greenwich mean time, but for water temperature, depth, and barometric pressure. I certainly paid enough for it for you not to doubt me."

"He's right," says the sixth guy to my right. "Your body's core, when it's cold, overreacts to changes in temperature. Like *super* sensitively."

"Wow, I never knew that." I turn back to Anson. "So, you're saying that the felt effects of the outside conditions depend on our condition inside?

That we have different reactions to external stimuli based on our internal states?"

"I guess that's how a doctor and scientist would put it, yes," he says in a mocking tone. "But I'd just keep it simple and say that you're a wimp."

Another wave of laughter, this time at my expense.

OUTSIDE IN AND INSIDE OUT: A TALE OF TWO PEOPLE

Bruce

I race across town to make my 8:00 a.m. team huddle in time. My clinic's patient list features some truly sick folks, and I know I'm in for a challenging morning. But the swim has left me bubbling over with positive energy, ready to face the day.

Bruce Spiller is a long-haired, handsome, well-read, witty, but cynical car mechanic, a lanky guy nearly exactly my age who also is a road bicycle enthusiast. A guy who thrives on high adventure, getting his dopamine surges from a range of risk-taking activities, including high-speed motorcycle racing, bungee jumping, sex with anyone and everyone, and occasional forays into cocaine use and inhaled heroin. Often these activities go hand in hand.

Bruce's life began to fall apart a bit before I met him, when, in his early forties, he developed bad elbow pain related to his work as a mechanic, a severe case of tendonitis that was preventing him from working with his dominant hand. From the moment he presented to me, we hit it off, amicably competing with each other with ironic witticisms. But whereas mine were benign in nature, his were characterized by a biting nihilism and bleakness that began to concern me.

Over the course of treating his tendonitis with a variety of strategies, I was struck by both the severity and unresponsiveness of his pain and the fact that he consistently responded to the problem in catastrophic—and at times hostile—terms. He quickly became one of my most draining patients.

"You gotta give me some stronger stuff, Dean. This elbow is literally *killing* me. I haven't worked in *four months*! I'm gonna lose my apartment, my car, my clients. I'm gonna be unemployed, homeless. The physical therapy you sent me to is pure bullshit. The injections are bullshit. The orthopedic doctors are bullshit. This hospital is bullshit. My life just sucks, and you gotta do something about it."

Bound by his business being a cash-only operation and his status overseeing the work of a few undocumented immigrant mechanics, he had never reported enough taxable income to enable him to go on temporary disability and give the elbow the rest it needed to heal. And while his father left $90,000 to him in his will, Bruce always described this nest egg in negative terms.

"My father was a total asshole to me. And he's still torturing me from his grave. It's because of this damn inheritance that I can't get disability or get on Medicaid. Too many assets, they say. So, I'm stuck having to keep working and getting care at this dump. I have no other options."

In reality, he was rapidly spending this money down to fulfill any one of his dopamine-fueled urges. It became clear to me that these costly and risky escapades represented futile attempts to treat a deep-seated and chronic depression. A depression he openly acknowledged he suffered from but refused to take antidepressants for because of a false belief that they would damage his liver. A liver already undermined by the chronic hepatitis C that often comes with the kind of lifestyle he had been leading. His experience with psychotherapists was uniformly negative, describing them as "overqualified dunces who don't give a shit. I am so *sick* of their superficial advice. Just thinking about them makes me want to vomit."

As his untreated depression worsened, his life began to spiral downward through an ever-deepening whirlpool powered by external events and compounded by internal turmoil and struggle. Each external event amplified his psychic suffering, and his psychic suffering further amplified the physical pain he felt and the disability he experienced. A high-speed motorcycle accident left him in the hospital with multiple fractures, including one that resulted in self-described incapacitating knee pain. His recovery was complicated by use of opiates and stimulants he obtained from the street, an increase in the numbers of days he spent in bed, and a growing sense of hopelessness.

"I can't even ride my bicycle, Dean. The only form of exercise I could once do, now—because of this knee—I can't even do anymore. That used to give me a rise, even a bit of happiness. The man upstairs—you know who I'm talking about, the one I don't believe in—he's clearly got it in for me. I can't escape it. Why me? My elbow is *destroying* me. And my knee is so bad, I'd rather cut the whole leg off. And to top it off, my girlfriend—you remember—the Norwegian one you once labeled a *femme fatale*? Well, she finally had enough of me and moved back to London. Permanently. No matter where I turn, I remain just a barely walking piece of shit. Worthless. What's the point? There's no way out. And yes—the cocaine gives me sixty minutes of pleasure. So, get off my back about it."

Against my advice, he spent $15,000 down Highway 101, at Stanford University, trying to fix his elbow tendonitis with injections of a novel substance that had only recently been FDA-approved. The procedures failed miserably.

"Now I am $15,000 poorer, and my pain is fifteen times worse."

This was followed soon thereafter by a car collision. Unrestrained by a seat belt, he struck his breastbone against the steering wheel. The trauma not only led to a sternal fracture but also to an arrhythmia in the underlying heart, an additional problem we would find ourselves having to actively manage over the subsequent years.

"Now my heart is like an old man's, and I'm not even fifty yet."

"Bruce, I've long said that your heart is broken and that your spirit is broken. Your injuries are real, and your pains are real, but the amount of *suffering* you experience is disproportionate and reflects a much deeper pain. Your limbic system—your reptilian brain—has been on such high alert for so long that you're drained of all emotional reserve. So now you not only feel the aftereffects of trauma, but you have a deep and long-standing depression, which colors every other event you experience in profound, persistent, and unbearable ways. And this ramps up your suffering even more. You're in a terrible cycle, I admit. We have to interrupt this cycle, because what's been going on these last few years isn't working. You've got to admit that. I consider this a true emergency. So, I think it's time we stop chasing down the physical ailments and their cures and face the tiger head-on. But in radically different ways. If we do that, if *you* do that, I can tell you with confidence that there is a light at the end of this tunnel. That I am truly hopeful on your behalf."

"How can you be so sure?" he sneers.

I don't answer him right away. I first release a long breath.

"Okay. How can I be sure? I haven't told this to any of my other patients and not even to my colleagues. But I will tell you because it is real, and it is true, and I feel you need to hear it. A few years ago, I suffered from a major depressive episode that lasted nearly a year. So, I absolutely know what you're going through—not specifically, but more generally. The utter hopelessness. The suicidal thoughts. The 'no way out' thinking. The nihilism. The desperation. The inability to get out of bed. The complete lack of motivation, even to make a cup of tea. The constant, pointless search for relief—any relief—in any form. And never finding it. The *absolute certainty* that this shit is your life and always will be. And it's simply not tolerable."

"You got that right. Nail on the head." He pauses and says, with genuine concern, "I had no idea you went through that."

"Yeah, I did. It was awful. I'm not telling this to you to get your support, but thank you for that. I'm telling you because I also know firsthand that it can get better. That *you* will get better. Major depression is, in part, a biologic thing, and it is an emergency that requires we change the biology, so I want to stress to you how important medications are in this. Any concerns you have about them pale in comparison to the alternative of staying this way or—God forbid—getting worse. I know this firsthand. But there's more. What happens for many people who have depression is that we become our own worst enemies in the process, and we decide to let biology be our fate. Biology is not fate, it is just a state, and it can change. Make different moment-to-moment choices and you can get better—if you suspend disbelief and just trust and engage in a serious reboot of how you deal with the bad things that happen in your life. And whether and how you choose to appreciate the good things that come your way. And realize that you have so much to offer the world and so much to still enjoy. And, yes, that you have been through a helluva lot, but that you are resilient. You can find ways to tap into all of that."

He looks at me suspiciously. "You said *radically* different ways. What, are you gonna send me to Nepal? How can I climb up the mountain to see the guru with this bum knee and bad heart?"

"I'm not talking about a pilgrimage. But you're on the right track. I'm referring to an internal journey. One that you either can do on your own or with some help. As you wish."

I share with him what little I know about meditation and mindfulness-based methods as paths to recovering from trauma and coping with depression. We discuss Peter Levine's *Waking the Tiger*, which teaches us ways to restore calm in our limbic systems after we have been traumatized and retraumatized. I recommend the CD collection of Pema Chödrön, who teaches us that it is the avoidance of, and aversion to, feelings of sadness, despair, and pain that inevitably accompany life that generate ongoing suffering. That, paradoxically, only by deeply feeling pain and loss, by truly experiencing and then accepting them, can we find the self-compassion and inner strength needed to heal. And open up new ways of making different choices in our daily lives. Finally, I recommend he join the weekly Dharma Punx meditation group, one that involves people our age, some of whom are also dealing with recovery from drugs.

"I know that's a lot to throw at you. I'm just giving you some options to consider, not giving you homework or telling you what to do. But if you're open to what I'm suggesting, just pick one of them and go for it. And then do it with a welcoming heart."

For once, he is silent.

"Okay, you've worn me down. Lemme do the CDs. I can do that from my bed."

"All right, then. You have a CD player and headphones? Good. Then allow me to buy the CD set for you. Look out for a box from Amazon in a few days."

"Geez, Dean. That's kind of you."

"Well, don't let this gift be given in vain."

Two months later, he's back. For the first time in a while, I had been looking forward to a visit with him, now hoping to learn what he had gleaned from the CDs.

"So, what did the wise and benevolent Aunt Pema teach you?"

"We can talk about the CDs later. I made this appointment because of this," he declares, pointing to a place on his neck just under the angle of his jaw. "It just popped up."

Not surprising. He has found a way to sidetrack our foray into alternative methods to address his mental health problems by refocusing on physical complaints. I have no choice but to respond to his direct request. There is no use forcing a plan on him that requires personal commitment to a different path.

I examine his neck and identify a two-centimeter lymph node on the left side, mobile and nontender. No other nodes are palpable.

"It's just an enlarged lymph node. We see these all the time. That lymph node drains the mouth and throat areas. Often a sign of a throat infection or tooth problem. They usually go away in two to three weeks. Let me have a peek inside."

I look deep into his throat with a wooden tongue blade. All good. I survey his teeth, tapping each with the tongue blade to identify the painful one. Nothing. His gums and tongue also appear normal.

"Looks clean as a whistle in there. Come back in three weeks if it's still there or if it's bigger. And let's talk about the CDs at some point, okay? But before I go, just tell me how you're doing. I mean in your heart and your spirit."

"The heart's still ticking, and the spirit's still pining."

"Well, if it's ticking a regular beat, I'd say things are looking up for your heart. And regarding your spirit—well, pining is better than feeling nothing. Pining is a yearning, a sign of desire. It's a prelude to feeling a drive, a motivation. I also see that as a good thing."

"If you say so."

The three weeks arrive, and he doesn't show for his appointment. But three months later, he's back. He starts in on his suffering. The endless circles of victimization, with no way out. I can't tell if he's listened to a single CD. I am not sure I can take it today. I've got to shift gears and snap him out of it.

"How's that lymph node?"

"Oh, I forgot all about that," he responds, brushing his hand against his neck.

"Well, let me have a feel. Please hop up on the table."

The lymph node is still there. While it is no larger, it is firmer and no longer mobile. These are not good signs. The next few days involve an open lymph node biopsy. Then a diagnosis of squamous cell cancer of the head and neck. Then surgical procedures involving the removal of the lymph node, a search for a primary source, and an exploration for metastatic involvement in nearby structures. The primary lesion is identified at the very base of the underside of the tongue, so small as to be nearly invisible on external exam. It too is removed. Exploration of the other lymph nodes reveals no additional involvement. Cause: a sexually transmitted infection with human papilloma virus (HPV), the virus that creates genital warts and can result in cervical cancer in women. It is now showing up as head and neck cancer in middle-aged, sexually active males who were exposed to an infected partner through oral sex. The "Michael Douglas" cancer.

"It's now our number one head and neck cancer," the chief of surgery, Dr. Bill Schechter, tells me on the phone. "It's dwarfing the numbers we used to see from tobacco. And it's happening in youngish men. It's a tragedy. We need to get the word out."

I miraculously expedite Bruce's entry onto the sophisticated and high-tech cancer conveyor belt. As soon as he recovers from the surgery, he undergoes rounds of chemotherapy. Then he submits to a brutal but necessary oral surgery procedure: complete dental extractions. This is required so that he can withstand the high-dose radiation treatments that some head and neck cancers respond favorably to. Without extractions, the teeth become terribly infected and pose a serious risk to the patient. He undergoes the extractions and then a full course of radiation.

Now a fifty-year-old male with a history of elbow and knee problems, cardiac arrhythmia, hepatitis C, depression, and locally metastatic head and neck cancer, status post–successful and uneventful surgery, chemo and radiation treatment, Bruce is a cancer survivor whose prognosis is relatively good, all things considered.

But he suffers terribly. He truly is miserable. The radiation—not unexpectedly—led to a thickening and degree of scarring of the overlying skin of his neck that he describes as "disfiguring." His salivary glands have wilted, so his mouth is perennially dry, "like the fucking Sahara Desert." And the mucus he sporadically produces is a near-solid, gummy substance that he is unable to fully clear. He claims his roommate—who pays part of the rent—is going to bail on him because she can't stand the phlegm he is constantly hacking up. He shows me the archive of mucus photos he keeps on his iPhone, concrete evidence of his secretory suffering. His appetite and his ability to swallow have also been undermined, and he loses weight. His boniness, his temporary toothless state, and the straggly goatee he has grown to cover his neck scarring have combined to make him feel "hideous," a "modern-day Elephant Man," making it impossible for him to show his face in public. The dentures made for him, he says, are "worse than the wooden ones made for George Washington."

He vilifies every physician involved in his cancer care, the very ones who went all out to protect his health: the ENT doctors who have had no effective advice for the war against his mucus, the medical oncologist who toxified his body with chemotherapy, the oral surgeon who robbed him of his pearly whites, the dentist who "can't fix a cavity to save his life, let alone make well-fitting dentures," but especially the radiation oncologist—widely recognized to be the most patient-centered and caring specialty in the cancer care spectrum. She is simply "a butcher."

I try to validate his anger while defending my colleagues. He refuses my referral to our cancer survivor support group.

Over the next few weeks, he falls into a deeper depression, starts using cocaine and opiates again, and involutes even further. Despite received state-of-the-art cancer treatment, he suffered only more. I realize that his cancer care and his medical care in general—in the absence of the kinds of professionals and types of alternate tools that could help him address the ailments that afflict his spirit and his heart—will never meet his needs, will never alleviate his suffering. He needs support and guidance to recruit the internal resources to enable him to respond in very different ways to the adversity that is hitting him from the outside. For him, as for all of us, emotional states are an important determinant of whether and how much we suffer from what life throws at us, whether we accept our present state with grace, and even whether we can overcome our fate and craft a more affirming future.

I return from a short vacation and read through my unopened messages and lab results in the electronic medical record, hoping to catch up on any happenings involving my patients. Reading a message sent by our most experienced nurse practitioner, I learn that Bruce had dropped by the clinic with a range of complaints. Upon evaluation and a review of my prior notes, she determined that his depression had worsened. Now he was expressing more concrete suicidal ideation. She determined that he represented a danger to himself and informed him that he needed to go to our psychiatric emergency services (PES). He flat-out refused. She felt she had no choice but to call the institutional police to escort him to PES, where a psychiatrist would decide whether to place a 5150 seventy-two-hour hold on him to further evaluate his risk for suicide and attempt to craft a treatment plan to mitigate this crisis. That was a week ago.

I decide to phone him.

"Bruce, I just got back from vacation and read about your eventful visit to the clinic last week. I am sorry to hear you've been struggling so much. Tell me what you've been going through and what happened that day."

"What happened is," he starts in, his speech pressured, "that I am *never* setting foot in that fascist hospital again. They handcuffed me. Can you believe it? They roughed me up and actually *handcuffed* me. That little know-it-all witch says I'm not safe to go home and says I need to go to PES. 'Thank you, but no thank you,' I tell her. Next thing I know, three uniformed goons walk into the room, and they just take me down. The fucking San Francisco General Gestapo. My shoulder still hurts. They handcuff me and 'escort me' to that hellhole. Where I tell the psych people at least five times that it was no suicide gesture. Just my way of expressing myself, sharing with another human being the extent of my suffering, for crying out loud. Can't a person do that? Then they talk among themselves, they make their phone calls, do their paperwork. Eight hours later, they release me and I'm back home. Complete and utter bullshit. I came for help and all I got was a WWE takedown. That's the last time I show my face at your so-called health care facility."

I communicate regret and sorrow that he was traumatized that day as well as concern about his emotional well-being. I try to talk him down from this decision, to no avail. I tell him I will always be here if he changes his mind. I encourage him to reconsider getting professional help for the depression and, at a minimum, to get into the CDs I had given him.

"I've barely gotten out of bed since I left the hospital," he admits. "Not to mention doing any exercise. If only I could do some exercise . . ."

I suggest swimming. "I guarantee you that if you feel like your mood is a one out of ten before your swim, after your swim, you will score higher. And if you do it every day, the mood will inch up and up. Just give that a shot, okay?"

"I'm so bony now, I am freezing all the time. I wear three sweaters in my own apartment. I can't enter a frickin' pool. Plus, I look like a skeleton. I am not showing up at a pool in this state. I'm a freak."

"Bruce. You yourself just said how important exercise is for your mood. You've told me before how biking would make you happy. Swimming can do this for you. I swim every day. It keeps my mood up and prevents my own depression from coming back. You can do this. I have an extra neoprene vest, you know, real wet suit material. It'll keep your core warm and make you look like a weight lifter. I will send it to you in the mail. And not just to show you that we care about you. I know it's hard, that it feels impossible. But take it one step at a time. And soon you will see the light at the end of the tunnel, the one that I see for you."

Winifred

Winifred is next up on my schedule. We've been an item for over twenty years. At age sixty, she has twenty-one problems listed in her electronic medical records' problem list. Not just the usual chronic conditions, such as hypertension, asthma, and urinary incontinence, but also sickle cell anemia and literally every one of its attendant complications.

Sickle cell anemia is an inherited condition, more common in people of African descent, which results from a single mutation on the gene that produces the protein hemoglobin—the chemical transporter of oxygen located in abundance within our red blood cells. Individuals who inherit a copy of the mutation from one parental chromosome do not manifest illness. In fact, they have an evolutionary advantage: their red blood cells are protected from the potentially fatal malarial infections so common in parts of Africa. But those who inherit the mutation from both parents suffer from sickle cell anemia.

Life for those with the disease can be a nightmare filled with intermittent or frequent pain crises, each of which can result in a prolonged hospitalization.

Winifred's medical record is peppered with dozens of such hospitalizations over her many years. And her chart reveals that she has also suffered from the more chronic complications of this disease—all of them, in fact. Avascular necrosis of the hips and shoulders, wherein the ball-shaped ends of these long bones collapse due to oxygen deprivation. Resultant joint replacements. Detached retinas and visual deficits from the delicate retina not receiving sufficient nourishment. A gallbladder that needed removing because of an infection due to the strange stones created by the liver's breakdown of the deformed hemoglobin molecule. The self-destruction of her spleen due to the pooling of sickled red blood cells. And small blood vessel changes in her legs that have left her with peripheral vascular disease, a condition that causes pain with walking and, when it progresses, limb pain at rest. Untreated, it can lead to gangrene. She has had three bypass surgeries to ensure that blood flow to her legs remains precariously intact. Twenty-one serious, active medical problems. And seventeen daily medications, many of them needing to be dosed two or three times a day.

On paper, she is a medical disaster.

In person, however, she is not only a resilient medical survivor but a person of warmth, humor, and love. And inspiration.

I enter her room.

"Hey, baby. It's been too long," she teases me. "How come you only wanna see me every three months? Don't you know I got real problems?"

She slowly stands up and pushes her walker away so we can exchange our usual warm hug. She smells like coconut. Like a balmy day at the beach, the ocean waves gently lapping at my feet.

"You'd spoil me if I saw you any more than that."

"Aw, ain't you crafty with your flattery? But I know it's just 'cause you lazy."

"You deserve the flattery, Winifred. But tell me how've you been."

"It's been tough, I can't lie about that. But I'm doin' good now. You know me."

"Yeah, I do know you. What's been happening?"

"Well, I had another one of those retinal detachments. Again, in my right eye. My better eye. It got all flashy and then all red and blurry. So, it got me real scared. But I went back up to my friends in 4M, you know, the retina doctors? They been operating on me for as long as I known you, even before your twins was born. They know me real well, and they take me serious when I complain about something."

"Yeah, I know. You've been through the wringer and back with those eyes. What did they say?"

"Like I said—that I had a retinal detachment. And that I needed another surgery. My fifth one, if memory serves. The sickle cell just keeps them eyes on their toes. So, I went through with it, and it went fine. But that wasn't the thing. They said, after, that I had to lie on my stomach—*flat*—for four whole weeks. I had to eat on my stomach. Pee into a bedpan on my stomach. They said I needed to keep my head down so that gravity would pull the retina down, so it'd heal right. This is my first time outta the house since I got off my stomach. I didn't even go to church."

"Oh my God, Winifred. How did you get through that? It must have made you nuts."

"My close friend, you know the lady I do the craft shows with? She came over and set me up right. Put a table down in front of me so I could do some crafting for a few hours a day. My vision was good enough for that, thanks to my doctors. So, I made some new stuff we gonna sell up at the fair in Sacramento in October. And my son, he set me up with his iPad. I never thought I'd say this 'cause I hate how people are always on them phones, but that iPad got me through a lot of hours on my stomach."

Remarkable woman. Not a resentful bone in her damaged body.

At the close of my next visit, on the morning of Christmas Eve, she reports to me a vague pain in her left thigh. Thinking it was likely a problem associated with the hip replacement she got two years ago, I start ordering up the hip x-ray. But I decide to do a quick exam to make sure her distal pulses are intact. Her foot is cool, and I can't feel a pulse wave either on the top of her left foot or behind the anklebone. There is only a faint pulse behind the knee. Damn it. She has probably clotted off her bypass graft in her upper leg, at the groin. Again. I recheck for pulses with a handheld Doppler ultrasound and determine that thankfully there is still a trickle of blood flowing. She's going to quickly need another procedure with a wire and balloon to open up the graft, or maybe a major surgical revision of that graft.

I gingerly break the doubly bad news that she needs an emergency procedure to open up the plumbing. And that she will be spending Christmas in a hospital room—and maybe even New Year's. I really hate when the rituals that mean so much to my patients need to be disrupted by an emergent health problem. And she always has people over to savor her Christmas pies.

"As long as Dr. V. is here to do the surgery, then it's okay. And I am just thankful that you found it in time. I almost wasn't gonna mention it. I musta known it coulda been serious. And I already made my pies, so folks just gonna have to enjoy them without me. Maybe I'll invite a few of 'em over to share some with me here."

"Winifred," I say, almost moved to tears by her positive attitude. "You are so inspiring in how you react to bad news. I've always wanted to ask you: How is it that, no matter what bad thing happens to you, you always find a way to see the bright side? You don't seem to let anything dampen your spirits. Is it just how you're built? Or is it that you just decided one day that you want to face the world that way? I want to know because maybe I can learn something from you that I can share with my other patients, some of whom are really struggling with their health problems. I mean struggling *inside*."

"You right about that, baby." She smiles. "I don't let these things get me down. I can't afford to. But to answer your question, I think it's a little bit of both. Maybe I am built a little different than some people. But I had tried it the other way, and it wasn't any good. And so, I had to learn how to take what gets thrown at me different."

"Tell me more."

"When I first got the sickle cell—when I was a grown child—my life was awful. I suffered terrible. You can't imagine the pain I had. And I felt like I was a victim. And that it was unfair. And of course, it *is* unfair, especially when you a child. But when I was a younger woman, and I kept suffering, that was when I got into lots of bad ways of responding. I started the drinking and the yelling and the complaining. No one wanted to be around me anymore. Even my fiancé left me, sayin' I was no good. And my health got worse and worse, I just got sicker and sicker, and I was real miserable. I kept asking myself, *Why me?* It wasn't till my grampa talked some sense into me that I changed my outlook. He always was a happy guy. He had a real hard life, but he was always smiling. I did love him so."

"What was it he said to you?"

"I remember it like it was yesterday. He says,

'Winnie, you only got this one life. And I can tell you this life is gonna be full of bad times, full of good times, and full of a lot of nothing times in between. You got a disease, it's true, but you also got a lot of gifts and blessings. You can let life crush you like a giant wave, or you can let it gently wash over you, with you still standin'. So, you gotta choose how you wanna see your life and how you wanna live your life. Ain't no one can choose that for you. Ain't no one gonna snap his fingers and make it all good. Just like there ain't no one to blame for the disease you got. I'm not sayin' *just be happy. I'm saying it's okay to ask for help, and it's important to take care of yourself when you sick, but take care not to make yourself more sick by only thinkin' and talkin' and feelin' bad 'bout how sick you are.'*

"That advice really stuck with me. The couple of years after that, he helped me change how I react to bad things and see all the good things I wasn't seeing. He didn't do nothing for my disease, but he did a lot to make sure it didn't take over my life. If not for him, I think I'd be suffering like some of your other patients. Yeah, I'm sick, and sometimes I'm real sick. But because of him, I ain't over-suffering. So, if you asking me for my advice, I say: tell your patients exactly what my grampa told me."

SEEING RED

About fifteen years ago, I suffered from a severe episode of major depression that lasted nearly a year. It manifested as a combination of physical incapacity and the darkest of moods. For my family and my closest friends, the only ones to whom I disclosed it at the time, nothing could have been more unexpected and atypical than to see me so deeply mired in an entirely helpless and hopeless state. To hear me unable to express any enthusiasm or interest in anything other than the inner pain I was experiencing, this inescapable journey in an indescribable hell. Always someone planning the next adventure or devouring up the latest novel by whichever author I was into at the time, this new me was a stranger to them and to myself. I had fallen into the bottomless and terrifying pit of depression. And I had lost myself.

It was a loss that without a doubt felt permanent. A loss of my very identity—my personal identity as a man, a spouse, and a father; an athlete and a musician; an avid reader, a friend, a jokester, and a conversationalist. Now I couldn't even get myself to say a word to my five-year-old daughter as I drove her to kindergarten, let alone joke with her or sing to her. And—when things got so bad and so dark that I felt I couldn't care for my patients, and I had to go on temporary disability—a loss of my professional identity. I was convinced that my entire career, all I had worked so hard to cultivate over the prior two decades, was over. That my reputation as a doctor, an educator, a scientist, a colleague, was now permanently sullied. That our financial future, and that of our children, was a disaster. I felt as if I were at the edge of the cliff. These projected losses compounded one another, and my endless ruminations around them—futile attempts to salvage something from the wreckage—not only solidified my depressive state but amplified my suffering by adding a hefty dose of anxiety into the mix.

Simply put, I was a mess. I spiraled further and further down the vortex and found myself seeking relief in fantasies of suicide. Every building I saw became a possible platform for jumping. Would it be tall enough? I began to squirrel away leftovers from my antianxiety prescriptions, keeping them in the event that I would reach the point of no return. Lying to my wife and my doctor about them. Doing so became my only source of comfort. I came that close.

I was drowning. And I could no longer even see the surface of the water.

But Ariella, my spouse, didn't give up, talking me through and challenging my endless ruminations. And my children, only an occasional presence in my room, tried to provide me with encouragement. My twelve-year-old son Eytan printed out two messages in large font, taping the first to my wall:

You can't control the wind, but you can adjust the sails.

And the second to my door:

When one door closes, another one always opens.

And my doctors didn't give up. Eventually, through an alchemy of story and science, described in the prologue of this book, I began to recover.

REENGAGEMENT

As my recovery began to take hold, I started to return to playing sports. I started with a game of pickup basketball, feeling a hint again of what it meant to be alive. While I hadn't played for over a year, that day, I was playing better than ever. Until I felt someone behind me whack my lower leg hard with a baseball bat, a trauma accompanied by a loud popping noise. I crumpled to the ground, looking behind me and quickly realizing that, in fact, no one had hit me. I had ruptured my Achilles tendon. A ruptured Achilles is no small affair. Surgery, bedrest, physical therapy for weeks and months. Maybe I would be able to jog after six to nine months. Not a great way to accelerate a recovery from major depression.

But this injury became a blessing because it was the reason that I entered the water. I had hated swimming. I was an awful swimmer. The water was cold. It went up my nose. I could only swim two laps, and then I was done. But I knew that one of the paths out of my depression was to return to exercise—preferably daily—something that had always kept my mood up. And the only exercise I could do with a healing Achilles repair was something in the water, where gravity wouldn't work against me.

Every day, I went to the university pool. I hated it. But every day, I got a bit stronger, a bit better. And with each day, I began to hate it less. By the end of the month, I was swimming for half an hour, one kilometer. And I noticed that my mood, inevitably very bad before my swim, was slightly but consistently better after it, something that seemed to last through the rest of the day. And that any day that I delayed my swim was a day accompanied by depressive thoughts and feelings. So, I committed to swimming early each morning.

Now my talk therapy began to take. I began to set goals and make progress in meeting them. I joined a twice-weekly meditation group and was actually able to concentrate enough to meditate. I read Peter Levine's *Waking the Tiger* and learned about a therapeutic modality known as *somatic experiencing*. I engaged in a few sessions that had me focusing on the pleasant external stimuli in my immediate environment, naming and describing the positive physical sensations that they elicited. A way to retrain a mind that had become conditioned to experience all external stimuli as noxious, a way to gently steer the body to react differently to one's environment. An attempt to rewire the brain. I listened to Pema Chödrön's CDs and, rather than avoiding the pain I had been experiencing, I took her advice and deeply felt it, felt the loss that it represented, and grieved over that loss. And I tried to accept it, as she teaches, with compassion for myself. But now, paradoxically, feeling this pain head-on and accepting this loss did not destroy me. I began to believe I might be able to move on.

THE JUNCTURE OF THE ELEMENTS

Mood—especially the chronic mood state—is a determinant of the stories we tell ourselves and the stories we tell others. Mood states are a powerful influencer of how we experience life and how we experience disease. Yet despite their power, mood states remain a mystery. How much of our mood states has to do with biology and genetic predisposition? Was Winifred endowed with an ability to face adversity with an affirmative outlook, and Bruce cursed with a genetic predilection to be overcome by adversity? Or was Winifred nurtured by her grandfather in such a way as to enable her to positively self-regulate her mood, and Bruce so traumatized by an abusive father that he became unable to confront life's many challenges as anything other than a form of amplified suffering? How do these two competing theories—the first related to inherent biology, the second to external exposures—interact? And how might these interactions inform how we as clinicians work to reduce suffering among our patients?

Well into my recovery, I exit the locker room of the Dolphin Club for a swim and am hit with the bracing cold winds already blowing through the gap in the mountains of the majestic Golden Gate. As the Central Valley of California heats up during the day, this singular opening in the coastal mountain range serves as a conduit for the elements, rapidly funneling inland the moist, cool air that sits over the Pacific. I look out from the little viewing deck. The flag is pointing west to east, as rigid as cardboard. The buoys are vigorously bobbing, and the open water, partially protected by the semicircular pier, is dotted with whitecaps. I descend the stairway. Each step forward feels daunting, bringing me that much closer to the frigid water. Encouraged by veteran Dolphin Club members, I had jettisoned my wet suit a week prior, motivated by a desire to avoid the verbal tormenting reserved for wet suiters, but even more so by the suggestion that my daily swim would become more invigorating, perhaps even addictively so, if I swam without one. I arrive at the windy, cold beach, crowned with my orange swim cap and bespectacled with my mirrored goggles, quite dreading what's to come.

A much older, early-bird swimmer pulls herself out of the water, through the breaking waves, and up the little sandy beach.

"What's the mood of the Bay today?" I ask.

"She's mighty. She's dominant. She's cold, and it's blowing. The waves roll you. Almost can't keep your head down and direction straight. Plus, she's ebbing pretty good—"

"Sounds overwhelming. You're supposed to be comforting me, you know, not scaring me."

She starts up the little steps to the deck, shouting back to me with a smile.

"You didn't let me finish. It's also *glorious*! Sometimes you have to fight her. Other times, just go with it."

I enter with purposeful, bold steps. I feel the tide already pulling me out toward Alcatraz. When the frigid water reaches my belly button, I dive forward and start in with a crawl. It is shockingly cold. Breathtakingly painful. Every cell in my body is screaming for me to get out. But I know that after about a minute, if I push forward, I will begin to acclimate. "One hundred strokes to heaven" is how we try to reassure the newbies at the Dolphin Club.

I force myself to exhale, and I start the count in my head. Nine, ten, eleven. I concentrate on the feelings the water makes on my bare skin. No, it is not cold. It feels more like a full-body attack of pins and needles. The waves toss me about, in no logical pattern. I shift to a rapid breaststroke, bobbing above the cresting waves to keep my bearings, keeping away from the pier. I let myself be taken along, just a piece of laundry in nature's washing machine, getting tumbled and spun to be cleansed. I give in to the power of the water, propelled by the interactional and oppositional forces of this unique juncture of air, land, and sea. The elemental interactions between body, mind, and spirit. The mysterious relationships between bodily disease, emotional illness, and spiritual suffering.

Ninety-three, ninety-four, ninety-five. The hostile exposures have passed. The internal suffering was minimal. I have survived to be able to enjoy, and I tread water for a moment. I see the span of the Golden Gate Bridge in the distance, the same bridge from which I was going to leap only six months prior. I holler out into the open air, an expression of release. Perhaps, even, of joy. I swim on.

CHAPTER 15

Flags and Statues

I T IS 7:00 ON A MONDAY MORNING, AND I AM DRIVING TO CLINIC. I AM listening to a radio report on the status of the immigrant children recently separated from their parents at the US-Mexico border—children placed in temporary detention centers, with no end date or clear plan in sight. I imagine the fear that must have gripped these children as they were ripped from their parents' arms, and the isolation, solitude, and growing despair they must be feeling as they await a disposition from this purgatory and try to envision an unknown future.

And I imagine the emotional state of the parents—the anxiety, pain, and anguish as they brood over the fate of their children. How soon will they see them again, hug them, put them to bed? Will they *ever* see them again? And the fear and desperation as it becomes apparent that, for some, applying for status as refugees may no longer be a realistic means to obtain asylum in the US. And their distress when they realize that the one portal through which they had hoped to find safety for their families has been closed. As I wonder about the human impacts of this traumatizing and intensely stressful experience on their current lives, I reflect on the downstream effects of this experience on the future health and well-being of these families.

RUNNING MY LIST

I arrive to my clinic and engage in my preclinic mini-huddle with my medical assistant, herself an immigrant from Central America. I tell her about the radio news story and my musings regarding trauma and its health implications. We review the patient list for our morning clinic, discussing trauma and its relevance to our daily work. She and I point out to each other the names of those patients we are aware of having been exposed to prior or current trauma in ways that we believe have impacted their health. Of the fourteen patients on my list, we name six. We commit to checking in with each of them on this subject during this clinic session and to exploring for exposures on the remaining eight, to make sure we haven't missed any.

One of the patients on my list is unknown to me and, feeling the stress of what will be a busy and hectic morning, I express to my medical assistant my displeasure that this patient was added to my fully booked primary care roster for the day.

She tries to mollify me.

"Don't worry, Doctorcito, she was just an urgent care, simple drop-in patient. She's just coming in with one problem. I told them not to do it, but one of our nurses put her into your add-on slot because she needs some reassurance. She's been seen a few times here already, and they tell me she's anxious. So, she's gonna be quick."

I give her a wry smile.

"Having worked here for over twenty-five years, I can tell you that when I hear I've been scheduled a patient who will be 'quick and easy,' my antennae pop up. And a giant red flag appears before my eyes."

She gently elbows me in the ribs.

"Oh, Doctorcito, don't be such a pessimist! Just tell yourself, 'She will be quick! And I will be quick!'"

I glance back at the list and see that this patient is thirty-seven years old and that the complaint typed onto the printout by the office clerk is *Right Breast Pain*.

"Unilateral breast pain. Interesting . . . Okay. We'll see who wins this game. You may be right."

CUTTING CORNERS

My morning is intense, and I move along at what feels like rapid speed. But somehow, by midmorning, I am more than thirty minutes behind. I enter the room of the "quick and easy" and "single problem" patient, hopeful that I can take advantage of our fifteen-minute visit to cut corners and catch up, at least somewhat. She is here with another woman who appears to be a friend. I quickly introduce myself, and the friend says she has come to translate. I thank her and tell them I speak Spanish. I sit down, open my computer screen to her medical profile, and start the visit.

I ask the patient directed but largely unrevealing questions about her breast pain—its location, its severity, its characteristics, and so on—while I try to multitask by scrolling through the computer to see the records from her prior visits. I make three quick observations. The first is that she does not sound or appear anxious at all. Rather, she is pleasant, calm, and inquisitive about the cause of her breast pain. The second is that, when responding to my questions, she frequently makes eye contact with her friend as if looking to her for support and validation. And the third is that she has made five prior visits to our hospital for this complaint. The first was four years ago, when she was seen in the OB-GYN clinic and was given Tylenol. The latter four have been within the last three weeks: first to the ER, then to the OB-GYN clinic again, and then twice to the triage nurse in my clinic. Something about these small observations makes me want to start over with my questioning, this time without multitasking.

"I'm so sorry—I've been looking too much at my computer and not at you. Can you tell me again how it all began?"

She smiles.

"It's okay, Doctor. Like I told the other doctors, it first started about four years ago, and it was in both breasts. But the right breast was always much worse, and it was a constant pain. Back then, I went to see the nice lady doctor upstairs, and she asked me a lot of questions and examined me. But in the end, she said she wasn't sure why I was having pain. She told me she sometimes sees people who have this kind of pain. She gave me a pain medicine and told me to wear a special bra."

She looks at her friend, who nods in a comforting way.

"Then what happened?" I ask, making an effort not to look at my watch.

"Well, it seemed to work pretty well. The pain stayed there on the right side, but it was less. And the pain in the left side just went away completely."

Again, she looks at her friend.

"So, you stopped taking the Tylenol—the pain medicine?" I ask with a touch of annoyance and impatience.

"No, that's the thing. I have been taking it all along. But about three weeks ago, the pain came back, really, really bad. The last few days have been unbearable." She begins to tear up, but she collects herself and remains calm.

"In both breasts?"

"No, just the right side."

"Are you having any fluid or discharge coming out of the nipple?"

"No, Doctor."

"Have you felt any unusual lumps or bumps?"

"No, Doctor."

"Has anyone in your family ever had breast cancer?"

"No, Doctor, *gracias a Dios*. But my sister has some kind of blood cancer and is very sick. Do *you* think this could be cancer?"

"No, I don't, but I'm not sure what it is just yet. Does the pain change, depending on the time of the month? Like where you are in your cycle?"

"No, Doctor, it is a constant pain."

I pause. I seem to have ruled out the easy things. So, I begin to wonder whether the breast pain could be a result of some sensory or nerve-related issue, like a pinched nerve, or shingles.

"Does the pain involve the entire breast or only a small part? Or does it also include any part of your back and right side? And any rashes on your skin?"

She draws a perfect circle around her breast and gives me an anxious look. "It's my entire breast. Nowhere else."

"Does the pain feel like a shooting or electrical pain, or like a shock or vibration?"

"No, Doctor. It stays, like a bruise or a toothache."

"Hmmm. . . . Have you ever had any trauma to your breast? Has anyone ever hit you on the breast?"

Again, she looks to her friend.

"No, Doctor."

I feel I am getting closer, that I may be on to something.

"Are you in a relationship with anyone?"

"Yes, I have a husband. We live together with my two children."

"Does your husband treat you well? Do you feel safe at home?"

She visibly relaxes and smiles at me and at her friend.

"Yes, I am very safe, Doctor. He is a very good man."

"I'm so glad," I respond, and I mean it, even though it means I am coming up empty. But sometimes a dead end opens up new possibilities. I begin to see a light at the end of this tunnel. Breast pain in pregnancy is not uncommon, especially in early pregnancy.

"Is there any chance that you could be pregnant?"

"It's not possible, Doctor."

"How can you be sure you are not pregnant?"

She doesn't respond but looks at her friend, who chimes in.

"I believe they took out her uterus, Doctor, because she was having heavy bleeding. It was in a different hospital."

I stop, roll my chair back, and survey the scene. I am fresh out of ideas. So, I decide to shift gears and do the physical exam. Perhaps I will become enlightened by what I find. But mostly I need to buy time to think some more.

"Well, okay then, let me examine you and see if we can figure out what's going on. Please hop up on the table here, take off your top and bra, and put on this robe, with the open side to the front. I will pull out the curtain, turn my back to you, and do some typing onto the computer until you are ready."

"Yes, Doctor."

She disrobes, and I do a complete breast exam, including a careful skin exam and a search for lymph nodes. I try to express discharge from her nipple, but it is dry. I systematically examine the area for tenderness, and she winces in pain in a distribution that involves the entire right breast area. Her left breast is not tender, and she has no tenderness to the touch anywhere else. I note that the distribution of her right breast pain is more aesthetic in nature than anatomic, more consistent with how laypeople perceive where the borders of the breast are than with how and where pain perceived by the nerves of the chest or pain emanating from the breast tissue gets distributed.

I ask her to put her clothes back on and return to her seat.

"Do you think it is cancer, Doctor?"

"No, I don't feel anything unusual. Everything seems totally normal, actually. And you are very young to have cancer. And you have no family history of breast cancer to make me worry."

I scroll through the computer and see that four years ago she had a normal mammogram.

"Your prior mammogram was normal, but we should probably get another one, just to be on the safe side."

"Yes, of course, Doctor."

I look at my watch and realize that our fifteen minutes are up. I consider my options. I could keep chiseling away, looking for a gratifying answer to this clinical but largely unconcerning mini mystery. Or I could just document the thoroughness of my evaluation, order the mammogram, and leave it up to her new primary care physician—with whom she has an appointment scheduled three months from now—to try to figure it out, assuming the pain persists. She doesn't seem to be suffering *that* badly, I tell myself. So, I move to wrap up the visit, aware that doing so will not be that satisfying for either of us. But sometimes that's just how it's got to be.

But then that red flag appears in front of my eyes. I have noticed it appear whenever I put my own needs and stress ahead of the patient in front of me. I have learned that when this flag flies, I should be careful to double-check my thought process and ensure that I have closed all the loops.

Just one such loop is bothering me: that near-perfect circle she drew around her breast, that nonanatomic circle of tenderness I felt during my own exam.

"I just have one more question for you before we wrap things up, Ms. Martinez. And I ask this of all my female patients because we have learned that it can contribute to a lot of health problems. It's a sensitive question, and it may be upsetting. But it's important that I ask."

"What is it, Doctor?"

As gently as possible, I ask, "Can you tell me if, at any point in your life, you were a victim of rape or abuse? As a child or as an adult? Or did you ever witness any violence here or in your home country?"

She looks down and away. Then she looks to her friend in an imploring sort of way.

This reaction, so different from the others, makes me realize she probably is a survivor of rape. I patiently wait, but there is no verbal response.

The friend breaks the silence. "*Estas bien*, Yelva?"

The patient nods.

"Let me answer for her. Yelva was brought here about ten years ago by an American man who said he would marry her. But instead, for over three years, she was basically a prisoner in his apartment, and he forced her to have sex with hundreds of men. He made her into a sex slave. She was a victim of human trafficking. But she is safe now. Now she has a husband who is from her own country and who is very good to her."

Well, that is worse than I had expected to hear. I close my eyes and try to imagine what her life was like and take a deep breath.

I realize I need to change my tone to tailor my communication to her specific needs. Away from that of a bureaucratic and hyperefficient doctor going through his diagnostic checklist and toward a compassionate and gentle physician with whom she can feel safe and secure.

"I am glad you are safe now. And I am so sorry to hear that that happened to you. That was awful."

"Thank you, Doctor. Yes, it was awful for me. It was terrible."

"Did the other doctors you saw about your breast pain know about this?"

"No. You are the first one to ask."

I am only somewhat surprised to hear that.

"Yet somehow you survived that time. And you seem to be functioning fine except for this breast pain. Do you have nightmares about the past?"

"I used to, but not since I am with my new husband."

"Well, it's good that you haven't suffered from nightmares this whole time. I am wondering something, though. Do you think those awful experiences affect how your body feels?"

Yelva looks to her friend and then back to me. "I don't know. What do you think, Doctor?"

I carefully consider her question. It's only been about one hundred years since Western medicine fully validated the notion that trauma and prolonged states of extreme duress can lead to serious physical and psychological symptoms in their aftermath. These range from mental health to physical health problems, including higher rates of panic disorder and depression, chronic diseases such as diabetes and heart disease, as well as difficult-to-treat physical symptoms such as chronic pain syndromes. First described in military survivors of World War I, *shell shock* was once believed to be a syndrome unique to active military experience and exposure. As a primary care doctor in a public hospital, I have witnessed firsthand how a diverse array of traumatic circumstances can have significant health consequences. Because of the high prevalence of prior trauma in our patient population, our clinics aspire to deliver what has become known as *trauma-informed care*.

"Well, I am not sure. We should try to decide together. Do you think it is possible that the trauma you went through—being forced to have sex against your will, being a sort of slave—do you think that the experience and memory of that may be a *cause* of your breast pain? Because that kind of trauma can come out in the body many years later in all kinds of ways."

She looks away and presses her right breast, gently massaging it as she considers my question.

"I suppose it is possible, Doctor," she says in a near whisper.

"Well, I believe that might be what is happening to you. I am not saying that the pain is not real, or that you are not truly suffering from what you are feeling in your breast. It just means that you are not quite healed from that trauma. And that your suffering may be deeper than just in your breasts. That your body is expressing this suffering through your breasts. Which maybe makes sense because your breasts were a part of what was taken over by the men who forced you to have sex with them."

She looks at me in silence, the palm side of her open hand still pressing down on her breast.

I continue, "But the good news is that understanding that the past trauma may be the cause of your breast pain gives me ideas about how to help you heal. To reduce your breast pain and even to heal yourself in a deeper way. Are you open to hearing some of those ideas?"

She remains still, with her hand over her breast, a partially chiseled statue sculpted into a hand-over-heart, Pledge of Allegiance pose.

I am sure I have just overwhelmed her with too much information. I apply the three-second rule, giving her time and space to respond. But she remains statuesque.

"I know I just said a lot of confusing things about the possible cause of your pain. Can you tell me in your own words what you *understand*? I want to make sure I explained it all clearly."

She looks at her friend, who nods.

"Well . . . you said you think my breast pain is caused by what happened in my past. And that if I trust that you are right, you think you can help me to heal."

"That's exactly right," I respond, visibly impressed.

I roll my chair forward, closer to her.

"Now tell me: What do you *believe* about what I said?"

"I believe I can trust you. I believe you may be right."

"I am really happy to hear that you are so open to this possibility. I feel optimistic for you because you seem to be so strong and so capable. These events in your past did not destroy you, but they are causing you pain."

"Well, I have my children to live for. I have to be strong."

"Yes, you must be. But it must be hard. I have three children of my own, so I can understand where that strength comes from and how hard it can be to stay strong. One thing I am puzzled by, though, is the timing of all of this. Usually, when we see this sort of pain come and then go away and then come back again, it means that something happened during those times to trigger or set off the pain. Something that brought back to the body the hidden memories of the trauma."

She removes her hand from her breast and gives me a blank stare.

I go on.

"You said that the sexual trauma started ten years ago and ended seven years ago. But that the pain started about four years ago. Do I have those dates about right?"

"Yes, Doctor."

Despite my ticking watch, I keep chiseling, deeper and deeper, chiseling away at the stone to try to recognize the form of the sculpture taking shape.

"When did you have your uterus removed?"

"About five years ago."

She begins to tear up again and turns to her friend.

"That was a *very* difficult thing for her, Doctor."

"Tell me why it was so difficult, Ms. Martinez."

She finally breaks down, sobbing in near silence, shaking her head from side to side.

I hand her a tissue box and let her release her emotions before I continue with my questions.

But she takes the initiative, speaking between the involuntary gasps that can follow a cry.

"My children are my pride and joy. I wanted to have more children. I loved my babies. And my daughter . . . really wanted to have a little sister. She still asks me every day why . . . she can't have a sister. Now my little boy is asking me the same thing. But I can never have children again."

"That must be so hard for you. Tell me—did you breastfeed your children?"

"Yes, I did. It was so sweet."

"It must be a very special feeling. My wife has told me how special it can be. And you miss that feeling, the feeling of holding your child to your breast. Ms. Martinez, can you remember if your uterus was removed *before* or *after* your breasts started hurting?"

She stops sobbing, wipes her eyes, and looks at me.

"I think . . . I think it all started right after the surgery. Yes. *After* the surgery."

"This is all beginning to make sense. I think having to have your uterus removed made you feel that one piece of your womanhood—your motherhood—was taken from you. This loss brought back silent memories of the trauma from ten years ago, when different parts of being a woman were taken from you. And all these losses are painful, but this deep pain in you comes out as pain in your breasts. I know I am a man, and I can't possibly know what a woman feels, so I am only suggesting this idea. But does any of that sound true to you?"

"Yes. Yes, it could be possible, Doctor."

"Have you ever told anyone about your trauma?"

"Well, I told the police and the lawyer, yes."

"But have you ever told anyone else? Family or friends? Or a therapist?"

"My husband knows. Well . . . not all the details. But he knows I was raped. And Elena knows." She motions to her friend. "I have told her everything."

"But you have never spoken with a therapist or counselor about it?"

"No, Doctor."

I turn to Elena and ask, "You seem to know her well. Do *you* think my idea about the pain coming out in her breasts sounds right to you? The hidden memories of the rapes and the surgery, and her sadness over not being able to have more children?"

"Yes, Doctor. That does make sense to me too."

What was but a block of stone—a simple complaint on a paper printout—is now becoming a well-formed and complex sculpture: a strong immigrant woman with a history of profound and repeated sexual trauma, a woman who has been suffering in silence, a now infertile mother whose hand covers her breast—at times drawing a circle around it, at other times shielding it.

"Well, it makes sense to me too. And it is important that we may have figured it out. Because there are ways that we can help you and things you can do to heal and recover."

I proceed to describe a menu of options ranging from seeing a therapist in our Trauma Recovery Center for talk therapy, to receiving a treatment modality for post-traumatic syndromes known as *somatic experiencing* that can rewire the brain to respond to sensory inputs with positive bodily sensations, to guided meditation and other, newer innovations designed for those with prior trauma. She is open to trying them all.

"Let's start with the therapist in our clinic, and she can review all these options with you in more detail. Like I said earlier, I am hopeful that by finding the treatment that fits best for you, you will heal. And your breast pain will fade away."

"Yes, Doctor. I hope so too."

While I haven't figured out why her pain so suddenly returned three weeks ago, I tell myself I have done more than enough to set her up for success and more than enough to hand her off to her new primary care physician. But I find myself compelled to continue participating in this process, to know if and how she heals over time or to support her if she deteriorates. That longitudinal care experience is the mother lode of primary care, the source that fills me up. While my patient load is full, I decide to make an exception.

"We will need to follow you to make sure you are getting on the right track and that you stick with that treatment plan. Healing is often gradual and can take time. I know you have a new doctor appointment coming up in three months. I want to offer instead to become your new doctor, if you would like, so I can work closely with you in your recovery. If you would prefer not to have a male doctor, I totally understand. I won't take it personally. The new doctor is a female doctor. So, you have a choice."

She pauses, looks to Elena and then back to me, and says kindly, "I think I will wait for the new woman doctor."

"That's fine. If it's all right with you, I will tell her about our conversation today so she can check in with you by phone before your first appointment with her."

"Of course, Doctor."

She places her hand back on her breast, but this time, it appears to me more a sign of gratitude than of self-protection.

"Thank you for your kind attention, Doctor."

"Yes," says Elena. "Thank you for helping Yelva. And if you ever want to reach me, Doctor, here is my business card."

I glance at her card:

ELENA SANCHEZ
ADVOCATE
LIBRE LEGAL AID SOCIETY
SAN MATEO COUNTY

"Wait. Are you a friend? Or are you working with her on a legal matter?"

"I am sort of her case manager. We are representing her in her court case. She has a U-1 visa and now is applying for a U-3 visa."

Because my wife is a legal aid attorney with expertise in domestic violence cases, I am clued in to the fact that a U visa is a special visa that can be granted to an immigrant who has been a victim of a crime in the US that resulted in physical or mental suffering. A result of the federal Violence Against Women Act of 2000, its focus is on protecting victims of sex trafficking and domestic violence and enabling law enforcement to investigate and prosecute such cases.

"Oh, I see. I know what a U visa is. But what is a U-3 visa?"

"It's for her son," says Elena. "She is trying to get her son out of El Salvador. Victims of sex crimes can sometimes get their children into the US. It is urgent that we get her this visa."

"I'm confused. I thought her children lived with her."

"Her two little ones do. But she also has a sixteen-year-old son who lives in a village in El Salvador. He is in serious danger. The largest gang there has been recruiting him for a long time, but he has refused to join. It was fine for a few months, but three weeks ago, they threatened to kill him if he didn't join, and they threatened Yelva's sister too. So Yelva came to us to help her get him this visa so he could get out. Then, four days ago, her son called her again and said that things have gotten really bad. And that he and his aunt have no choice but to escape to another town. He said they would be in touch soon. She hasn't heard from either of them since."

I look at Ms. Martinez. I half ask and half tell her, "So the breast pain suddenly came back when you first heard that your son was in danger?"

"Yes, Doctor, it seems so."

"And then the pain became unbearable four days ago, when you learned he had to escape to save his own neck?"

"Yes, Doctor, that seems so too."

"And you have not heard from him?"

"No, I have not. But I am praying."

"Is this the same sister who is suffering from the blood cancer?"

"Yes, she is very ill, and now she can't even see her own doctors."

"Wow. You are dealing with a lot of really heavy stress and fear right now. I am not at all surprised you are in pain. In fact, I am amazed at how strong you have been throughout this series of ordeals. And that you can even think straight and get the legal help you need. We can provide you with medical and emotional support that can help you be as effective as possible as you work through this. And help you recover from it once you have made it through."

"Thank you, Doctor."

"Good. And finally, let me offer to you and Elena that if there is anything I can write to the court to support your application for the U-3 visa, I am willing to do so."

"Thank you, Doctor," they respond in near unison.

"Ms. Martinez, thank you for sharing your story. We accomplished a lot today. I will be thinking about you and hoping for your son. Please go to the front desk to get an appointment with our therapist so she can help you stay strong. She is very busy, but I will make a request to squeeze you in as soon as she can. And you will get a postcard with an appointment for that mammogram, just to double-check."

I exit the room to see my medical assistant giving me back a wry smile of her own, half-jokingly tapping her watch at me.

"Don't give me that look," I say. "Give me this instead."

I approach her and motion for a high five. Our palms slap together, echoing in the hallway.

As I turn toward the next room and the waiting patient, I turn back to her and whisper, "I won our little game this time. I'll tell you about it later."

She responds with characteristic sass. "That's not really fair, Doctorcito. You set the rules of this game. You can win this game anytime you decide you want to."

I pause to consider her claim. I have learned the hard way not to expect that my best efforts will influence whether good or bad things happen to my patients. But perhaps, in some cases, my medical assistant is not so wrong. It's more a question of which game one is trying to win.

CHAPTER 16

The Frequent Flyer

Patron of your beloved city,
O San Francisco, saint of love,
Co-sufferer in searing pity
Of all our griefs, whom from above
Birds would alight on, singing feeding
Within your hands—hands pierced and bleeding
With Christ's own signs—who, stigmatized
As dupe and clown, apostrophized
The sun in its blistering starkness
As brother, and the blistered moon
As sister, and who blind at noon,
Opened your heart and sang in darkness—
And where it was, sowed light, look down.
Solace the sorrows of your town.

—Vikram Seth, *The Golden Gate*

THE SUN HAS RISEN OVER SAN FRANCISCO AND THE BIRDS ARE AL-
ready singing. It's the start of New Year's Day in the year 2000, the
morning after my team's busy night on call. This is the last call cycle of my
month as the attending physician on the wards for this year. My resident,
interns, and medical students together admitted ten new patients, and I

need to meet them all and make sure everything was handled correctly. And we need to check in on our eight old patients.

My senior resident, Hurstley, an overly jocular guy, especially when he hasn't slept overnight, starts us off.

"For our next act, we present one of our most frequent flyers, Jan Taggert. This is her ninth hospitalization at our fine institution in the past year. Dr. Jadhipur, why don't you give Dr. Schillinger the abbreviated version, since I presume he has met her a few times over his career here and since we all know her so well."

I interrupt the flow. "Yes, you are right. This unfortunate woman follows me every time I attend on the wards. Unpleasant as they come, as hopeless as they come. Every time she gets admitted, we all just become witnesses to the unfolding of an unremitting real-time tragedy."

The intern Jadhipur sidesteps my comment and keeps the tone lighthearted. "It would be my honor, Dr. Hurstley."

"I do know her well, Amar, so you can speed-walk us through it. We have a lot on our plate this morning."

"Certainly, Dr. Schillinger. Ms. Jan Taggert is a *lovely* and oh-so-personable twenty-six-year-old marginally housed, HIV-negative woman with a twelve-year history of intravenous drug use, including methamphetamine and heroin, with a habit primarily financed through prostitution."

"Go on," I say, thinking about how I will need to pull him aside afterward to address his hardened outlook.

"Past medical history includes tobacco use, sexual abuse as a teenager, and in this year alone: two episodes of right-sided endocarditis, one episode of pelvic inflammatory disease due to gonorrhea and chlamydia, four brief admissions for incision and drainage of skin abscesses, and a recent five-day admission for cellulitis of the left arm."

"Just tell me what brought her here this time, Amar."

"Well, she is an unreliable historian due to uncooperativeness. She reported being in her usual state of health—which is not something to write home about—until three days ago, when she presented with intense left shoulder pain and fever. Of note, she reports not having used any IV drugs for three months. She denies any acute trauma to the shoulder and reports no domestic violence. She also denied chest pain or abdominal pain until yesterday when, presumably, she went into acute opiate withdrawal and started experiencing abdominal cramping, vomiting, and diarrhea."

"And the physical exam?" I ask impatiently.

"Physical exam last night was significant for a peak temperature of 39.4 degrees and tachycardia to 112. She was a disheveled and irritable woman who appears much older than stated age. She was alert and oriented times three until she was given methadone in the ER, after which she became somnolent but arousable. I'll cut to the chase: she had a warm and erythematous area over the right shoulder, which had a range of motion very much limited by pain, even with passive range of motion. Pain was elicited at thirty degrees of abduction; she refused further movement. I was unable to perform the drop-arm test due to her subjective pain. Skin exam revealed multiple old track marks throughout, with evidence of recent injections into her axillae. Laboratory evaluation revealed an elevated white blood cell count. A shoulder x-ray was unremarkable and, specifically, did not reveal any evidence for osteomyelitis."

"And your assessment and plan, Amar, please?"

"Our assessment was that of a young IV drug user with a septic joint, likely due to *Staph. aureus*. We also consulted the Orthopedic Service to ask them to tap her shoulder joint and obtain additional cultures. We started her on IV vancomycin and gentamicin to both cover the septic joint as well as possible endocarditis. She also received 50 mg of oral methadone last night and another 50 mg about an hour ago, a dose based on my review of her opiate requirements during the prior hospitalization. She did not submit to my examination this morning and refused to even answer my questions. Orthopedics reportedly came by very late last night and tapped her joint, but I haven't found their note in the chart. Our hope is that we can quickly punt her to their service, since maybe she'll need surgical drainage of that infected joint."

"Good luck with that. I appreciate your optimism, though, Amar. Okay—nicely done, team. Now prepare to be charmed, and let's go in. But before we do, let me ask our medical students: What do you make of her report that she hasn't used IV drugs for three months?"

One of the medical students steps up.

"Uhhh. Well . . . Amar did say he found evidence that she was shooting up in her underarms, and she sounds like she is having symptoms of heroin withdrawal, so it seems doubtful. I'd say she's still using, but not sure why she'd lie to us. It doesn't help her in any way to lie, does it?"

"That's right. Our former chief of the Medical Service and God of All Diseases Infectious, Dr. Merle Sande, used to preach: *Once a shooter, always a shooter.* This case was obvious, but I have seen cases when a patient with a very distant history of IV drug use comes in with bad low back pain and swears up and down that he hasn't used in over a decade. And his doctor believes him. But then he comes back a few days later, paralyzed from the waist down from an epidural spine abscess from shooting up, with the bacteria having lodged themselves next to the spinal cord. Bad business. So never forget that if someone has a history of IV drug use, you should have a high suspicion that they may still be using. I know that sounds super cynical, but know that I don't mean it to be. People can and do change. You just can't always tell who. I'm just making sure you don't ever make that kind of mistake in the future."

I knock and enter the room of the frequent flyer, bringing my team along. She is covered from head to toe by a white hospital bedsheet, looking like a corpse in a morgue.

"Good morning, Ms. Taggert. It's nice to see you again. Although, with you all wrapped up in your cocoon like that, I can't really see you. Do you mind if we pull back the sheet so we can talk to you and take a closer look at that painful shoulder of yours?"

She croaks from under the sheet, "Go away! All of you. Leave me alone. I was asleep."

"I know how hard it is to get any sleep around here, and I appreciate that you're exhausted. But despite what you may think, this isn't a hotel. It's a hospital. And we are doctors who need to talk to you and examine you now."

"You gonna give me pain meds?"

"I'm sorry, but I can't communicate with someone whose face is completely covered and whose voice is muffled."

Whipping off the cover sheet from her face, she yells, "I said, are you going to give me pain meds?!"

The frequent flyer that breaks out of her cocoon is no monarch butterfly. What is revealed bears no resemblance to a twenty-six-year-old woman. Before us lies a sweaty, elderly-looking woman with a gaunt, wrinkled face, greasy, long, stringy hair, and nasty teeth, some of which are blackened and jagged. In the one year since I last took care of her, when she was already looking awful, she has aged an additional ten.

"Thank you for coming out of your cocoon, Ms. Taggert. I'm Dr. Schillinger. We've met a number of times before, over the last few years."

"I don't recognize you for shit."

"That's a lovely sentiment. Don't worry, I won't take it personally. I've probably changed. As have you. To answer your question regarding pain medications: yes, it's a possibility. Along with a lot of other things we'll need to decide on, with your cooperation. Can we count on you to work with us to help you get through this? Because it sounds as though, based on what Dr. Jadhipur just told me, you might have another serious infection. This time in your right shoulder."

"You guys are a bunch of fucking *geniuses*."

"What a piece of work," mutters Hurstley audibly.

I place a restraining hand on Hurstley's arm. "Whether we are or aren't geniuses doesn't change my question. We are here to serve your critical health needs, and quite frankly, we're all you've got. So let me ask you again: Can we count on you to help us help you get through this?"

"Whatever . . ."

"Well, as the leader of this team, I'll take that as a yes. And, to be clear, we not only want to help you get your shoulder back in order but also really want to give you every opportunity to get your life back in order. Which, as best as I can tell, means helping you kick heroin and speed. It's tough—if not impossible—to live a normal existence when those drugs are a presence in your life."

"Good luck with that, Dr. Genius."

"Funny. I just said that to Dr. Jadhipur about something else. I'm actually in the business of waiting for luck to hit, of never giving up. Of always holding out hope. And I have that hope for you. Maybe this time's the charm."

"That's nice. Aren't *you* charming. But what about those pain meds?"

"Let's start with my examining you and we'll take things from there."

She's got no chance in hell. Luck has nothing to do with her trajectory. She's a hard-core user with no plans to kick. She's on a one-way train to certain death. She's already had her eight lives. This is her ninth. Her body isn't getting any younger, and she can't keep bouncing back. It's only a matter of time.

I manage to get my stethoscope onto her chest.

"I do hear a murmur over the left sternal border. Please, Ms. Taggert, roll a bit to your left side. . . . Good. No radiation there. Okay . . . now lean back again and let me just listen to your neck. Right. I'm hearing a little something up here in the carotids too."

I point to a spot on the right side of her neck.

"Amar, take a listen here."

Pulling the stethoscope out of my ears, I step back from the frequent flyer and, assuming a professorial tone, I address the entire team.

"As I'm sure you know, the absence of a murmur in no way rules out endocarditis. So, we always cover with antibiotics until we rule it out, which requires about forty-eight hours for the cultures to come back. As we're doing now. But the *presence* of a systolic murmur in an IV drug user with a septic joint—as we have here—is quite concerning for acute bacterial endocarditis. It's often impossible to hear these murmurs when you examine someone down in that loud ER. That's why we do these post-call rounds. Two sets of ears are always better than one."

I turn to the frequent flyer.

"What I'm saying to my team, Ms. Taggert, is that the previous infections you've had involving your heart valves make them really vulnerable to getting infected again. I'm worried now that you have a newly infected heart valve that also sent some of the bugs to your right shoulder. We're giving you some good bug juice now to treat it, but we need to get a picture of your heart today—an echocardiogram. You know, that test where they put warm jelly on your chest and rub a wand over your heart?"

She pulls the sheet back over her head. "Fuck this."

"Indeed. Very well put. Fuck this. I'm hoping the antibiotic treatment for the shoulder will also take care of any infected valve. One step at a time, though, okay?"

She pulls the sheet back off her head. "Just examine my shoulder so we can get this over with. Then get me my pain meds."

The next day, I inform the patient that the echocardiogram revealed an infected aortic valve. She receives the news with characteristic disdain. I let her know that today is my last day on service, that I will be handing her care off to a colleague, and that I wish her the best of luck. Her outcome will have nothing to do with luck, of course.

A few months later, I run into my intern Amar, and he tells me that our mutual patient ended up needing to have her shoulder surgically drained and that she received four weeks of IV antibiotics for the aortic valve—the full course. He had recently heard from a colleague that she had subsequently been readmitted for heart failure, as her aortic valve had been damaged by the last episode of endocarditis. And that, as a result, she is going to need cardiac surgery up at the university hospital to repair the valve. But that he isn't sure they will do it, given her active IV drug use. Receiving this news, I felt no emotion. These were just clinical facts.

Fifteen years later, I walk into the clinic room for a new patient visit. Strange. My patient panel has been closed for five years. I shouldn't be seeing new patients unless I personally schedule them in. I push away the resentment I feel at—yet again—having to go the extra mile without having agreed to.

"Thank you for seeing me. My other doctor, she was sweet. But she left to work at another hospital. So, I asked my nurse who would be good to take over for her. My nurse said you were special. She told me you were full up, but she did me a favor and snuck me in."

The middle-aged woman smiles. "So here I am, whether you like it or not. I hope that's okay."

"Not a problem. It's always helpful to have someone who can advocate for you. And Nancy is the best at that. I always end up loving the folks who she manages to squeeze onto my schedule against my direct orders. Meaning—*you* are the one who must be someone special. Well, enough from the Mutual Admiration Club. I took a quick look at your computer records and have a feel for what's been going on over the last year or so. You've really been through the wringer. What can I do for you today and moving forward?"

"Well, I've been having really bad fatigue for about six months. It all started after my latest surgery. I had a mitral valve and aortic valve repair—my third time, actually. They say I have nine lives! But this time, I developed a sternal wound infection. It was really ugly, and I was in the hospital for almost three months. And ever since I got out, I've felt exhausted. The cardiologist says my valves look fine and my heart is pumping fine, so that's good. And my prior doctor said the infection definitely cleared, so it's not that. But it's gotten really bad. I have an eleven-year-old daughter that I have to wake up for, 'cause I have to drive her to school for—ugh!—a 7:50 start, and I'm so tired when we wake up at 6:00, it's *painful*. Then I have to rush to get to work—I'm apprenticing as a tattoo artist three days a week—but most of the time, I feel like I need to just drive back home and climb back into bed. I force myself not to, but then I am fast asleep by 9:30 at night."

"I see. It's good that you have shifted your sleep cycle appropriately. But your question is why you are so tired, despite that. I read that your valves had been damaged by IV drug use, is that correct?"

"Yeah, that's right. I really *fucked* them up. Oops, sorry! I mean I messed them up. But now, supposedly, I am fit as a fiddle."

I really like this woman's spirit. I can see what Nancy saw in her. Something weird about the way she said she'd "fucked up" her valves, though. Like a déjà vu.

"Well, you've shown it's never too late to change. In terms of getting to the bottom of your fatigue, I need to ask you an important question. Before I do, I want to tell you I am not judging you one way or another when I ask this. So you can be perfectly honest. When was the last time you used?"

"No, it's good and right that you ask. I've been clean for over nine years. Nine years and two months, to be exact. I actually am a counselor and a sponsor at NA now. I'm really proud of that. It's amazing and challenging work."

"Wow. Congratulations on both fronts. How bad was your habit?"

"Oh, it was bad. I was an absolute mess. Heroin, speed, prostitution, homelessness, withdrawal, going in and out of the hospital, in and out of jail. And then back out to start the cycle all over again. Twenty years of my life down the tubes. In some ways, it's all a blank. But in other ways, I remember specific details. Mostly, I remember the acts of kindness I received. I did spend *a lot* of hard times in this fine institution."

She giggles and goes on.

"I guess in some ways—to be fair—this place saved my life. Although I absolutely *hated* being here most of the time."

Jan Taggert. Jan Taggert. That is her name. Her clinic card actually says she's Jan Taggert. If I squint and imagine her with greasy long hair, some bad teeth, and a mean disposition. . . . Oh my God.

"Ms. Taggert, what years were you at your sickest? I mean, when were you being hospitalized here the most?"

"Well, up until my daughter was born . . . so probably from 1998 to 2006. Roughly. It's kind of a blur."

"That's crazy. I *know* you. I was one of your doctors then. Probably four or five times. You were really sick. Valve infections, joint infections, abscesses, you name it."

She laughs. "Weird. Yeah, a lot of doctors took care of me during that decade. Dozens probably, if not hundreds."

"You're right. You were here so much you were known as one of our frequent flyers."

She laughs again.

"But have you met any of those doctors again, now fifteen to twenty years later?"

"My cardiologist says he maybe remembers me, but other than that, and maybe you—I guess—no."

"Well, I distinctly remember you. And I have to tell you, I am blown away to see you here. What an honor to become your doctor again. And under such different circumstances. To be honest, I never thought you'd live to make it, let alone show up here in my clinic as my patient. Most times, you were a woman banging on death's door. As one of your doctors, I felt pretty powerless back then. But seeing you now—maybe I misinterpreted."

"In some ways, you're entirely right. I have undergone a real change. In other ways, though, I was the same person then that I am now. NA has taught me to see both sides of the equation."

"Yes, I can see how that would both be true and even helpful. Man, we tried really hard to help you get clean. I mean, we must have had dozens of conversations with you about kicking, and you must've talked to dozens and dozens of our substance abuse counselors trying to motivate you to choose a new path and get treatment. But you were like a wall."

"Yes, I can be stubborn."

"Are you comfortable telling me your story of recovery?"

"This is what we do at NA all the time. Telling stories as a means to reinforce our ongoing process of recovery and heal ourselves. And to encourage others to find and tell their own stories so they can begin to recover and even heal. I never get tired of it."

"I'm all ears."

"For me, it was a couple of events, I think, happening close together. The most important one was the birth of my daughter, Ella. I was using heavily then. I was jailed and they took her away from me for nine months. It actually happened here, on the maternity ward upstairs."

"Wow, that must have been hard. What happened next?"

"As I started having more visits with her, I fell in love. She was so fragile. I started to fantasize—just little images, really—about being clean and becoming a *real* mother for her."

"Becoming a parent can be a very powerful thing."

"Exactly. Then, one day, after I was out of jail, I got hospitalized here again—I can't remember for what—and, like always, a substance abuse counselor came to my bedside. And somehow, maybe she was different from all the others, or maybe I was in a different place. Well, either way, she was very special. I got real lucky that day because she was the one assigned to talk to me. *Really* lucky. I'm still in touch with her, actually. She was a former user and a victim of childhood trauma too. She said stuff to me that I really could identify with, and she took the time to listen. Not only the time but also the *interest*. She was genuinely interested in me. She wasn't just going through the motions. You know what I mean?"

"I do. Absolutely, I do."

"So, with her help, I got into Walden House, a residential treatment center for drug users, and I got on methadone. That was another lucky break, 'cause Walden House usually has a long waiting list. Or maybe the hospital just convinced them that I was a desperate case."

She laughs again.

"Like many things, it was probably a mix of luck and effort. Including effort on *your* part," I say.

"True . . . that's true. So anyway, for the first time in a long time, I had a roof over my head, a regular schedule, and no overwhelming need to get my fix. It's not that my life became perfect. Just that I finally had the time and space—and a sense of safety—to try to put the pieces of my life back together."

"That makes sense."

"Yeah. And with each month that passed, CPS let me see Ella more and more. Which locked me in on my plan to truly recover. And like I said, once I decide on something, I'm really stubborn. I actually was able to get off methadone, and I religiously attended NA. And, yeah ... so I got Ella back before her first birthday. And I started working as a waitress. I saved up some money and got some of my teeth fixed and then was able to get better waitressing jobs."

"And you say you're becoming a tattoo artist?"

"Well, I already am an artist—ever since I was little, I've been a good visual artist. I have a website if you wanna see some of my stuff."

"Absolutely. Show me after."

"So now I'm trying to make some money off of it. It's going really well. In about a month, I'll get my certificate and can start getting paid."

"And your daughter, Ella. How is she doing?"

"She's doing great. She's gonna be a sixth grader. I try to be a good mom, and she's a really good girl. We're like close friends. We've been in therapy together on and off, which has really helped us both, in different ways, of course."

"Ms. Taggert . . ."

"Call me Jan, would you?"

"Okay, but only if you call me Dean."

"That's fair," she laughs.

"Jan—I can't tell you how inspired I am by your story. But more than that, how inspired I am by your *spirit*. I think—actually, I know—that I had no inkling of what was inside you all this time. Or *who* was inside you, hiding under the sheets that you would always cover yourself with."

"I know, I just wanted to sleep my life away. Being high or sleeping. Those were my two go-to places."

"You mentioned the important role that the counselor played in your recovery. What do you remember about the doctors and nurses during that time? About how we treated you? I ask because we are always trying to figure out how to do a better job taking care of our patients, and people who use IV drugs can be very challenging for us."

"Most of them were just shadows passing before my eyes or faceless voices around my bed. Some of them could be really mean. Although I'm sure I was totally unpleasant to deal with back then. But there were a few times I can remember when a doctor or a nurse was particularly kind to me. A comforting word. Being physically gentle with me. Asking me what I needed and really listening. Letting me stay an extra night in the hospital when they could have sent me out. Those little acts of kindness gave me hope. Most of the time, though, I felt subhuman. I hated myself, and I think many of you guys hated me too. But those special moments made me feel human; they gave me an ounce of self-respect. Just enough to go on."

"Yes. I can imagine how that would be important. If you were teaching a bunch of doctors and nurses about how to care for people with severe substance use disorders, what advice would you give us?"

"Hmmm. No one has ever asked me that before. Gimme a minute here. There's probably a lot I'd say."

"Take your time."

She is so genuine, so down-to-earth. So engaged and engaging.

"Okay. Got it. I think the top three things would be: First, make sure you hire drug use counselors who've 'been there and done that,' who can speak from a place of true experience. Second, never give up on people; you never know when we're ready to turn the corner. And third, be kind to people, treat us with compassion so we can be reminded that we are human, even if we seem otherwise."

She looks up at me apologetically. "I'm sorry, Dean. But I can't honestly say I remember you from those days. But I'm sure you were good to me."

"I don't know about that. I can say that I was never mean to you, but I can't say that I ever was especially kind either. Nor did I show you the compassion I should have given the awful trauma you experienced from a young age. I probably was, like you say, one of those shadows simply passing before you. I have learned a lot since then."

She laughs from her belly this time. "Well, I'm glad I was of some use, then . . ."

"Very funny. Actually, not so funny. Look—thank you for sharing your story with me. I'm going to shift gears and get back to your fatigue in a minute. But before I do, I want to go out on a limb and ask you something. It's a favor, actually. But I think it's aligned with the work you do at NA and with your sentiment about being of use, so maybe it's the kind of favor that gives back."

"Now I'm all ears."

"Every year, I work with a colleague to put on a large national course for doctors and nurses on the care of medically and socially marginalized patients. You know, one of those big three-day courses in a fancy hotel in San Francisco?"

"I actually wouldn't know, but I can imagine. Go on."

"Point well taken. Well, these courses are one way that doctors and nurses stay up-to-date on new things happening in our field. Usually, the courses are on one organ system or another. Like Updates in Cardiology. Or the Latest and Greatest on Schizophrenia. Ours is the only course to give updates on both the diseases that commonly affect poor and marginalized populations—like hepatitis, HIV, heart failure, diabetes, asthma—as well as describing the common social problems that these patients often confront—like food insecurity, illiteracy, homelessness, sexual trauma, substance use. And then we put it all together, showing how the social and the medical interact, and what we can do about it as clinicians in our offices and hospitals, as well as in our communities."

"I get it. That's very cool that you do that."

"Yeah, it's been a success for each of the first three years we've done it. Anyway, one of the things I am proudest of in the course is that every half day, we do something pretty different: instead of the usual PowerPoint, fact-based lectures, we switch things up. We have an expert talk about something important, but as a personal narrative. Sort of like an 'up close and personal' window into their journey in medicine through the storytelling format. It's meant to be inspirational and to build a sense of community among the learners, which is really important if you're going to work in a place like this. To try to prevent burnout."

"I can see how that could help you guys, yes."

"Well, this year, we've been talking about having one of those slots filled by a patient. A patient telling his or her story. We've talked about how it has to be someone special, because this can be a challenging group. We need someone who is articulate and honest about his or her experience, someone who doesn't hold back. Someone who has a lot to teach us. Someone who can show us not only how social marginalization can generate illness but teach us how resilience can produce recovery. And what role we can play in that trajectory."

"Okay. . . . So are you asking me to do that?"

Six months later, I am onstage with her, sitting on director's chairs in front of two hundred clinicians. We each are holding a mic in our hands.

"Thank you for sharing your story with all of us. It is a very moving story, and it gives me hope. I am sure we are all inspired. Now, here you are, over fifteen years later, speaking to a bunch of doctors and nurses from around the country. Let me give you back the floor to teach us—to give us your advice, based on your experiences—about how to better care for people with severe substance use disorders."

"I'd be glad to, for whatever it's worth."

"It's worth a lot. It'll be priceless, actually. So, what advice would you give us?"

"Well, you asked me this once before, so I've had some time to think about an answer." She turns to the audience. "I think the top three things would be: First, make sure you hire substance use counselors who have truly been there and can speak from a place of real, lived experience. Second, don't give up on people. Even if we say we don't need your medical help, we do. And even if we seem to not appreciate your acts of kindness, deep inside, we do. So, third, show compassion to people like us. We are human beings who need to be treated with kindness. We are not monsters that need to be shamed or punished for our sickness. Trust me, we already carry enough shame. We may be obnoxious and unpleasant; we may be taking up a lot of your time. All that can be true. But I guess I'd say always try to remember that it's not about you. Remember that *we* are the ones who are really suffering. What we need from you is that you witness and acknowledge our suffering. And remember that we *need* your help. Your medical help and your kindness are critical. What you're doing is not a waste of your time. Even if we're not ready to accept your advice, we need to hear it. Because one day, if we're lucky, we will be ready. I was kept alive by people like you so that one day I could hear it. I am so grateful that I am here today speaking with you, that I am well again, and that I can enjoy my beautiful eleven-year-old daughter. I thank you all from the bottom of my heart."

Ms. Taggert receives a standing ovation from the doctors and nurses who have been listening to her, rapt, in the downtown hotel's conference ballroom. Her session receives the highest ratings of any of the twenty-four talks delivered for the course.

What a wondrous woman.

CHAPTER 17

Smoke and Mirrors

HANDS AND DOORKNOBS

As my afternoon clinic begins, Mrs. Beatrice Johnson is, as usual, on time and already waiting for me in my exam room. A seventyish-year-old African American woman with salt-and-pepper hair tightly held up in a bun, she sits in her wheelchair, her lap covered by what appears to be a home-made quilt, and beams a smile up at me.

"Hello, Mrs. Johnson, so nice to see you again. That is a gorgeous quilt. Did you make that?"

"No, those days are over. My sister made this one for me because I always get a chill when I wait for the van to pick me up to take me here."

I recall that Mrs. Johnson has to take a long paratransit van ride from her apartment in the Sunnydale projects located just off Highway 101 on the way to the airport, in the outskirts of San Francisco. She was born in the South, but her family moved to San Francisco's Fillmore District in the '40s, as did many African American families. Her piece of this great migration was a result of families like hers escaping the Jim Crow laws of the South, pursuing job opportunities associated with the massive, war-related shipbuilding industry. Many found lower-cost rental units to live in, including those recently abandoned by families of Japanese descent who had been forcibly removed as part of the Japanese internment. Quickly becoming the vibrant African American center of the city and the undisputed home of the West Coast jazz scene of the '50s and '60s, the Fillmore District became known as the "Harlem of the

West," where Miles Davis, Dexter Gordon, Dizzy Gillespie, Billie Holiday, and Ella Fitzgerald were frequent performers. The streets were home not only to jazz clubs but also to churches, barbershops, and small, locally owned grocery stores and food joints. Despite its flourishing cultural life, the district was targeted for redevelopment in the late '60s—funded largely with federal dollars—with the rationale that the neighborhood was the city's sore thumb of urban blight and that the government had to "clean up the inner city."

What has subsequently been termed the *Negro removal* project resulted in the destruction of thousands of low-rent apartment buildings and homes, leading to the permanent displacement of over eight thousand people, mostly African American. The city's promise to relocate these families back to the Fillmore was never kept; housing costs had jumped in response to redevelopment, and the promised boom in the local economy to support former residents never materialized. Mrs. Johnson, by then a young woman, was one of the displaced. She found herself going from living a "life at the top" in the Fillmore to living her life at the bottom—in the Sunnydale projects.

"But I used to be the quilt maker in the family. I learned it from my grandma, and then I taught it to my youngest sister. She's at home most days now and has the time to make these. I just wish one of my grandkids would take it up. You know . . . to keep it going. Because, well, with these fingers, I just can't anymore. I don't need to tell you that."

She takes her hands out from under the quilt and places them on her lap. They are textbook examples of how advanced degenerative osteoarthritis looks: the fingers unable to extend, the little bones of the distal joints bloated like doorknobs, the intrinsic muscles that give the back of the hand its shape atrophied. Those hands—more like a Gothic rendering of human claws—rest on the lap of this gentle lady.

Mrs. Johnson has eight grandchildren and raised four of them on her own after one of her daughters succumbed to the crack epidemic of the 1980s.

"Yes, well. It is wonderful that you were able to pass this craft on to your sister and that she could give the gift back to you in this way. But don't give up on those grandkids. Sooner or later, one of them will appreciate the combination of creativity and calm that quilting can give them. And they'll come looking for you."

"Now you're talking like a quilter yourself, Doctor."

"No, not me. I find my peace in other ways. But how are you doing otherwise?"

We review the status of her arthritis-related pains, pains resulting from the kind of joint damage that had made walking—even with her four-point walker—impossible for nearly two years. We then discuss her mood, as this level of chronic pain and immobility can be emotionally devastating. She reminds me that the two-year anniversary of the death of her husband just passed. A World War II veteran who received his care at the VA hospital, he had been a companion for her every appointment with me. A gentle man, he had always shown her the respect she deserves. When I learned that he had once been a GI fighting the Nazis on the European front, I told him that I was here today only because of men like him—soldiers who had sacrificed everything to liberate my father from a concentration camp. I had told him it was an honor to be able to return the favor by taking care of his wife. I could tell that touched him and stuck with him. As a dedicated caregiver to her, he had enabled me to do my job better.

Mrs. Johnson continues, "But this year, I think I'm okay. This year, I was sad for only a few days, and it passed. There's so much hustle and bustle in the house, I am too busy just trying to keep track a who's comin' and who's goin'!"

I then ask her about the status of her breathing. She also suffers from emphysema, the gradual disappearance of lung tissue resulting from tobacco smoke exposure, a progressive illness that literally takes one's breath away, slowly but surely. She had adamantly denied ever smoking, but she had lived with a lifelong smoker. Her husband, like so many soldiers, had become addicted to the cigarettes handed out freely by tobacco companies, courtesy of the US Army. Frank had died of emphysema. A horrible way to die, like drowning in open air.

"For the first time," she says, "I think it hasn't gotten worse. At least not since the first anniversary of Frank's death. I'm not sure if it's my lungs just deciding to gimme a break for a change, or if it's because I am doing less due to me being stuck in this wheelchair."

I hold my tongue because I know that the cause of the stabilization of her lung disease is the absence of tobacco smoke in her environment related to the death of her husband. She likely knows this too, but it is too painful to admit.

"Ahhh, who knew that being in a wheelchair could improve your health?" I sarcastically quip.

She laughs the laugh of an ex-smoker, a laugh that ends in a classic coughing spell. I give her some tissue and she spits some phlegm out and rolls the tissue up in a knobby, clawlike hand.

Her vital signs show that her blood pressure is high; I ask her to roll up her sleeve so I can repeat it. I confirm it is elevated. This is the second visit in a row with an elevation, so we discuss increasing the dosage of one of her four blood pressure medications. She begrudgingly agrees.

I quickly do my charting, refill her five oral medications for arthritis, hypertension, high cholesterol, and diabetes, plus two inhalers for her emphysema, and remind her that it is flu season and that she needs a flu shot. Before I am finished with my sell job on the need for the flu vaccine, she has disrobed her right shoulder, taking her cardigan half off, leaving only a tank top.

"I always dress right for the doctor. I been doin' this too long to get all layered up."

"I do appreciate that, Mrs. Johnson."

I poke my head out the door and ask my medical assistant to get the flu shot ready.

I pop back in, grab her chart, start to say my goodbyes, and move to make my way out. I've spent twenty minutes with her in what is a fifteen-minute visit slot. Not so bad.

She interrupts me midsentence.

"You know. It's funny. This same shoulder has been really hurting. It makes it hard for me to even lift my arm to brush my hair. I stopped using it, it hurts so much. Probably my arthritis, right? Now it's in my shoulder too."

We physicians call this the *doorknob complaint*, a patient complaint that arises the moment the doctor grabs hold of the doorknob to exit the room and end the visit. We dread these doorknob complaints because, apart from interrupting one's clinic workflow, they tend to be especially time-consuming and—for reasons that are not entirely clear—often reflect more serious pathology relative to other complaints discussed in the earlier, structured portion of the visit.

In general, the shoulder is an oddly behaving, yet critical, joint. Disuse of the shoulder as a result of pain and associated lack of prompt diagnosis and treatment can lead to a frozen shoulder, a poorly understood phenomenon in which all mobility is lost, often for many years. Leaving Mrs. Johnson, even temporarily, with no legs to walk on and only one arm to lift with is not an option. So, I let a breath out to release my mini-frustration, put on a concerned look, and say as kindly as I can, "Let me have a look."

Shoulder pain is the fifth most common complaint in primary care, but many primary care physicians are simply not comfortable with the inner workings of what they perceive to be a region of the body requiring an orthopedist. I, on the other hand, like many other internists, developed particular areas of specialty expertise, and the diagnosis and management of shoulder pain had become one of mine.

I do a cursory shoulder exam on Mrs. Johnson to rule out a rotator cuff tear. I determine quite quickly that she has point tenderness at the right acromioclavicular (AC) joint, the fixed joint that connects the tail end of the collarbone to the curved hook of the shoulder blade, a juncture that lies just above the miraculously mobile shoulder joint itself. The AC joint is the part of the shoulder girdle most commonly affected by degenerative osteoarthritis, and AC joint arthritis is one of the more common causes of shoulder pain in primary care settings. So, it all makes sense. I don't want to give her any anti-inflammatory pain medications for this, as these can worsen high blood pressure. Fortunately, AC joint arthritis is remarkably responsive to low-dose steroid injections, so I offer her one. She agrees, and I ask my medical assistant to bring in the injection tray for me to use before she gives the flu shot. Two minutes later, I am through, and I tell Mrs. Johnson that the injection can take forty-eight hours to kick in. I show her a few shoulder exercises I want her to do once the pain recedes, so as to avoid frozen shoulder syndrome. I schedule her for a nurse visit in eight weeks to follow up on her blood pressure and tell her to let that nurse know at that time if she still is suffering from the shoulder pain. I finally can leave the room, still feeling good about what transpired between us.

SOLDIERING ON

Two months later, I am cruising through my afternoon clinic, feeling a rare rush of satisfaction for being on time with every patient. I am nearly done.

Only two patients left. This means I not only will be home for dinner with my family but that I may even be able to make the dinner. As my medical assistant places my last patients into their rooms, I drift to the central hallway to gloat over my afternoon schedule, congratulating myself for the unusual efficiency with which I managed my busy day. Like a sports fan repeatedly enjoying the highlights of a game he knows his team already won.

But I am foiled again. A handwritten name has been penned into my last add-on slot: Beatrice Johnson. Next to her name is a yellow sticky note:

PLEASE STOP BY TRIAGE RE BJ—SUE.

I have a minute before my next patient is ready, so I trot down to the nurse triage room.

"Whassup, Sue?"

"I just put Mrs. Johnson back into the waiting room. She's still complaining about pain in her shoulder. I wouldn't have added her on, but I've known her for fifteen years, and she's not a complainer. She is one of the founders of our Grandmothers Who Care group . . . that group of Black grandmas we were able to bring together to support each other around the loss of their children during the crack days and the stress of needing to care for their grandkids. She is one tough cookie. But she was in tears when I tried to get her to move her shoulder."

"No problem. Thanks for picking up on that. Just let her know I'll see her once I finish up with these last two, okay?"

Fifteen minutes later, I see my medical assistant wheeling the quilt-covered Mrs. Johnson into one of my exam rooms. Her torso is twisted in such a way that I can see from down the hallway that this stoic lady is indeed in a great deal of pain.

I finish with what had been my last patient of the day and glance at my watch: 5:35 p.m. My medical assistant lets me know she's off now and that I'm on my own. Clinic is winding down. I thank her and grab Mrs. Johnson's chart, knock, turn the doorknob, and enter.

"Hello again. Oh, poor you! You look miserable. So, I didn't cure you, despite all my fancy needles and magic potions? Tell me what's going on."

She attempts a smile but puts her left hand out, beckoning for me to wait a moment. She lets out a series of wet coughs, and with each cough, she winces in pain, favoring her right shoulder.

I hand her the tissues.

"Take your time," I say. "I am here. And you made it here. We're in no rush."

She relaxes her body and catches her breath.

"It's this damn shoulder. It's worse. I still can't lift it. But now it hurts even when I don't move it."

"Did the injection help, even for a short time?"

"You want the truth, Doctor? No. Not at all."

"Darn. I am sorry. Have you been able to do any of those shoulder exercises?"

"Are you kidding? I can barely sleep. Every time I try to roll over, I'm in agony."

I wonder whether I could have been wrong about the AC joint and whether this could be degenerative osteoarthritis of the shoulder joint itself, a very painful problem that requires joint replacement. Or an infected shoulder joint. I glance at her chart: no fever.

"Wow, okay. Let me take a look again." I gently withdraw the right side of her same cardigan, again revealing the tank top.

"I'm sorry, I haven't been able to change my clothes for a week."

"It's okay. It's fine."

But it's not fine. Just next to the AC joint, I see a walnut-size, multicolored, oozing nodule emerging from her collarbone. It has a fetid odor. I put my gloves on and slowly work my way from her midline down the length of the collarbone, gently pushing and prodding the bone as I proceed. As I approach the nodule, she again winces in pain, and tears well up in her eyes.

Damn it. I realize it's likely a *Pancoast tumor*. A rare cause of shoulder pain, a Pancoast tumor is an aggressive type of lung cancer arising in the upper lobe of the right lung that can present with shoulder pain, although typically with no pain with shoulder movement. But in her case, eight weeks prior, her shoulder had hurt when she moved it because the tumor likely had already invaded the collarbone. It is not surprising that I had misdiagnosed it, and the fact that she presented with bone pain meant that it had already been inoperable at that time. But I still feel guilty, and I vow to do right by her moving forward. Because, damn it, now the cancer is eating through that bone and is eroding out of the skin of her upper chest.

"Are you able to see this? This spot that is so tender?" I ask as I point to her AC joint.

She gingerly rotates her arthritic neck down and to the right, and her eyes follow suit. "See what?"

I detach the little mirror from the clinic wall above the sink. I sit beside her and place my finger on her distal collarbone as I hold the mirror in front of her.

"This painful bump. Can you see it now?"

"Oh yes. Yes, I do. What is it? It looks *awful*," she says to my reflection in the mirror.

"I think this bump is the reason you are in so much pain. I noticed you coughing a lot when I came in. Have you been coughing more since I last saw you?"

"Seems like that's all I do. Cough and cry, cough and cry."

"Hmmm. That is worrisome. Okay, look, you were honest with me. Can I be honest with you?"

"Doctor, after seventy years, I can't stand any beatin' around the bush."

I say to her reflection in the mirror, "I am worried that you have a cancer in that right upper lung. And I am worried that this lung cancer has grown through to this shoulder bone next to that lung and that this cancer is now pushing its way through your bone to your skin. And it's really painful when it does this."

She turns to try to look at me directly. I put down the mirror and roll my chair across from hers.

"And so, what do we do now?" she asks, her chin jutting forward in a show of courage.

"Well, now I wheel you over to x-ray to see if there is a spot or two or three in your right lung. And get x-rays of that shoulder too and of a whole bunch of your bones. In other words, we need to find out if my guess as to what is going on is right. As you know, I've been wrong before, so maybe I'll be wrong again."

"And what if you're not wrong? Then what?"

"Well, either way, we'd need to get a piece of this lump and take a look at it under the microscope. If it shows you have lung cancer, then I think we would need to treat it with radiation. Radiation can shrink the tumor and reduce your pain. You'd take those treatments every day or so for a number of weeks. And sometimes we can add chemotherapy too. But that's getting a bit ahead of ourselves."

"I see."

"Like I said, I'm here. And you're here. So, let me take you down to x-ray to take some pictures of this beautiful lady. And let's take this thing one step at a time, okay? Together. Let me just call my wife to let her know I'll be getting home a bit later than usual, and then off we go."

A MIDSUMMER NIGHT'S PROJECT

Summer 1969. Buffalo, New York. The Ferry Grider housing project. I am almost four years old. It's hot. I'm wearing a wet, white tank top, unhappily sporting the fresh crew cut my father forced us boys to get each summer to avoid the louse-borne diseases that killed so many in his concentration camp.

"Typhus!" my father would spit out at us whenever I tearfully questioned him as to why he had to shave off our hair.

I am splashing with my older brother in the little blue, plastic swimming pool my parents had placed in the small, chained-in communal front yard. I am still wearing my cheap, but oh-so-special, Pro-Ked lookalike high-top sneakers, because I never take them off. Sometimes I stand on one foot atop the chains between the poles, trying to balance myself like a surfer riding a wave.

I was born and spent my early years in these housing projects. My parents, highly educated but newly immigrated, spoke five languages between them but could only afford federally subsidized public housing. My mother was scared of mentioning to others that she originally was from Chile. She had cried when, in 1963, as a young couple, they had moved here from Jerusalem. From the "Joyful City" of the promised land to the capital city of the Rust Belt. From her sunny apartment overlooking the Judean Hills—made from the glowing, off-white Jerusalem stone—to a sterile and garbage-ridden compound composed of red blocks of brick surrounded by other blocks of brick amid a sea of urban decay. For what? To pursue the American dream?

My father, ever since his liberation at the hands of US soldiers and his recovery from tuberculosis and hepatitis at the hands of US physicians, had vowed someday to move to America and become a doctor. A survivor of a world war in Europe in 1945 and an anti-Soviet revolution in Hungary in 1956, he had emigrated to the only country that would accept him: the young nation of Israel. But this was just a placeholder for him: just another war-torn country getting in the way of his reaching his ultimate destination—the land of freedom, peace, self-determination, and prosperity—at least for some.

So now we are in Buffalo. He is doing his residency training in urologic surgery and is rarely home. His take-home pay is $250 a month. My mother tries to fill the gaps teaching Hebrew part-time at the local Jewish day school, but they pay a pittance. So, we are stuck here for now. But she knows it is only temporary.

My brother and I jump into the little blue pool under the watchful eye of my Hungarian-only-speaking grandfather, a benign, silent presence in my early childhood. The sounds of televisions spill out from the windows above us, accompanied by the ever-present cigarette smoke. The night before, our parents had let us stay up very late to watch Neil Armstrong descend the staircase of Apollo 11 and step onto the lunar surface. My father had rejoiced, "This country can do anything!" Like many, I will never forget witnessing that moment in human history.

The other TV image I can recall—my earliest—is of the five overlapping rings of the Olympics accompanied by the majestic Olympics theme song. Mexico City. Black athletes standing with raised fists on the medal podium below American flags, the US national anthem playing. What was everyone so upset about?

A man and a woman yell at each other from our neighbors' apartment, and I stop splashing.

"It's Mr. and Mrs. Mills. . . . Just ignore them," my newly buzz-cut older brother says, surprise-splashing me in the face.

"Not fair! Time-out!" I splash back hard and fast.

About once or twice a month, my parents would go out for the evening, leaving us boys under the tender loving care of our next-door neighbor, Mrs. Mills. The moment they left, she would plant her oversize body in the only soft armchair we had, just in front of the open kitchen of our small apartment.

Always wearing her see-through nightgown and once-fluffy slippers, and crowned with curlers, she'd immediately light up in one hand and open a can of beer with the other. And do it again. And again. All this while balancing a big bag of orange Cheetos in her lap. That was her official babysitting posture. While I don't remember her ever raising a finger to help us, I still can remember watching in awe as her pendulous skin would waddle each time that she lifted her right arm to take a chug of her beer.

But most of all, I was amazed by the void of her mouth, by its absence of any teeth, a dark and gaping hole encircled by an orange halo of Cheeto-dusted lips.

"Can you actually chew food with no teeth, Mrs. Mills?" I would ask, as only an almost-four-year-old can.

What she lacked in dentition was more than matched by the vocalizations that came out of that mouth.

She'd first take a puckered suck on the orange-dusted cigarette end and then growl, "I'd have no problem chewing you up, little boy!"

She terrified me.

And then there was Mr. Mills. He would make only rare appearances during our babysitting sessions, pounding on our door until his wife was able to rock herself back and forth enough times to gain the momentum needed to catapult herself from the armchair. Nearly falling forward off the chair, she'd just manage to right herself while somehow deftly placing her can of beer on the floor on her way up. Then she'd slip and slide over the linoleum floor to open the banging door. She'd stand at the threshold, blocking her husband from entering with one blubbery arm cast against the side of the doorjamb, the other on her hip. She'd just stand there and get an earful from him. His face red and full of pockmarks, his hair slicked straight back, his big shoulders and biceps bulging from his white T-shirt, his voice booming, he'd spew forth a jumble of slurred words from another edentulous mouth. All I could discern was that he was yelling at her. Had we been bad? Was she not supposed to be here with us? She'd yell right back, using words I couldn't always understand. She'd slam the door on him, bolt it shut, and slip and slide toward the kitchen, stopping to pivot in her slippers before slowly backing into her armchair, muttering to herself in that incomprehensible language. We knew we were not supposed to talk to her after one of those screaming matches.

We were poor, for now. My older brother, jealous of the toys his school
friends had, had begged my mother to buy him a Big Wheel, a low-riding
plastic tricycle with an oversize front wheel and a hand brake on the right
that would make you do a 360 if you yanked on it at top speed. On the frequent occasions during which we accompanied my mother on her shopping
errands, he'd spend his time just staring at the Big Wheels in the discount
department store.

After putting him off for days and trying to mollify him with indirect answers, she finally admitted, "Donny, I am sorry. We just don't have enough
money to buy you a Big Wheel. Maybe next year, for your birthday."

Undeterred, he naïvely countered, "But why don't you just go to Kmart
and buy some money?"

I can't imagine what my mother paid Mrs. Mills to watch over us, if that's
what you call it. A few hours here, a few hours there, perhaps a dollar each
time, at most. Mrs. Mills was my mother's go-to coverage, including during
the day when she had to leave us to work her part-time job. As a result, our
apartment—my bedsheets, my towels, my shirts, everything—always bore
the unmistakable smell of Mrs. Mills. What I now recognize to be the stale
stench of deep-seated tobacco residue and spilled beer, mixed with the sour
odor of lifelong poverty, combined with a hopeless sense of entrapment.
Those two people would never leave the projects.

WHAT ARE THE ODDS?

With some primary care heroics, I manage to schedule Mrs. Johnson to receive daily radiation therapy for stage IV lung cancer over the course of the
subsequent weeks. But now I need to find a way to get her there and back
with consistency. I gradually discover that many medical transport companies are averse to daily routes to and from the Sunnydale projects, because of
both its isolation and—they tell me—the risk it exposes to their drivers and
vehicles. I scoff. I go down the list my social worker gave me and speak to a
representative that is movable on the issue, and after a personal appeal to her
humanity related to reducing the horrible cancer pain that a kind little old
lady is in, I get her to agree to supply Mrs. Johnson with the daily transport
service she requires.

Two weeks later, I receive a call from the Radiation Oncology Department technician telling me that Mrs. Johnson has made it to only about half of her radiation treatments.

"She missed hers today. And since she doesn't have a phone, I can't ask her what happened," she tells me. "I think the radiation's been helping her with the pain, but not as much as it could. After the two-week mark, we tend to discontinue radiation treatment with this kind of noncompliance. It's not benefiting her that much, and it's a slot that we aren't offering to another patient who could take full advantage."

"Don't go there, please," I plead. "When's her next appointment?"

She shuffles some papers. "Tomorrow at 2:00 p.m."

"Okay. What do you think the chance is that she'll make it tomorrow?"

"What is this? Are we rolling dice in Vegas?"

"C'mon, I'm just trying to figure out what to do here. I'm not gonna hold you to it."

"I'd say two out of three."

"That's not bad. Please page me at 2:30 tomorrow. Either way. If she comes, I'll come up and speak to her. If not, I'll figure this out some other way."

I search through her chart and confirm that she has no phone number listed. Instead, I find the phone number of the transport company, hoping to find out what's happening from their perspective, but I can only leave a message.

At 2:30 the next day, the transport tech pages me. Mrs. Johnson is a no-show. I ask her to give me Mrs. Johnson's home address, and I scratch it onto a piece of paper. I leave the hospital around 5:30, walk to the parking garage, and get into my sparkling new red Honda Civic hatchback. Instead of going straight home, I meander through the city streets in rush hour and slowly merge onto Highway 101 South toward the airport. I'm going to make an unannounced home visit in the Sunnydale projects.

RETURN OF THE GREATEST GENERATION

Over the years, I had gotten to know Frank Johnson and his war stories fairly well. And a bit about what happened after. When the twenty-five-year-old Frank returned from World War II as a victorious soldier, one of many in

"the Greatest Generation," he looked first for a job, then for a woman to spend
his life with, and finally for a place to live in with her and their future family.
He quickly scored on all three, first finding work as a barber in a local shop
and then meeting a lovely girl, eight years his junior, in the same building he
lived in. While he had found a small, low-rent, one-bedroom apartment in
the Fillmore District, it was not the kind of place one brings a new wife to.
So, he asked some of his war buddies and found out that Daly City, a small
coastal city bordering San Francisco to its south, was a place where many
returning veterans were making a fresh start, a place where new homes were
popping up at very low cost for people just like Frank. And he was turned on
to the newly formed Veterans Administration (VA), established under the
GI Bill. He had heard that as a returning veteran, you could get a mortgage
with help from the VA.

With two exceptions. First, the Federal Housing Administration, which
helped to finance the development of Daly City, had enforced deeds with re-
strictive language that forbade the resale of property to Blacks. This 1950
covenant on property in Daly City is quite clear on the matter:

> The property . . . shall never be occupied, used or resided on by any person not
> of the white or Caucasian race, except in the capacity of a servant or domestic
> employed thereon by a white Caucasian owner, tenant or occupant.

So, Frank looked to the east a bit—to South San Francisco. Not a new
development, South San Francisco, known as the Industrial City, offered
lower-cost houses that might be within their reach. Especially with the VA
behind him to help returning soldiers with their mortgages. But the VA
had also adopted racial exclusion programs enacted by the Federal Housing
Administration and previously determined to be constitutional by our Supreme Court. Specifically, he discovered that government funds could only
be used to insure mortgages for individuals who were not African American, including for returning veterans, irrespective of income, wealth, or
assets. Without mortgage insurance, no bank would lend to a future home-
owner. This represented a particularly insidious form of redlining, one
sponsored by the state.

In essence, no African American could buy a home. And owning a home is the essence of the American dream. The consequences of these exclusionary housing laws and practices were not only felt in the short term but have had long-term effects. A house purchased in 1950 in a Daly City development cost around $15,000. In 2022, the average sale price of such homes is over $1.1 million. That kind of money and that kind of wealth can dramatically change the trajectory of a family. And when aggregated across families, it can transform the destiny of an entire community.

So—back to Frank and Beatrice. The couple had no choice but to stay in the Fillmore District, splitting their time between Beatrice's family's larger two-bedroom apartment and, when privacy was needed, Frank's one-bedroom apartment. After holding off for nearly a decade so they could save up a little money, they had two children. Space was cramped and was a challenge, but they were happy. They were part of a vibrant community located in one hub of the city's multifaceted cultural and social life.

But then, with the urban redevelopment of the Fillmore District, they found themselves one of the unlucky ones. They were displaced, along with Beatrice's family. They had nowhere else to go but the Sunnydale projects, a development created at the beginning of World War II to house the influx of shipyard workers. That much I knew. But at that time, that was all that I knew.

PASSAGE INTO A FOREIGN LAND

I slowly crawl down Highway 101, leaving the city behind me, exiting the highway to my right just as Candlestick Park and the Bay appear over my left shoulder. The sun is setting behind the mountain range to my right, and the pastel-colored homes of South San Francisco appear in the distance. Dusk is settling in as I slowly wind my way up the long road to an open area filled with windswept, high, dry, and yellow grass. As I drive on through this eerie wilderness, I enter what can only be described as a large institutional compound. One dotted with rectangular, gray and yellow two-story structures made of concrete. Too many to count. Cell blocks almost. A corner store appears— the Little Village Market—what I later learn is the only store for miles. I see a woman exit the store, holding the hand of a boy who looks about five years old, his free hand trying to pour a bag of Red Hot Cheetos into his mouth as she drags him along. In the woman's other hand is an open twenty-ounce bottle of beer and a lit cigarette. She glares at me as I drift past in my shiny red car, presumably a defiant response to my glaring at her.

I drive by cell block after cell block, repeatedly stopping to try to see the building numbers to orient myself so I can locate Mrs. Johnson's building. There are no streetlights anywhere. Each time I get out of my car, a different man appears, stepping out from behind one of the cell blocks. They each wear a flat-billed baseball cap (is it the same cap each time?) atop a shaved head, and each is dressed in black and smoking a cigarette. They each look at me as if I need something, projecting a strange combination of threat and offering. I see two little girls on tricycles bumping their way down a garbage-strewn hill. Other than these two and the men that haunt the shadows of each block— these Sunnydale guardians in uniform—the streets are empty of people. Only a few beat-up cars dot the curbs.

A young man in a cap approaches me just as I am bending down to get back into my car. An unlit cigarette dangling from his lips, he gives me an upward head flinch.

"Whassup?"

I abort my entrance into my car and stand back up to face him.

"Yes, hello. I am looking for Mrs. Beatrice Johnson. I need to see her. I am her doctor. I work at San Francisco General Hospital."

I flip him my hospital badge and open my bag to show him my stethoscope, as if somehow this will safely pave the way to the destination I am in search of.

"Yeah, Mrs. Bea. I know her. Nice lady. Keep goin' and take a right at the end here. She in the second building on the left."

"Thanks. Have a good night."

"Yeah, you too."

Despite his clear directions, I feel disoriented as I slowly drive away. The usual signposts that signify that I am in my city, that I am in California, and that I am in the US are simply nowhere to be seen. I feel as though I am in an entirely foreign country, a brutal land that operates under different rules, rules unknown to me.

THE HOME VISIT

I inch my car forward, and, shining my flashlight out my window, I spot the numbered building and then the lettered door that correspond to the address I have scribbled down. A light is on in the ground-floor apartment. I park on the street, get out, and slam the door shut, double-checking that it is locked. I spot another man, a large man, appear from behind the building's corner and start to come my way. He too has a shaved head but is not wearing the cap. I pause for a moment but then decide to proceed to the front door, tobacco smoke wafting my way. I pull back the screen door and knock. No answer.

I knock again and hear a woman yelling, "Tyreke, go see who at the door. But don't open it!"

I hear the shuffling of feet from inside, and I wait. It feels as though it is taking Tyreke forever. The soldier is getting closer. Am I wrong to feel scared?

A boy who looks about eight years old shows his head out the little window beside the door. He's looking me up and down.

I shout through the window, "Tyreke. Please tell Mrs. Johnson that her doctor is here."

I hear him run to the back of the apartment.

"Auntie, there's a white man who say . . ." But his voice fades away.

The large man with the shaved head has reached the doorway. He is older than the others and older than I am.

"You her doctor?"

"Yes, sir. Mrs. Johnson's doctor. I need to talk to her, to see how she is doing."

He puts out his hand. "Cornelius."

"How you doing?" I respond, shaking his hand. "I'm her doctor, like I said."

He moves me aside and proclaims to the door, "Bea! . . . Bea! Your doctor's come. Open up! Mary, open up for her! He needs to talk to Bea."

He turns to me and says, "Be just a minute."

A woman whom I presume to be Mary opens the door. She is younger than Mrs. Johnson, has thin tubes in her nostrils, and pulls a small oxygen tank on wheels behind her.

"You her doctor?"

"Yes, I am. Are you Mary, her sister?"

"I am. I heard some nice things about you."

"You gonna let this man in, or we gonna do this out on the porch?" Cornelius asks.

"Well, come on in, then. And I guess you can come in too, Cornelius. Assuming you wanna hear what he has to say . . ."

We enter the small apartment right into the kitchen. A round table with a red-checked plastic tablecloth is surrounded by four unmatched chairs. The kitchen is clean.

I hear Mrs. Johnson calmly speaking in the back of the apartment. And then she appears in the hallway to the kitchen, quilt on her lap. Tyreke pushes her forward in her wheelchair. She's wearing a nightgown, but the shoulder nodule is covered with a large square of white gauze and tape. She is much thinner than even three weeks prior.

"Ain't this a surprise!" she beams. "Doctor, I believe they used to call these visits 'house calls.' I don't recall getting a house call for over sixty years. I think it was the measles."

She is again bent in that awkward torso position that shows me she is still in pain.

"Well, you've always come to me. I figured that it's high time I visited you. Is that okay? I couldn't reach you by phone. So, I thought I'd just check in on you in person."

"Of course, of course."

She slowly turns her head to the side and yells, "Janelle! C'mon in here. It's my doctor! He's with Mr. Jones. Please come make us some tea."

Cornelius quickly moves one of the chairs aside. Tyreke wheels Mrs. Johnson into the space at the table.

"Do sit down, Doctor. It really is so nice of you to come. I am sorry we don't have much to offer you, but I hope a cup a tea will sit nice with you? You too, Mr. Jones."

Mary slowly approaches the table, oxygen rolling behind her.

I can't help myself. I turn to her.

"I'm sorry. But is someone smoking in the house? I only ask because cigarette smoke and high-flow oxygen don't mix well. It can cause an explosion at worst or a fire at best."

Mary rolls her eyes.

"No. But all our neighbors—up above us and on each side of us—smoke. We been smelling that smoke for years, even after Bea's husband, Frank, passed. I quit fifteen years ago, but a lot a good that did me. I still have the emphysema. And little Tyreke, he got asthma bad."

"It's not that bad," says a young woman, presumably Janelle. She looks about eight months pregnant. "It's gettin' better, and you know it."

Tyreke looks back and forth between Mary and Janelle, whom I assume is his mother. She pours us some hot tea into nonmatching cups placed on saucers of various colors and sizes.

Mrs. Johnson takes over the conversation with her characteristic tranquil voice.

"I'm not the only one who's sick in the household, you know, Doctor. Mary's got emphysema and is chained to that oxygen all day and night. Janelle has the sugar diabetes now that she's pregnant, which is not good for the baby. And little Tyreke, my handsome grandson, he has asthma, like my sister said. He missed lots of school this year already. Seems like everyone is sick around here. Except for Mr. Jones here. He's gentle, but he's strong as an ox," she says with a smile, patting the back of Cornelius's hand.

"Well, Bea, you yourself know this ain't no place to raise a family. At least not a healthy one."

Mrs. Johnson nods in agreement, wincing in pain.

"Mr. Jones is a bit of an expert on the subject, Doctor. He even convinced the *San Francisco Chronicle* to talk about it. Tyreke, honey, can you grab that old newspaper I keep in that bottom drawer over there?" she asks, pointing her knobby index finger at the area under the sink.

"Bea, he don't wanna see that."

"Actually, I do. This is the first time I've ever been to Sunnydale. I want to read what was written about living here."

Tyreke hands the newspaper to his grandma. Mrs. Johnson hands it to me, showing me a full-page story with photos of the Sunnydale buildings and an abandoned and decrepit playground. She points that knobby finger at three circled paragraphs.

"Here it is, Doctor. Read what they said, and it's thanks to Mr. Jones."

I take the paper in my hands and shoot a glance at Cornelius.

"That's right. Read it out loud, Doctor. Mr. Jones is a real fighter, he is. And he is an eloquent man."

Mr. Jones whispers to me that it isn't he who was quoted but another Jones from Sunnydale. Nonetheless, as the dark envelops Sunnydale projects, I read to the little group gathered around the checked table:

Most San Franciscans never see Sunnydale, unless they play at the nearby Gleneagles golf course or get lost trying to avoid traffic on Highway 101. Afraid to come in after dusk, the cable guy makes only morning appointments, and Muni bus drivers often refuse to enter after dark. Garbage isn't picked up regularly. In Sunnydale, many residents subsist on the change they make from underground businesses, like stores run out of their apartments that offer junk food and cigarettes, haircuts and pirated DVDs. Because of Sunnydale's isolation, underground stores are popular. There is no post office or coin-operated laundry, no grocery stores or even fast-food restaurants. Residents shop at the Little Village Market, a convenience store located near the entrance to the development that is stocked with harsh cigarettes, junk food and cheap booze. Others are afraid to go into the store because there is always a large group of men loitering outside. Unlike most of San Francisco, in Sunnydale, you can't really walk to anything.

Though the housing is designed to be temporary, residents stay for decades. A combination of factors—geographic isolation, extreme poverty and a lack of access to social services—make it virtually impossible to leave Sunnydale. There are no stepping-stones to something better, no road map for how to get out. Parents want to encourage their children to go to school, where they could get an education and a better job, but they get robbed at the bus stop.

"People hide and catch you off guard. The kids hang out in front of the bus stop and usually are up to no good," said 55-year-old Cornelius Jones, who runs an underground barbershop in the development. "Then at night, the place isn't even lit up." He knows a woman who refuses to let her son take the bus home from school because he will get hurt before she gets home. So the boy stays with relatives until she can pick him up.

"We don't have role models," said Jones. "We don't go to Harvard. We barely have police. We have to take care of ourselves. This is like a concentration camp. There is no way out unless you die."

I put the newspaper down and look at Mrs. Johnson.

"You were right. Those are some powerful words."

I take a sip of my tea and go on.

"Mrs. Johnson, I heard you've missed a number of your radiation treatments. Does the medical van just sometimes not show up because you live in Sunnydale?"

She starts to answer but is seized by a coughing fit. Cornelius places his hand on her back to support her.

She catches her breath and starts up. "Sometimes they show up; sometimes they don't. And other times, they do come, but the driver tells me that he can't bring me back home, so he gives me the choice of getting in or staying home. Since there's no other way I can get home from the hospital, I choose to stay here with Mary and Janelle, and sometimes Tyreke. With the people I love."

Cornelius, seemingly offended, jumps in. "Bea, you gotta *tell* me when that happens so I can have a word with that driver. I tell you it won't happen again."

"Every time's a different driver, Mr. Jones." And then, in a quieter voice, "So it ain't no use."

Her statement hangs in the air, a declaration of personal powerlessness and communal forfeit around her own kitchen table.

"Mr. Jones is right," I retort. "This is not acceptable. I'll report the company to Medicare and Medicaid. That way, it's not a driver problem but a company problem. And that way I'm the bad guy, not you all. Will you let me do that?"

"You've always done right by me, Doctor. Why would I get in your way now?"

As I exit the apartment and descend the sidewalk toward my car, I see the lights of Daly City and South San Francisco twinkling off in the distance.

PRELUDE TO AN OBITUARY

Over the next several weeks, I make some headway on Mrs. Johnson's behalf. The transit company balks at my threat to report them and commits to consistent round-trips for her to complete her radiation treatment. The Radiation Oncology Department agrees to continue her treatments.

I check in on Mrs. Johnson a few times in the treatment room, and while she tells me that the shoulder pain is better, it is clear that she is rapidly dwindling.

Having orchestrated a successful completion of her radiation treatments, I make two more visits to Mrs. Johnson in Sunnydale. At my last visit, the pain in her shoulder is now unbearable, her coughing is worse, and her weight has dropped even further, despite the two cases of nutritional supplements I had brought her.

She and I are sitting alone around her kitchen table. We discuss the option of chemotherapy and the option of home hospice.

"I had a difficult life, Doctor. That's for sure. There's no reason to make it difficult at the end too."

I ask her if she wants to be in the hospital, at a hospice, or here at home.

"Like Mr. Jones said, there's no way out of Sunnydale unless you die. Well, this is my home. I've lived here, and I'll die here. Just help me go in peace."

I leave her a small bottle of long-acting morphine tablets and recommend she take them for pain every twelve hours, rain or shine. Or every eight hours if, after a day or two, she finds they provide inadequate relief. I tell her I'll be back in a week. I give her my cell phone number and tell her to have Mr. Jones call me if she needs more pain medication or anything else.

A few days later, at 8:00 a.m., my phone rings.

"Hi, Doc. It's Cornelius, Mrs. Bea's neighbor. She passed last night. Mary found her in her bed. Thank you for providing comfort to her in these last weeks."

CANCER'S ROOT CAUSE

As with many white families in the late '60s, my parents were able to get a mortgage on a house and we moved out of the Ferry Grider project. As the housing policy planners planned, we landed in the suburbs, in a good neighborhood with good schools. With my mother conveniently avoiding mention of her Hispanic heritage, we moved into a mostly white neighborhood named Williamsville, New York. We had benefited from the unique American privilege of not being Black, and we were behaving just as we were expected to. And we were able to buy a yellow-and-red Big Wheel that my brother and I would do 360s on, over and over down our driveway.

Over four decades later, and a few years after Mrs. Johnson's death, I am dropping my oldest son off to start his first year at Oberlin College in Ohio. A gifted upright jazz bass player, he was accepted to its highly regarded jazz conservatory with a partial scholarship. I help him outfit his dorm room, and as a last touch, we hang the giant poster of Charlie Mingus that I had bought him as a high school graduation gift, a semiabstract rendering of the great jazz legend playing his bass, notes cascading down and off his fingerboard like songbirds taking wing.

Since we still have three days before his school officially starts, I ask him if he wants to take a road trip to see my old haunts in Buffalo, a three-hour drive up the Lake Erie coast. Having heard my colorful tales of growing up in that remarkably unique and resilient city, he quickly agrees. After a wet visit to the still stunning Niagara Falls, we make a stop so I can revisit Ferry Grider, the project that had been my home for my first four years of life. It looks unchanged to me. Except now all the residents are Black. The opportunity to escape to the suburbs or to a nicer place in the city, to not be trapped amid other families of similar means and similar life trajectories marked by desperation, seemed to have escaped them.

But now I better understand how discriminatory federal and local housing and lending policies conspired with development policies marred by racism to ensure that the Ferry Grider project became filled with Black folk. That it was destined to become one blighted part of a predominantly Black neighborhood. That where and how the different colors of our nation live, and the extent to which the accumulation of wealth associated with home-ownership and its attendant social mobility are unequally apportioned, result, in large part, from a deep-seated and pervasive social malady—a form of state-sponsored segregation and racism—whose long-lasting effects are still evident. And how that reality and those kinds of environments, from which escape is close to impossible, shaped the health of Mrs. Johnson and those of her generation and continue to determine the health of generations after them.

The legislative and regulatory housing and development policies and practices that disadvantaged people of color have been subject to over the last century represent a cancer in the communal body politic. Our failure to recognize how these policies and practices generate social and health disparities—and our unwillingness to make amends for this failure—mean that this invisible cancer is allowed to systematically erode the very bones of our communities. But perhaps there is hope for Sunnydale. A recent private-public partnership in San Francisco, HOPE SF, sponsored by the Mayor's Office of Housing and the San Francisco Housing Authority, has generated master plans and fostered an associated community engagement process to reinvest and redevelop Sunnydale as a mixed-use housing development in partnership with a non-profit, lower-income housing development agency. Whether this new promise will be fully kept—over fifty years after the unfulfilled promise related to the displacement of the Fillmore District residents—remains to be seen.

A wise and experienced colleague of mine known by most as Dr. Dan—someone who has worked as a primary care doctor in the safety net for fifty years—shared with me that, sometimes, when a patient of his dies—especially a patient who has been socially isolated—he writes an obituary for them. Because he knows that nobody else will. After waiting a week to make sure no other obituary is published, he pulls together the bits and pieces of people's stories that he had gradually become familiar with, writing as if he were an intimate family member seeking to memorialize a loved one. He then pays to get them printed in the *San Francisco Chronicle*. This would honor both the patient and his relationship with that patient, as well as bring closure to a difficult struggle.

A week after I received the call from Cornelius informing me of Mrs. Johnson's death, no obituary had yet appeared in memory of Mrs. Johnson. So, I wrote one. But I never submitted it to the newspaper for publication. I have placed it here instead.

PART 3

Story as Catalyst

CHAPTER 18

Walking on Coals: Melanie's Story

DISEASE, AND THE SUFFERING THAT ACCOMPANIES IT, IS NEVER FAIR. But some patients' suffering is so unjust that it serves as a catalyst for broader change. A flash that sheds light on the immorality of the status quo, a spark that ignites a movement to prevent future suffering. About twenty-five years ago, I began caring for a lovely young woman of African American and Latinx heritage. She had a gentle way about her, and from the very beginning, she was open to discussing her life prior to her chronic diagnoses. A survivor of childhood trauma, Melanie struggled on and off with depression. She also had a lifelong addiction to nicotine and to sugar-sweetened beverages (SSBs). She described how SSBs were a special comfort to her, providing a lift to days that otherwise were weighed down by the blues. She told me that, when she was a child, her mother gave her SSBs with every meal and one more at snack time, and that her hands-down favorite was Hawaiian Punch Fruit Juicy Red. Her mother had always thought she was serving her a real fruit drink. But Hawaiian Punch, marketed as a fruit drink with particular targeting to African Americans and Latinxs, has only 5 percent fruit juice; the rest is high-fructose corn syrup and artificial colors. With four teaspoons of sugar in every eight ounces, she had grown up drinking sixteen teaspoons of sugar each day. Over ten years, she had consumed over 234 pounds of liquid sugar, over three times her body weight.

As an adult, she had graduated to 7UP, drinking three 7UPs a day, translating to twenty-seven teaspoons of sugar a day (7UP has nine teaspoons of sugar per twelve-ounce can). Like most Americans at the beginning of the twenty-first century, she was unaware that this degree of exposure to liquid sugar could lead to diabetes. Unfortunately, she had acquired type 2 diabetes in her late twenties. When I first met her, by the time she was thirty years old, she had consumed 2,860 pounds of added sugars solely from SSBs. Greater than a ton of liquid sugar. In this regard, she was no different from many lower-income young adults in the US, especially those of African American and Latinx heritage. Her ailments were, in some way then, unsurprising.

But to understand why Melanie acquired diabetes requires us to move beyond her individual dietary choices, zooming out to view the context in which she lived. Like the pioneering founder of modern epidemiology and public health, Dr. John Snow, we can begin to understand Melanie's story by looking at some city maps.

Melanie was born and raised in a rental unit in Bayview–Hunters Point in San Francisco, in zip code 94124, located in the southeast corner of the city (see Figure 1). Bayview has the largest concentration of Black residents in the city. It is also home to the city's only power plant and resultant environmental hazards. It also is widely recognized as the city's only "food desert"—devoid of supermarkets, but flush with corner liquor stores and fast-food joints, and lacking adequate safe spaces for recreation and physical activity. My hospital and clinic serve this zip code, its adjacent zip codes, and those of other lower-income neighborhoods, mostly populated by other people of color.

Despite the presence of San Francisco General Hospital (SFGH) and its associated community clinics, rates of hospitalization for consequences of uncontrolled diabetes—such as acute kidney failure, diabetic coma, and amputations—vary exponentially. Differences in rates are a function of differences in both the prevalence of diabetes in the local environment, on the one hand, and differences in the control of the disease via medical care, on the other. In the Marina District (zip code 94123) in 2009, which

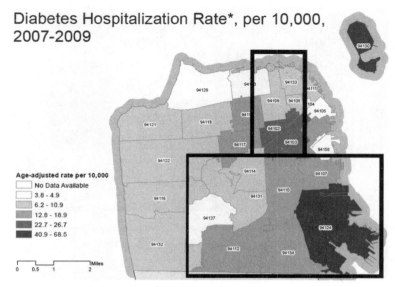

Figure 1. Rates of hospitalization for diabetes, by neighborhood zip code, San Francisco, CA, 2007–2009. Courtesy of the San Francisco Department of Public Health.

is not in SFGH's catchment area and is disproportionately populated by higher-income, mostly white individuals with private health insurance, only four to five individuals out of every ten thousand residents were hospitalized for uncontrolled diabetes each year. In contrast, in Bayview, between forty and seventy individuals out of every ten thousand residents were hospitalized for uncontrolled diabetes each year, a ten- to fifteenfold disparity. The inverted T shown in Figure 1 reflects the diabetes hot spots of San Francisco, delineating the borders between those neighborhoods that protect their residents from diabetes and those that promote diabetes among their residents.

These vast health disparities are a product of differences in social and environmental exposures that individuals and populations experience. In fact, type 2 diabetes is the poster child for how social and environmental conditions generate and promote disease. San Francisco, like most cities in the US, is socioeconomically segregated, and neighborhood environments vary in parallel. The inverted T pattern in Figure 1 is mirrored in the patterns of per capita income across the city's neighborhoods (see Figure 2). In 2009, the Marina residents' annual income averaged over $100,000 while those in Bayview averaged about $20,000.

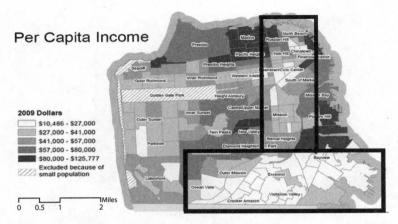

Figure 2. Ranges of per capita income by neighborhood, San Francisco, CA, 2009 dollars. Courtesy of the San Francisco Department of Public Health.

Similarly, the pattern of SSB consumption—now a known antecedent to type 2 diabetes—reflects this inverted T, with the highest consumers residing within the T, and the lowest consumers living outside it (see Figure 3). Similar patterns can be observed for other social predictors of type 2 diabetes, including food insecurity, fast-food outlets, trauma and violence, air pollution, unsafe spaces to exercise, and rates of physical inactivity.

The unhealthy social and environmental exposures occurring in the inverted T did not appear by accident. Rather, they are but one reflection of the legacy of racism in America, including one legalized form of racism: redlining. The map in Figure 4, printed in 1937, was created by the Home Owners Loan Corporation (HOLC). It shows San Francisco neighborhoods shaded with four different markers. HOLC maps were created by government surveyors during the 1930s that graded neighborhoods in and around 239 cities, where more "hazardous" neighborhoods were deemed risks to banks. Light gray represents "best" or "still desirable," medium gray is "definitely declining," and dark gray represents "hazardous." Banks used the maps to discriminate against people of color, denying home loans to residents of these locations. Such maps served as one means to deny people of color entry to higher-income, "whiter" neighborhoods outside the redlined areas while also preventing them from purchasing a home within the redlined areas—an investment that would have had long term-benefits for the individuals and the community. Today, those neighborhoods that once were in the redlined areas have lower incomes and

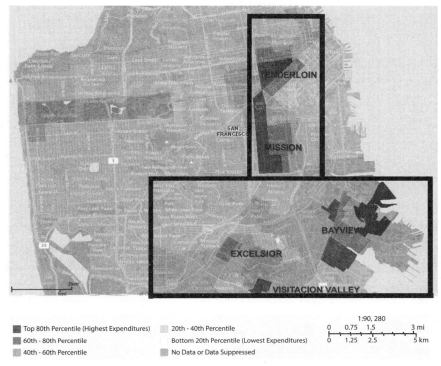

■ Top 80th Percentile (Highest Expenditures)	▨ 20th - 40th Percentile
▨ 60th - 80th Percentile	░ Bottom 20th Percentile (Lowest Expenditures)
▨ 40th - 60th Percentile	▨ No Data or Data Suppressed

1:90, 280

0   0.75   1.5   3 mi
0   1.25   2.5   5 km

Figure 3. Average daily sugar-sweetened beverage consumption by neighborhood in San Francisco, CA. Map generated using communitycommons.org, courtesy of Roberto Ariel Vargas, MPH.

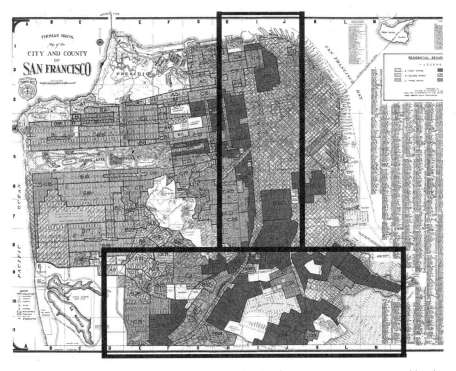

Figure 4. Modified map based on the color-coded map of San Francisco, CA, created by the Home Owners Loan Corporation (1937). Dark areas represent red-lined zones.

worse health outcomes. A recent study of diabetes-related mortality in King County, Washington, demonstrated that those who live in areas once deemed yellow or red have nearly double the rate of death from diabetes of those who live in areas once deemed blue or green. In other words, the health effects of redlining persist more than fifty years after the practice was outlawed.

Melanie grew up and lived in the epicenter of the T, in the heart of a low-income and historically redlined neighborhood. Her diabetes was poorly controlled. Despite my best efforts and hers, her disease slowly ravaged her body, leaving her with partial blindness, neuropathy that left her legs with painful tingling and an absence of real sensation, and worsening depression due to failing health at the prime of her life. She was soon unable to work.

At a routine follow-up visit one summer night in 2008, she waited for me in the clinic room with her partner and very helpful caregiver, Jean, by her side, as always. Before I entered, I pulled together my happy face. Melanie could be a downer, her depressed mood casting a shadow on most visits. After giving them both a warm hug, I glanced at her hospital card and took a quick look at her date of birth, as is my habit.

"Oh my gosh!" I exclaimed, trying to set a positive tone. "Today is your birthday! And you've hit the big four-oh. Wow. That's a biggie. Very exciting. Congrats. Happy birthday."

She gave me a shy smile, a smile that revealed the advanced tooth decay and gum disease so common in people with diabetes.

"How're you doing with it? I just turned forty last year, and, well, maybe I shouldn't tell you this, but it was harder on me than I thought it'd be. I hope you sail through it."

They both gave me giggles and nods of understanding.

She sat up in her chair. "Well . . . I've got a birthday present for *you*, Doctor."

"Really? That's how you do birthdays? I kinda like that idea."

"Well, not exactly," said Jean, glancing over at Melanie. "Just *tell* him already!"

"Okay, okay. Here goes: I did it! I quit smoking!"

"Really?" I was genuinely shocked. Smokers with depression are rarely able to quit. "That's fantastic! You have most definitely made my day. No, you've made my *week*!"

I had been working with her for over five years, trying every trick in the book to help her quit smoking. On average, having diabetes reduces life span by about eight years. But the combination of diabetes and tobacco use conspires to shave twenty years off one's life. In these cases, tobacco cessation is priority number one. If she could stick with it, this would be a real win, and I savored the moment.

"Well, really it was a birthday present to myself," she said. "Maybe next year, the soda will go too, but that's gonna be much harder. I still drink one or two 7UPs a day."

"C'mon, don't be too hard on yourself. Let's first honor your gift to yourself and celebrate that you quit smoking. And focus on not starting up again. You still have some work cut out for you there, especially in the first few months. So—what'd you do on your birthday?"

"Nothing really. Since Jean had to work today and because we had this appointment, we decided to take a rain check and celebrate on Saturday. But then Jean's gonna take me to do my most favorite thing: go to a water park. You know, the one near Concord?"

"Sure, I've taken my twins there. Amazing place. Great idea, especially since it's supposed to be ninety degrees in the East Bay this weekend. Good idea to get out of the fog."

"Yeah, I'm really looking forward to it. It must have been ten years since I've been to one."

"I just thought it would cheer her up," chimed in Jean. "She's been having a tough time."

"Thanks for letting me know. It sounds like the water park is exactly the right medicine for her."

I shifted gears and got down to the business of assessing her depressive symptoms, reviewing blood tests, assessing home blood sugar levels, adjusting insulin doses, rechecking her blood pressure, reviewing her medication adherence, and—as we did at every visit—checking her feet for the simple fungal infections that, if left untreated, can lead to foot infections and gangrene. An especially important exam for someone with poor sensation in her feet; an exam that, if done at every visit, prevents amputations. They looked clean and dry. I wrapped up what had otherwise been a run-of-the-mill visit with a person who has diabetes. Bread-and-butter stuff. I told her I wanted to see her again in two to three months.

❧

Three months after she celebrated her birthday, Melanie had a follow-up visit with me. Another evening clinic, since Jean, who had a day job, could only bring her to clinic in the evenings. I entered the room and found Jean, a heavyset woman in flowing flowery robes, alone, looking at me, tears welling in her eyes. She was in her usual seat, with Melanie's usual seat empty.

"Where's Melanie?" I asked. "Is everything all right?"

"I'm sorry, Doctor. I hope it's okay that I decided to come tonight."

"Sure it is. What happened?"

"It's too awful to tell you," she sobbed. "You remember how . . . how we were gonna go to the water park?"

"Yes, of course."

"Well, we did. But it turned into a nightmare. She had a great time, a *really* great time. I'll hold on to that memory. She must have gone up those stairs and down those slides thirty times, whooping and hollering all the way. But when we were going back to the car, she could barely walk. She wasn't in any pain, but her feet had swollen up like balloons. They had big bubbles and sores on the bottoms. They looked like they'd been burned in a fire."

"Oh no," I groaned, anticipating where this story was heading.

"Then I realized what had happened: she had been barefoot all day, going up those stairs in the ninety-five-degree heat, standing in those long lines on those flaming-hot stairs, with that sun beating down on that staircase. She never felt a thing. But she burned them really bad."

"Jean, that's horrible. Didn't she know to . . . ? Oh, I should've reminded—"

"Wait. That's not the nightmare yet. I brought her to the nearest hospital to get her burns treated. She kept saying she was fine and didn't need to go. But I saw what I saw, and it couldn't be good. And I couldn't ignore it."

"No, you definitely did the right thing, because a burn in a person with—"

"Well, I hope so. Because she . . . she . . . she never left that hospital. She first got gangrene in the left foot, and they tried to treat it with antibiotics. But it kept spreading, so they had to amputate her foot. It was horrible. . . . But it kept spreading even higher, and so they had to amputate the leg below the knee."

"Oh my God, I'm so sorry. I feel horrible."

"Thank you. I thought that would be that. We'd just have to deal with another challenge, just add one more to the hopper. Poor thing. . . . But then her right foot got gangrene, and so they put her on the schedule for another amputation of her *other* foot. But that night, she got real sick. They had to take her to the ICU; they said the infection had spread to her bloodstream, that she had blood poisoning."

"Oh, man. Yes, that sometimes happens." I listened in agony.

"I stayed with her till about midnight. The next day, her bed was empty. I thought they had taken her down to the operating room. But the nurse told me that she'd been kinda crazy overnight, that she had gotten out of bed, and that she had collapsed and . . . and that her heart just . . . stopped. They tried doing CPR on her, but she was gone. She had died. . . . And I hadn't even been there for her."

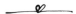

There were many systems-level breakdowns that led to Melanie's premature death.

Her own inadequate *health literacy*, a result of a dysfunctional educational system that leaves many in the dark when it comes to understanding their own bodies and is a barrier to gaining proficiency in the prevention and self-care of chronic illness.

My own failure to remind her of the need to *always* wear protective footwear, communication that would have improved her health literacy (had I not done that? I couldn't recall). And, relatedly, my health care system's failure to systematically provide, reinforce, and document successful receipt of such education for *all* patients with diabetes, and especially for those with documented diabetic nerve damage, failures due to what I have described as inadequate "organizational health literacy."

And our larger society's failure to confront the social and environmental drivers of the diabetes epidemic—in her case, the unfettered availability and consumption of SSBs—a communal failure known as inadequate *public health literacy*. To prevent the cycle of needless suffering and premature death, we would need to address these root causes.

Melanie's story, while dramatic in its contours, was not exceptional in its outcome. Different versions of the diabetic amputation story were being replicated all across America, the scope and scale of these battles being difficult to fathom. At the time of Melanie's death, the US had been waging a war in Iraq and Afghanistan for about a decade. During that time, about 1,500 US soldiers had lost limbs in combat. In that same period, more than 1 million US residents lost limbs to amputations from type 2 diabetes. Despite these numbers, we had yet to mobilize for a public health war against type 2 diabetes.

Thinking ahead, I committed myself to ensuring that Melanie's death would not be in vain. I would carry Melanie's story with me across policy settings as I tried to advance this cause. And I would retell her story to others—combining it with scientific data—to try to move them to action.

CHAPTER 19

Melanie Goes to the State Capitol

Medicine is a social science, and politics is nothing else but medicine on a large scale. Medicine as a social science, as the science of human beings, has the obligation to point out problems and to attempt their theoretical solution.

—Rudolf Virchow, MD (1821–1902),
founder of modern pathology

THE DIABETES CZAR

In 2008, because of my prior research into diabetes disparities and diabetes health care interventions in marginalized populations, I was recruited to serve as chief of the Diabetes Prevention and Control Program for the California Department of Public Health, to be the "diabetes czar," a position I held for five years. Because of budgetary limitations, the state could only support me in this role on a very part-time basis.

In this part-time role, the entire state became "my patient." My job—so I believed—was first to assess the severity of the problem and then determine the underlying diagnosis for, and the root causes of, the epidemic. Next, I was to synthesize an assessment of the problem, and generate and execute a plan that engaged the health system, governmental, business, and social sectors to confront the underlying causes.

At the time I began, one in nine California adults (11 percent) had diabetes, with double the rates among African Americans, Latinos, and Asian Pacific Islanders. The disease was costing the state $26 billion a year in public health care spending and lost productivity. Even though over 3.5 million adults in California had diabetes and another 9 million were estimated to have prediabetes (diabetes's predecessor), the US Centers for Disease Control and Prevention granted approximately $1 million a year to our program, roughly the same as their grants to Rhode Island and West Virginia. This meant we had 33 cents for every individual with diabetes or, if we included the 9 million with prediabetes, a little over 8 cents to spend per individual to prevent and control diabetes.

It was clear to me that the only way we could tackle the epidemic was to address the larger structural issues that lead to a diabetogenic society. But addressing these structural issues would require disrupting the existing equilibrium of power, a truism for all successful public health interventions. Changing how we transport ourselves, how we market and price unhealthy food and beverages, how we create and implement zoning laws for fast-food outlets, how we alert the public to unhealthy products, how we design our suburbs, and how we reengineer the sedentary workday—all would require herculean efforts of advocacy and political maneuvering.

It did not take me long to learn that even a Hercules would have a tough time successfully advocating for such change within this health department. In my first week in Sacramento, I got to know my committed and young program staff. I was then shepherded around to meet the department's branch and center directors. I began to observe the strict vertical hierarchy of the health department, so unlike the "in-the-trenches" and more horizontal functioning of San Francisco General Hospital. I was forewarned that, because the state of California was in the midst of a prolonged hiring freeze, there were some members of the leadership team who were perceived to be deadwood, including individuals who had been brought out of retirement to steer the aircraft carrier. Some individuals were considered to be "no people"—people who didn't, or couldn't, get things done or get out of the way to let others get things done. But I was inclined to give them the benefit of the doubt and tried to put my best foot forward as I met each of them.

Our program coordinator, my second in command, brought me to the office of the Division of Chronic Disease and Injury Control director, the number three person in the entire department. But before I was properly introduced, my right-hand woman had retreated back to our wing. It was clear she wanted no face-time with this guy, and so I was left to fend for myself. The division director, a short and balding man in his seventies, stood up from his chair, extended a small hand my way, gave me a limp handshake, and offered me a wry smile.

"So . . . you must be the famous Dr. Schillinger. Descended from his rarefied ivory tower to work where the real action is. Well, kudos to you for seeing the light and stepping into this role. It's not going to be easy, mind you. You can do great things here, Schillinger, if you have the skills and the temperament. Me? I single-handedly fluoridated California's water. Well, most of it. Try to top that, Schillinger, in terms of public health impact. And if you do, I'll tip my hat to you and give you the gold star."

"Yes, sir," I found myself replying. "I'll certainly do my best. And I hope to be able to learn from you and see you as a person I can turn to for advice as I try to tackle this diabetes epidemic. We've got a great team, but not a lot of experience or resources."

"Yes, yes, yes, of course," he satisfyingly responded, walking around his desk and warmly putting an arm around my shoulder. "I'm your man at the helm. And my door is always open.

"Let me tell you my secret, Schillinger," he continued in hushed tones as he inexplicably walked me to a corner of his office. "Look at this, Schillinger, and tell me what you see."

I followed his outstretched finger pointing to a coatrack bedecked with hundreds and hundreds of lanyards hanging from hooks like Christmas ornaments—colorful neck straps connected to laminated labels printed with his name, his title, his department, and a whole host of acronyms signifying whatever local, regional, statewide, or national public health conference he had collected them from.

I raised my eyebrows to appear duly impressed. "Wow, it looks like you have attended a lot of really important conferences over the years, sir. I never thought about actually collecting my lan—"

"No, no, no! This is not about me, Schillinger. Not at all. You misunderstand," he said to me in a singsong voice. "I have one word for you, Schillinger, one word that nicely sums up what all this means, what the secret is."

Then, a theatrical pause, making it clear that this was not the first time he had delivered his sage advice and shared his secret with a more junior colleague that he was taking under his wing. And making it clear that I had to drag this gem of a secret out of him. So I took the bait and read my line from his script.

"What word would that be, sir?" I asked, feigning curiosity.

"Community, Schillinger. *Community*. That's what it's about. About getting in there with the people," he said, punching his right hand into the palm of his left. "Mixing in to do your needs assessment [punch], keeping your ear to the ground [punch], keeping you honest [punch] and connected [punch]. That's the secret, Schillinger. Community."

He stepped away and folded his arms across his chest, performance complete, gazing lovingly at his lanyard tree.

"What do you say to that, Schillinger?"

I looked again at the coatrack adorned with lanyards and back at him to assess whether he was actually being serious with me. We looked each other in the eyes, and I noticed he had beads of sweat on his brow and that he was wearing a lanyard with his name, rank, and center printed in bold letters, slowly swinging back and forth over his heart.

On one hand, I found myself both offended and stunned by the sheer absurdity of his secret—his belief that attending hundreds of medical and public health conferences would in some way enable an authentic connection with "communities" that indeed urgently needed fully engaged public health leaders. On the other hand, I began to feel compassion for a man—someone who perhaps had made important contributions three decades prior—who now found himself embedded within, and even contributing to, an ineffective and ossified department.

"I can honestly say, sir, that I couldn't agree with you more. That your sentiment about serving the community by staying connected to the community, and really listening to what these communities have to say, is refreshing. And that it indeed is one of the secrets of success in public health. Thank you for sharing your reflections on that, sir. I anticipate that I will be coming to you a lot over the years for advice on how to best do that."

"Certainly, Schillinger, certainly."

Over the next few years, I never saw or heard from him again. By year four, he had retired, fading away to wherever old public health soldiers go.

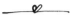

I teach a master's-level course in noncommunicable diseases at our global health school, and the diabetes epidemic plays an outsize role. Many of my students used to get confused when attempting to distinguish between type 1 and type 2 diabetes. This changed when I started explaining to them that type 1 diabetes—formerly known as *juvenile onset diabetes*—is a disease in which *the body attacks itself.* In type 1, one's own immune system (often that of a child or young adult) perceives the insulin-producing cells in one's own pancreas as "foreign" and destroys them. Insulin is like a key that unlocks the doors to the body's cells, letting the glucose in from the bloodstream to the muscles and the liver, where it can be used to fulfill one's immediate energy needs, or stored for later use. Without insulin, the body cannot transform the sugars we digest into the energy we need, and the blood sugar rises to dangerous levels. In contrast, I explain, type 2 diabetes—formerly known as *adult-onset diabetes*—is a disease in which *the body politic attacks the individual.* In an environment whose design is marked by an excess of added sugars and ultra-processed foods and a paucity of outlets for physical activity, the blood sugar rises. In response, the pancreas overproduces insulin. The body's cells, overwhelmed by this onslaught of insulin and high levels of blood sugar, gradually start changing the locks on their doors. As a result, the body becomes insulin-resistant, and the blood sugar rises to dangerous levels. With this understanding, it becomes clear that confronting the type 2 diabetes epidemic requires that we recruit not only the field of clinical medicine but also the field known as *social medicine.*

My battle for Melanie's health had been waged within the four walls of a county hospital—a battle that was being fought (often unsuccessfully) on behalf of similar patients by similar clinicians in similar ways across similar clinical settings, over and over again. It was time that we moved beyond this clinical model for battling the disease. Reversing the type 2 diabetes epidemic would also require social and environmental change, a type of change that would require political support.

My first attempt to carry forward Melanie's story of overexposure to SSBs, early-onset type 2 diabetes, and tragic death resulting from diabetes complications took place in the context of my state government position. This setting felt like the right place to move the needle on the type 2 diabetes epidemic, the right place to conduct social medicine.

FROM DOCTOR TO DICTATOR

As the son of an immigrant from Chile, I had been inspired by Chile's history of harnessing the political process to advance public health. In 2006, two years before accepting the position of director of the state's diabetes prevention program, I spent a semester working as a visiting professor at the University of Chile School of Public Health. My time spent there working as a doctor and learning about the country's public health history reinforced for me the potential for progressive social policy to improve the health of a population. But it also revealed the ways in which powerful interests view such policies as direct threats, and work to undermine their potential.

The School of Public Health had an atypically small faculty, one too modest for a university of this size and prestige. One afternoon as I was walking down the school's hallways, I discovered the reason. Affixed to a wall, a small, copper plaque read: *Dedicated to the Memory of the Physicians and Professors Who Lost Their Lives Under the Dictatorship*. Twenty-five or so names were listed. The plaque was dated 1991, only one year after General Augusto Pinochet had been forced to step down and nearly twenty years after the military coup that started his brutal dictatorship. That was in the early 1970s, at the time that then-president Salvador Allende was either assassinated by Pinochet's men or shot himself to prevent being murdered by them, depending on whose history one believes.

Allende had been a public health doctor who had trained at the University of Chile, studying social medicine and pathology under Max Westenhöfer, a mentee of Dr. Rudolf Virchow's, the father of the field of social medicine. This training was to profoundly influence Allende's career, one in which he started as a general doctor, subsequently evolving to become a public health advocate and leader, ultimately serving as a politician and then president. In 1939, as the nation's minister of health, he published *La Realidad Médico-Social Chilena* (*The Chilean Socio-Medical Reality*), which conceptualized illness as a disturbance of the individual fostered by deprived social conditions. It focused on common health problems generated by the poor living conditions of the working class: maternal and infant mortality, tuberculosis, sexually transmitted and other communicable diseases, emotional disturbances, and occupational illnesses. He concluded the book with the Ministry of Health's proposals for health improvement that emphasized social change on top of basic medical interventions: income distribution, a national housing program, and industrial reforms. During the 1950s, he introduced legislation that created the Chilean national health service, the first program in the Americas to guarantee universal health care.

In 1970, Dr. Allende won the popular vote in a three-way race and became president. He called for economic and social change focused on improving the conditions of the poor and decreasing the role of private property and of foreign corporations. As president, he nationalized the copper industry and advanced policies to distribute the nation's wealth in ways to promote social equity. He also sponsored the decentralization of health care by empowering local, participatory health councils that worked with social service sectors to serve the impoverished masses. Many Chilean doctors felt threatened by Allende's community health and health care policies, which focused on public rather than private care and thus meant less income for private physicians. Others were inspired by his ability to leverage social change to improve health and to leverage the discourse and logic of medicine to advance progressive social policy. And they joined the cause.

Allende's attempts to transform the Chilean economy, while popular with a majority of Chileans, were viewed as too radical by many powerful groups, including conservative factions in Chile and the US government. The dissatisfaction culminated in his death. With Allende gone, the next targets were the practitioners of public health and social medicine. Soon after the military coup, the dictatorship closed departments of preventive medicine, public health, and social science at the country's medical schools. Faculty members teaching these disciplines were summarily dismissed. Taken from their homes in the dark of night, many were tortured and others were disappeared, contributing to the ranks of the estimated forty thousand Chilean citizens

incarcerated or tortured, and the three thousand murdered during the Pinochet dictatorship.

The copper memorial plaque opened my eyes to the fact that the place
where I had been working was once the vibrant academic home for the growing field of social medicine in Chile and a hotbed for social activism. Perhaps it too was not a coincidence that, fifteen years after the dictatorship had
ended, I found myself working here. Because social medicine was about to
enjoy a rebirth in Chile.

———— ✐ ————

FROM DICTATOR BACK TO DOCTOR

In March 2006, my wife and our eight-year-old twin boys huddled around
the television in our small, high-rise Santiago apartment as the sun set, casting a deep red glow behind Cerro Manquehue. As if the Mapuche gods were
churning the lava within this natural pyramid, readying it to erupt and disrupt the status quo.

A formal ceremony dedicated to the handover of presidential power was
being held in a plenary session of the National Congress of Chile in Val-
paraiso. On the dais of the congress stood a short and somewhat stocky,
bespectacled woman dressed in a white pantsuit. Her infectious smile ra-
diated across the screen to the nation's twelve million viewers. The red,
white, and blue presidential sash was placed over her head as part of the
traditional, symbolic transfer of power. Incredibly, Dr. Michelle Bachelet,
a prior victim of torture at the hands of the military dictatorship, a former
exile from her own country, a physician trained in social medicine, and,
most recently, a minister of health, had just become the newest president of
the Republic of Chile.

Bachelet was a pediatrician who had been cross-trained in public health at
the University of Chile. Her father had been a pilot for the Chilean Air Force;
in the early 1970s, he was appointed by then-president Allende to run the
Chilean Food Distribution Office. When Pinochet seized power in the coup
d'état, Bachelet's father was detained at the Air War Academy on charges of
treason, where he suffered a fatal cardiac arrest. In 1975, Dr. Bachelet and her

mother were also detained in a notorious secret detention center in Santiago, where they were separated and subjected to interrogation and torture at the hands of Pinochet's henchmen. She was exiled for four years.

She returned to Chile and, after its transition to democracy, served in the Ministry of Health's West Santiago Health Service. By 2000, she had become Chile's minister of health, overseeing health reforms designed to reverse the health policies that Pinochet had implemented by re-expanding access to care. In 2002, having become deeply interested, formally trained, and well versed in military-civil relations, she was appointed Chile's minister of defense, becoming the first woman to hold this post in a Latin American country. While minister of defense, she promoted reconciliation between the military and victims of the dictatorship, culminating in the 2003 declaration by the army that "never again" would the military subvert democracy in Chile. True to her roots in social medicine, she subsequently put forward a progressive presidential electoral platform, which addressed many social and health inequities that had emerged during the Pinochet era. After being elected, she dedicated her presidency to executing a thirty-six-item plan in which a majority of the measures were aimed at improving conditions for the most disadvantaged social groups. She described her efforts as "creating a system of effective social protection which will meet the needs of Chileans from earliest infancy through to adulthood." This included free treatment in public hospitals for people over sixty, an increase in the lowest pensions of retired Chileans, a set of initiatives to promote gender equality, and significant investments in childcare and public education.

Six months later, I returned to California with renewed enthusiasm for my work, holding a belief that, under the right circumstances, governmental action to promote health by improving social conditions was possible. I carried this enthusiasm with me to the California Department of Public Health. However, at the time, this agency proved to be an inferior platform from which to declare, let alone wage, a war against diabetes. I gradually learned that working within the state health department, an entity of state government, one beholden to the governor and indirectly to his donors, felt like walking over endless obstacles in marshlike mud to, at other times, walking on coals. One misstep or false move, you burn; if your skin is too thin, you burn. And I had very few fans cheering me on to get to the other side.

At my term's midpoint, Arnold Schwarzenegger was governor. Since he was a champion of physical fitness, I believed he would be an ally in advancing statewide policy to prevent diabetes. In 2010, as his second term was coming to a close, he called in his closest health advisors to provide him with new ideas and guidance as to what he could do to improve the health of Californians. In advance of this meeting, I was consulted by one of these advisors, off the record. Sharing what we had learned from the war on tobacco, I suggested that levying a statewide tax on SSBs would lead to reductions in obesity, diabetes, and heart disease and save California a lot of money in health care costs. At that time, no municipality, state, or nation had ever taxed SSBs. As reported to me by an advisor who was in the governor's room when the idea was pitched, the governor—known for his anti-tax philosophy—was nonetheless intrigued by the idea. However, a lobbyist for the American Beverage Association was also present at the meeting. He reportedly approached the governor and asked him to first consider who the corporate sponsor of the Special Olympics was (answer: Coca-Cola). Eunice Kennedy Shriver—JFK's sister; the mother of Arnold's wife, Maria Shriver; and the founder and champion of the Special Olympics—the lobbyist suggested, would not be happy were such a policy to be pursued. The idea for an SSB tax was promptly dropped.

A year later, with Schwarzenegger out of office, I consulted with our new center director, a strong public health advocate and tested leader, about how best to proceed. With her agreement and support, I commissioned a crackerjack team to use sophisticated mathematical modeling to project the impacts of a penny-per-ounce SSB tax on diabetes and heart disease in California, including analyses of children, low-income populations, and racial and ethnic minority groups. And to generate estimates of money that would be saved by the state. We found that over a ten-year period, such an SSB tax would prevent about 20,000 new cases of diabetes in California, over 17,000 new cases of heart disease and 3,200 deaths. Of note, African Americans, Mexican Americans, and low-income individuals would enjoy more than twice the benefits of other Californians. Furthermore, the state would save $1.6 billion in health care costs.

Data in hand, I coauthored a California Diabetes Program policy brief that summarized our findings in language policymakers could understand and act on. I submitted this policy brief up the food chain, first to our center director, for departmental review. I received no response for six months. I made inquiries to her on a monthly basis, but these were left unanswered. When I finally heard back, I learned from her that the report had been coolly received by the higher-ups. Clearly disappointed, apologetic, and frustrated, she suggested I reframe the entire brief to be less about SSB taxes and more about *comparing different strategies* for reducing SSB consumption (e.g., anti-SSB educational campaigns, promoting water over SSBs, limiting SSB access, and finally, taxation). She thought this might make the brief more politically palatable to the department director and his audiences in government. As we had already lined up a number of health advocacy groups to carry the SSB tax message to Sacramento to advance policy, we worked feverishly to reframe the policy brief based on what little was known about these alternatives. A week later, I learned that my center director, my light in a sea of darkness, had unexpectedly left the department, having handed in her resignation for unspecified reasons. The word on the street was that she was felt to be too much of a "public health advocate" and too opinionated.

Within a month, I resubmitted the revised policy brief to the interim center director, a man whose former experience had been in communicable diseases, not in noncommunicable diseases like diabetes. And again, I waited. After an additional six months of email reminders and inquiries to his staff, I finally called him to find out what was going on. He gave me only minor feedback from a scientific standpoint. When I asked him whether I could affirmatively address these concerns and then release the policy brief, I was told it still needed to be reviewed by the department director.

"This policy brief—you know it could be a game changer for California, right?" I asked him.

No response.

So, I pushed. "Tell me: Will it ever see the light of day?"

A pause.

"You want my honest answer?" he asked.

"Yes, I do."

"The answer is: never."

"Okay. So . . . am I being censored?"

"Well, no, I wouldn't exactly call it that."

"Really? What *would* you call it?"

He didn't respond.

"Will I at least be allowed to publish this as a peer-reviewed scientific article, then, and not as a formal policy brief? It'll probably take a year or two to get from submission to publication, but at least it'll get out there."

"It can be published if you want, but your name cannot appear on that paper, nor can the California Diabetes Program's name. Under no uncertain terms. There can be no footprints that lead back to our department."

It was 2013, and I had been the California Diabetes Program's chief for five years. What had I accomplished? During this time, seven more of my own patients after Melanie had succumbed to amputations due to diabetes, as had tens of thousands more across the state. New data revealed that one in eight California adults (12.5 percent) now had diabetes. In other words, four hundred thousand more adults had acquired type 2 diabetes under my watch. I knew then that to declare and wage a war against diabetes, I needed to separate from a bureaucracy currently paralyzed by conflicts of interest and politics, and pursue an alternative strategy.

My decades of waging endless battles one individual patient at a time in my clinic—of trying to thread the needle between offering up modern medicine's miracles in the face of people's stories that often tell of the unhealthy social and environmental conditions that confound their ability to benefit from them—had taught me that we needed to do more, and do things differently. Reflecting on the war on tobacco, I first decided we needed to study the entities that represent the root causes of the epidemic and uncover and disclose the practices they pursue that perpetuate the epidemic. Identifying the myriad ways that US tobacco companies placed profit over public health had opened the door to public health regulations and other lifesaving policy changes. In the case of type 2 diabetes, much of the food and beverage industry was following a similar playbook, but few had taken them on. And drawing lessons from the war on AIDS, I realized that we needed a grassroots movement emanating from those disproportionately affected by the disease, people who could advocate for change from the ground up. Finding ways to bring in the voices of those at the margins—voices of patients like my own, and members of their communities—was sorely needed. And that we desperately needed to find a secondhand smoke equivalent, something that would motivate an average Californian to view diabetes as a *social and communal problem*, not just a health problem, something that would change the conversation away from *shame and blame* to a conversation in which we *reframe* the disease, *take aim* at the unhealthy environments in which we live, and *win the game* of transforming communities, so as to make the healthy choice the easier choice. Reframe, Take Aim, and Win the Game became my refrain.

CHAPTER 20

Melanie Goes to Court

REFRAME: MOBILIZING FOR A WAR ON THE HOME FRONT AGAINST DIABETES

In June 2014, the global diabetes scientific and clinical communities convened in San Francisco for the American Diabetes Association (ADA) meeting. Attended by nearly eighteen thousand health care professionals from 110 nations, featuring over a thousand presentations, and partially underwritten by 331 vendors and exhibitors, this meeting has grown exponentially in parallel with the diabetes epidemic.

A special symposium, entitled Public Initiatives to Improve Health, captured my attention. This session was the only one to address the larger social, structural, and environmental forces that are the engine of this global epidemic. Anticipating its popularity, ADA organizers reserved two conjoined ballrooms, with giant screens to amplify the images of symposium speakers. Stanton Glantz, PhD, the UCSF epidemiologist widely acknowledged to be a major force behind the war against tobacco, opened the session with "Lessons Learned from the Tobacco World." What could be more informative and inspiring than listening to Stan reflect on the guerilla war that he and others had been successfully waging over the last thirty to forty years?

However, only eighteen people, or only one of every thousand ADA conference-goers, attended the only symposium to discuss policy and public health approaches to confronting diabetes. Dr. Glantz and colleagues, in essence, spoke truth to no one. The dispiriting showing at the ADA's public policy symposium suggested a dangerous complacency. In an editorial in the *Journal of Endocrinology and Diabetes*, I proposed six causes for this complacency and highlighted lessons learned from recent sociomedical epidemics wherein scientific, clinical, public health, and lay communities overcame complacency to generate policy actions that saved lives. These included: 1) a false belief in the individual behavioral or genetic paradigms of type 2 diabetes causation; 2) a false belief that the causes of diabetes reflect the price of economic well-being; 3) cynicism and antipathy regarding the efficacy of public policy solutions; 4) the fact that some physicians and scientists are unwitting cogs in the wheels of the diabetes-industrial complex; 5) lack of a powerful and politically active advocacy community; and 6) the absence of a "second-hand smoking gun" equivalent. I made a call to action to mobilize for a war on the home front, one that would require physicians and scientists to lead the way by overcoming our own complacency in the face of the calamity in our midst.

To make the case, I pressed forward with hard facts:

- Between 2001 and 2016, as a result of the Iraq and Afghanistan wars, 1,650 US soldiers lost limbs in combat.
- In that same period, over 1.1 million US residents lost limbs to amputations resulting from type 2 diabetes.
- The number of home-front diabetes-related amputations was 666 times greater than that of the overseas front.

I added that, despite abundant evidence that clinicians, patients, and families fight thousands of life- and limb-threatening battles daily, the US clinical and scientific communities have barely begun to mobilize for a public health war against diabetes. This war would require us to confront and alter our diabetogenic economy and society—characterized by more sedentary work and lifestyles, food and beverage marketing and pricing that push diets engorged with processed sugars, and neighborhoods in which it is far easier and safer to drive than to walk or bike. I called for the development of new alliances across scientific, clinical, public health, business, and lay communities, and the creation of effective strategies that squarely confront the unhealthy social, economic, and environmental conditions that are the primary drivers of the type 2 diabetes epidemic. Unless we enhanced our single-minded, individual-level clinical approach with more holistic, population-level strategies that addressed the systemic and structural root causes of the disease, Melanie's story, and the stories of many of my other patients, would be destined to needlessly repeat themselves.

TAKE AIM: WARNING NOTICES ON SODA BILLBOARDS

Since the state health department was at the time not a conducive platform to go from "one to many" in the war against diabetes, I returned to my perch at San Francisco General Hospital and began to work closely with the San Francisco Department of Public Health and community coalitions to move forward local ordinances attempting to win some battles in the larger war. San Francisco has a storied history as an epicenter of political activism and social change, a city whose progressive politics have led to a forward-thinking municipal health department, whose work has often translated into progressive civic health policies. Often referred to as the *San Francisco model*, such policies have at times served as a harbinger for change across the US.

We began work on three city ordinances—one to ban sugar-sweetened beverage (SSB) advertisements on billboards, another banning such advertising

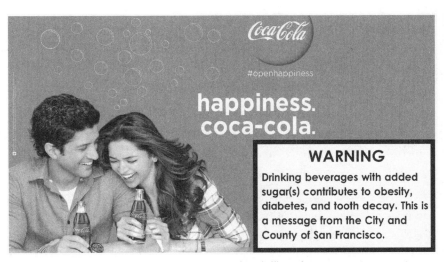

Sample sugar-sweetened beverage warning posted on billboard. *American Beverage Association v. City and County of San Francisco*, Civil Action 3:15-cv-03415-EMC (N.D. Cal. Aug. 24, 2015).

on city property, and a third prohibiting the city from spending money on SSBs. These initiatives thrust me into a new role, one that required integrating my clinical, public health, scientific, communication, and analytic skills in novel ways. Melanie and her story made a few appearances along the way.

In early 2015, the city considered whether to pass an ordinance that required billboards advertising SSBs to include a warning notice:

A clear, factual warning notice could be important in reducing disease rates among people with the lowest health literacy; low health literacy is an independent predictor of SSB consumption, contributing to daily SSB consumption of approximately 240 calories, or one sixteen-ounce soda, when compared to those with the highest health literacy. Studies suggest that warning notices can strongly influence consumer choices regarding SSBs and would increase the public's understanding of the risks of SSBs, providing a visible vehicle to advise people with (or at risk of) obesity, diabetes, and tooth decay. I provided expert testimony at a board of supervisors' hearing in support of this ordinance, providing scientific data about SSBs and diabetes, and sharing Melanie's story with members of the board.

The ordinance was passed and was scheduled to go into effect on July 25, 2016. It represented the first such warning notice in the world.

However, the beverage and billboard industries, in *American Beverage Association (ABA) et al. v. City & County of San Francisco*, promptly sued for a temporary injunction to block implementation of the law. Industry claimed its First Amendment freedom-of-speech rights would be violated were the ordinance to go into effect. They hired a scientist who until recently had served as the chief scientific officer for the American Diabetes Association—an engineer by training with no clinical experience and a long-standing science denier regarding the associations between liquid sugar and obesity and diabetes—to write their expert report. I was asked by the city attorney to author a fifty-page scientific report for the case, whose purpose was to describe and synthesize the state of the science regarding the associations among SSBs and obesity, type 2 diabetes, and tooth decay, and summarize the likely impacts of such a warning notice on public health.

We now know that the beverage industry was deep into its plan to create a false narrative around obesity and diabetes to deflect public attention from the likelihood that its products were causing disease. By creating what was known as the Global Energy Balance Network, the industry developed a communication machine that produced bountiful pseudoscientific content that "proved" how physical inactivity, and not the consumption of liquid sugar, was the cause of obesity and diabetes.

This court case would serve as a test of whether narrative epidemiology—the process of attending to authentic patient stories from the public hospital, reinforced by scientific data reflecting the aggregate of these stories—would defeat the industry's false narratives and pseudoscience. It would also begin to answer the question of whether patient stories from the public hospital are critical not only for doctors to hear but for policymakers to hear. And for all of us to hear.

WIN THE GAME: MELANIE VERSUS GOLIATH

On April 7, 2016, Judge Edward M. Chen presided over a hearing in the US Ninth Circuit Court. The boxing match began. It soon became clear that the city was outgunned, outfinessed, outdressed, outspent, and outmanned. Fifteen lawyers against two. Not a chance.

But then I recalled that the city had Melanie and her story on their side. In the expert report that I was asked to provide to the court, in addition to summarizing the science, I shared Melanie's story as one of a few case studies to illustrate the human toll of type 2 diabetes, expose discriminatory marketing practices that target minority communities (especially youths), and inform the court of the relationship between limited health literacy and SSB consumption. I wondered whether Melanie might serve as a humanizing factor that could influence the outcome of this case, generating meaning from her suffering and premature death, and shifting this war "from one to many."

Would the judge recognize that while the American Beverage Association had fielded fifteen lawyers, a million ghosts of Melanies were standing behind the city's two attorneys? Would he see through the shine and the gloss and the power, the falsehoods and the fabrication, and recognize how our society is mass-producing future Melanies? Could he envision the million victims who were not physically embodied in court that day?

In the hearing and expert reports submitted by the industry, their focus was on questioning the scientific veracity of the warning. Industry argued that it is unconstitutional for commercial speech to be infringed or "chilled" by compelled, noncommercial speech (e.g., a warning), particularly when the compelled speech is "misleading, false, or a subject of scientific controversy." The industry also claimed that consumers are likely to infer that SSBs are *uniquely* harmful, a conclusion they contended is not supported by science and therefore is unconstitutional.

The thrust of the industry's argument was that SSBs do *not* cause obesity, diabetes, and tooth decay; rather, they contended, obesity—and not SSBs—causes diabetes. Despite the medical research and studies, the industry had one goal in mind: profit. To reach that goal, they deliberately presented flawed research, marred by conflicts of interest and manipulated statistics. In essence, the industry made up its own story and dressed it up to look like real science.

In contrast, I provided real patient stories and supported them with sound science.

The city, based in part on the findings of my report and its associated patient stories, retorted that the warning is factually true and that causal relationships are supported by sound science.

WINNING THE GAME

In 2016, Judge Chen issued his decision. The court denied the industry's motion, stating that its arguments did not support their First Amendment claim. While Judge Chen recognized that an unjustified or truly burdensome warning notice might undermine their protected commercial speech, he stated that this does not hold if the warning is reasonably related to the State's interest in preventing deception of consumers. He further addressed the industry's claims that the facts behind the warning notice were controversial, concluding that controversy "cannot automatically be deemed created any time there is a disagreement about the science behind a warning because science is almost always debatable at some level." He concluded that, on balance, the SSB warning required by the ordinance passed the factual and accurate requirement.

This case represented a potential watershed victory in the public health war against obesity, diabetes, and tooth decay. While the decision required a careful analysis of the SSB warning ordinance and relevant legal precedents, the outcome hinged on scientific research, interpreted in the context of real stories from patients who have suffered the harms of overexposure, rather than the profit-motivated "evidence" used by big industry and their claims of future harms to their industry.

In my report, I described to the court many of the strategies the food and beverage industry employs to leverage science and countered by revealing the weaknesses in those arguments and presenting more compelling evidence, including narrative evidence from the public hospital, in support of the warning's accuracy. The outcome of this case demonstrated that the public health duty to warn can be reconciled with constitutional protections, without jeopardizing scientific integrity. Implementing such public health policies benefits all Americans but disproportionately benefits marginalized populations, including children, who are exposed to a disproportionate volume of SSB advertising and products and experience the greatest rates of chronic diseases. This landmark decision, were it to survive on the likely appeal, provided a pivotal legal precedent that could influence public health policy at local, state, and national levels related to communicating the risks inherent to SSBs and other disease-promoting products.

If the decision were to be upheld, it would mean that Melanie took on Goliath—the powerful $60 billion sugary drink industry—and won. But there were other rounds still to come in this boxing match.

CHAPTER 21

Melanie Goes to City Hall

BOXING IS A TWELVE-ROUND SPORT: TAXING SUGAR-SWEETENED BEVERAGES

In 2013, local health advocates and policy stakeholders started planning for a sugar-sweetened beverage (SSB) tax measure to be placed on the 2014 ballot. The San Francisco Bay Area had prior experience with such a measure: in 2012, the small city of Richmond, California, a former hub for shipbuilding during World War II, but now known mostly as a concrete wasteland of fast-food outlets, eight-lane roads, gas stations, and liquor stores, had introduced an SSB tax measure on its ballot. Richmond: one of the poorest cities in the state, a city of a little over one hundred thousand people, with the highest proportion of African Americans in the state (36 percent) and a high proportion of Latinos (27 percent), a city with one of the worst obesity and diabetes statistics in the nation. An unlikely place for a ballot measure on an SSB tax to succeed, given the ways in which the SSB industry has insinuated itself into minority communities. But one of the city's supervisors at the time, Dr. Jeffrey Ritterman, was a retired cardiologist and a practitioner of social medicine. And he was simply sick and tired of all the premature heart attacks, deaths, and amputations he had seen in a lifetime working in Richmond. And he wanted—no, he needed—to do something about it.

The Richmond vote was to be the first toe in the water of public opinion and, as such, a critical litmus test for the nation—a test the American Beverage Association (ABA) simply refused to fail. The ABA outspent the pro-SSB tax coalition thirty-five to one, pouring over $2.5 million into their campaign, representing $23 per resident of Richmond, and $100 for every child under age eighteen. The theme of their campaign was that an SSB tax would hurt African Americans most. Every billboard and every TV ad hammered this message home: African American consumers would be hurting; African American businesses and storeowners would be hurting. A simple message about pocketbooks. In the end, the measure went down, although the fact that it garnered 33 percent of the vote was an inducement for the future.

We now know that blocking taxing SSBs not only in the small city of Richmond but around the globe is the SSB industry's number one priority. Internal Coca-Cola documents uncovered and disseminated by WikiLeaks exposed the corporation's "public policy risk matrix and lobby focus" for Coca-Cola Europe. This powerful and informative visual representation provides insight into how the industry understands current threats to its bottom line. It graphs the potential business impacts of a broad range of policies,

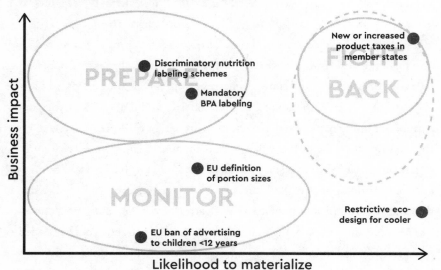

Public policy risk matrix & lobby focus

Adapted from an original Coca-Cola Europe graphic, released via WikiLeaks. Coca-Cola Europe public policy risk matrix and lobby focus; SSB taxes are positioned as most likely to materialize and most likely to generate significant negative business impact. Credit: WikiLeaks.

and the likelihood to materialize for each one. Any policy that maps onto the upper-right quadrant of this graph represents significant jeopardy and, as such, is in the bull's-eye of the industry's lobbying efforts. The only policy at the outermost upper-right quadrant—having both significant potential business impacts and higher likelihood of materializing—is taxing SSBs.

MELANIE WINS A ROUND

In 2014, Berkeley and San Francisco placed an SSB tax on their local ballots. The stakes were high, and polls suggested that the voting public was evenly divided. This ambivalence was due in large part to industry's well-financed campaigns to dishonestly frame the tax as a "grocery tax," falsely claiming that the tax placed on distributors of SSBs would be passed on to consumers not through vendors raising the prices of SSBs but instead through raising

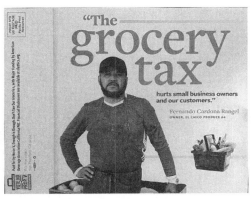

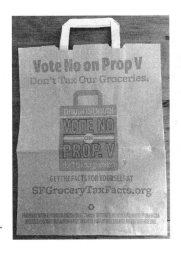

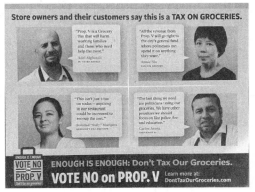

the prices of staple foods and fresh produce. They paid off storeowners in communities of color—the communities hardest hit by the diabetes epidemic and the neighborhoods from which my patients come—to disseminate this false narrative, making it appear to be authentic and valid.

A critical influencer of public opinion—the *San Francisco Chronicle* editorial board—had yet to make its decision about whether to endorse the SSB tax measures in the Bay Area. Before they made their decision, they invited key informants from industry and public health to each make their case. I found myself in a downtown office presenting to the board and taking their questions, speaking as a primary care physician at San Francisco General, a public health expert in type 2 diabetes, and a concerned parent of three children. While my presentation was peppered with impactful scientific facts and statistics, I conveyed to them what it was like to be a doctor at San Francisco General Hospital facing the diabetes epidemic. And I told them Melanie's story.

I couldn't tell if my appeal had won them over. A few days later, I received a call from the *Chronicle*. Apparently, I had made an impression on the board, and they invited me to submit an op-ed related to the upcoming SSB tax vote—one that would summarize my presentation in under eight hundred words. In my op-ed, I shared stories of caring for the ever-growing number of diabetes patients at San Francisco General.

Subsequent to their key informant meetings and the publication of my piece, the *Chronicle*'s editorial board endorsed the SSB tax measures. The outcome of the 2014 vote was mixed: Berkeley passed their measure with a majority. But San Francisco—where the measure included language mandating that any associated tax revenue must be allocated solely to promote public health—required a two-thirds majority to pass. While an impressive 63 percent of the public voted yes, the measure did not garner the votes needed to pass.

MELANIE BLANKETS THE MEDIA

Emboldened by the preliminary evidence from Berkeley that suggested that SSB consumption had rapidly declined after the new tax took hold and that reductions were disproportionately greater in low-income and minority communities, three California cities—Oakland, Albany, and San Francisco (again)—each placed SSB tax measures on their municipal ballots in 2016. This time, no city placed any restrictions on how the tax revenue would be spent, and so only a 50 percent majority was required.

The *Chronicle* again turned to me to provide at least a modicum of a counter-narrative to the ABA's well-financed communication campaign regarding the "grocery tax" and its claims that an SSB tax was economically regressive. This time, after having one of their most experienced journalists shadow me in clinic for a day, they published a three-page feature story entitled "San Francisco Doctor Fighting Diabetes Epidemic Backs Soda Tax." While the article contained a few quotes from me, the words featured, the photos included, and the opinions voiced were largely those of my clinic patients. My patients told their own stories of sugary drink overconsumption (and, at times, addiction) as well as the resultant complications of diabetes from which they suffered. Just as Melanie would have communicated had she still been alive. And, most importantly, contrary to the title of the article, it was my patients who were the ones quoted as backing the SSB tax. It was my patients who eloquently reframed the SSB taxation discourse as a fight against the "regressive disease" of type 2 diabetes— one that disproportionately affects low-income communities and communities

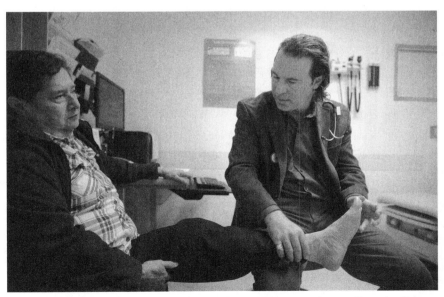

Photo from 2016 *San Francisco Chronicle* article on SSB taxes and controlling the diabetes epidemic. Courtesy of Lea Suzuki / *SF Chronicle* / Polaris.

of color due, in part, to excess exposure to SSB marketing, easy access to such products, and limited access to local healthy alternatives—rather than an economically regressive tax policy.

The text accompanying this image from the *San Francisco Chronicle* article read:

> On a recent morning, one of those patients was 66-year-old Bayview resident Ruth Arrozco. Like most of Schillinger's patients, diabetes is just one of her many diagnoses—she also has had pancreatitis, kidney stones, and depression.
>
> Arrozco said she used to drink a couple of sodas a day, but has cut back to one a week. She said she thinks soda contributed to her getting type 2 diabetes and supports a tax on it.
>
> "So people wouldn't buy it," she said, matter-of-factly. "If someone sees it on sale, they want to get it, just like cigarettes and alcohol."

JUNK FOOD AND JUNK SCIENCE

The 2016 election, as a potential harbinger of change, was to be a critical one not only for the Bay Area but also for the rest of the nation. As the elections drew near, the sugary beverage industry flexed its media muscles, doubling down on its misinformation campaign, including casting doubt onto the relationship between sugary beverages and disease. I decided that, as a scientist and academic physician, I had a responsibility to do more to ensure that the truth about SSBs and disease became widely known. I was holding on to a scientific analysis that evolved out of the report on the sugary beverage warning notices I had previously authored on behalf of the city, an analysis that could lend further evidence that SSBs can cause obesity and diabetes. It was also one that would expose the industry as merchants of misinformation and doubt. If this study could be published to coincide with the upcoming elections, it might get picked up by major media outlets and help inform public opinion regarding SSB taxation.

A week before the election, *Annals of Internal Medicine*, a top-ranked and highly respected medical journal, published my study, "Do Sugar-Sweetened Beverages Cause Obesity and Diabetes? Industry and the Manufacture of Scientific Controversy." In the paper, I described how the outcomes of recent regulatory initiatives, tax measures, and nutritional guidance designed to curb SSB consumption have hinged on the question of whether SSBs are a proven cause of obesity and/or diabetes. The SSB industry opposed such initiatives, characterizing the case for causation as scientifically controversial. My team had carried out a systematic review to determine whether experimental studies that found no association between SSBs and obesity- and diabetes-related outcomes (so-called negative studies) were more likely than positive studies to have received financial support by the SSB industry. We identified whether articles were independently funded or were funded by—or had author(s) with financial conflicts with—the SSB industry. In the end, we discovered that studies with industry-related financial conflicts of interest, when compared to studies that were independently funded, had over *thirty-fold greater odds* of finding *no causal relationship* between SSBs and metabolic diseases. While industry-related conflicts of interest, such as those in the pharmaceutical industry, have long been known to influence the results of scientific research, the scale of the influence of the sugary beverage industry far outstripped that of other industries (which typically generate a relative risk for industry-friendly bias of two- to threefold). The SSB industry appeared to be uniquely manipulating contemporary scientific processes to create controversy and advance their business interests at the expense of the public's health. They were creating their own story and ignoring those of my patients.

Our study garnered a significant amount of local and national media coverage at a critical time with respect to the upcoming SSB tax vote. In addition to the *San Francisco Chronicle*, the *New York Times*, Reuters News Agency, the *Independent*, and the *Los Angeles Times*, among others, disseminated our findings and conclusions. It didn't take long for the American Beverage Association to strike back. In a letter to the journal that smelled of industry propaganda but was somehow deemed publishable by the editor of *Annals of Internal Medicine*, Maia M. Jack, PhD, vice president of science and regulatory affairs at the American Beverage Association, applied the same methods that Big Tobacco previously used when irrefutable evidence emerged related to the health hazards of tobacco and secondhand smoke. In a predictable fashion, she characterized the American Beverage Association as a good corporate citizen that was interested in the public's welfare, one that had an obligation to study its products' "efficacy and safety." She also tried to discredit the science behind our findings. And she attempted to discredit my team—the scientists who carried out the study. In this regard, and on behalf of the American Beverage Association, she accused me of having a so-called intellectual conflict of interest, stating: "Intellectually motivated biases are as important as financial conflicts of interest." In essence, she contended that my scientific study, by virtue of being motivated by an interest in responding to the stories of my patients and of their communities with respect to over-exposure to SSBs and resultant diabetes, was as faulty as I contended their profit-motivating studies were. This false equivalency was astounding.

MY DAUGHTER MICA, MELANIE, AND THE MIRROR

A few weeks earlier, I had received a call from the San Francisco Department of Public Health informing me that Mayors Ed Lee of San Francisco and Libby Schaaf of Oakland had decided to endorse their respective cities' SSB tax measures and that they planned to announce their support in a public event to be held on the steps of San Francisco's city hall. I was asked to join them as they made this announcement and to speak for a few minutes to provide the medical and social justification for their support. I gladly accepted.

The public event was to be held at 9:00 a.m. on a morning in which it was my turn to drop my nine-year-old daughter, Mica, off at her school, Buena

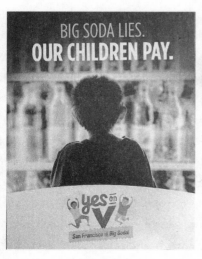
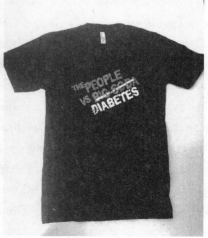

Vista Elementary. Because dropping her off in the Mission District would make it difficult for me to arrive back at city hall in time, I decided that having her by my side at the event not only would provide her with an educational experience in civic engagement but also would provide me with an important prop: she would serve as the visual metaphor for the community of children we all would be advocating for on that day.

Wearing a THE PEOPLE VS ~~BIG SODA~~ DIABETES T-shirt, Mica stood by my side at the dais as we listened to the two mayors say their pieces. She then stepped forward with me up to the podium as I spoke to the crowd on behalf of my patients, our community, and our children. The TV cameras rolled. Standing on the steps of city hall, I chronicled Melanie's clinical trajectory, telling the gruesome story of her untimely and preventable death shortly after her fortieth birthday, a death due in part to the sugary beverages that, as a low-income girl and then woman, she was destined to be overexposed to across her life span. I asked the crowd to help me honor the memory of Melanie and the thousands of others like her in San Francisco and Oakland— especially people of color—who have died or suffered needlessly as a result of the overconsumption of SSBs.

I closed by focusing their attention on my daughter, describing the effects that SSBs were having on our youth. I reminded them of the fact that only two decades prior, a case of diabetes in a child doubtless represented type 1 diabetes, an autoimmune disease in which the cells that make insulin are destroyed. In other words, "a non-preventable disease in which *the body attacks itself* for reasons we do not understand." But that now, especially among children of color, a case of diabetes in a child was more likely than not to reflect type 2 diabetes, a metabolic disease that historically had only affected the very old, a disease in which a body exposed to large doses of unhealthy foods becomes resistant to its own insulin. In other words, "a preventable disease in which *the body politic attacks the child* in entirely predictable ways." With my arm around Mica, I urged them to seize this moment to protect all of our children from the secondhand smoke equivalent of today by voting yes on the SSB tax measures.

That afternoon, while I was teaching medical residents in our clinic, my cell phone rang. Buena Vista Elementary was calling, which was very unusual. I stepped out into the hallway to take the call.

"Hello?"

"Dr. Schillinger, yes—hello. This is Principal Micky Sanchez from BV. I'm sorry to disturb you. But I need to check in with you real quick. It's about Mica."

"Yes, of course." I swallowed hard. "Is everything all right?"

"Yes, she's safe and sound. She's sitting just outside my office, actually. But she's gotten into a bit of trouble over here."

"Really? That's not like her," I responded in disbelief, certain that she had been unfairly accused of some wrongdoing. "What's going on?"

"Well, we caught her going off campus alone, which is strictly prohibited at this age."

"Wow. She knows not to do that."

"She was caught crossing Valencia Street . . . coming back to school from the corner store during recess."

"Oh, well, that's not cool. I'm really surprised to hear that. Thank you for telling me. I'm sure when she gets home, her mother and I will—"

"Well, that's not all, actually. We looked in her backpack and found that she had a bunch of drinks and some candy bars. Junk food is also not allowed on the school campus. So that's two strikes."

This was making at least some sense now. Ariella and I had caught Mica red-handed a number of times over the past few weeks, finding dozens of candy wrappers stowed away in the recesses of her many-pocketed, zebra-striped backpack.

"Okay. Let me speak to her. But before I do, can I ask you two important questions, Principal Sanchez?"

"Yes, of course. Shoot."

"What kinds of drinks was she bringing back to school?" I asked, wincing in anticipation of the answer.

"A bunch of Vitamin Water. It seems to be very popular with the kids these days."

I was well aware of its popularity. I was also aware that the Coca-Cola Company, which owns Vitamin Water, had recently been sued by the Center for Science in the Public Interest (CSPI) for false advertising. Silently acknowledging that their messaging around the health-promoting attributes of their products was misleading, to say the least, Coca-Cola had settled the case, forking over a large sum of money to CSPI to fund public messaging and education to counter the health claims of SSB companies.

"And what was your second question?"

I pictured my daughter standing by my side on the dais at city hall, knowing that our defiant image and righteous message would be broadcast over the local news stations in a few hours.

"Can I ask if . . . if . . . well. How should I put it? Is she still wearing the black T-shirt with the words THE PEOPLE VS B̶I̶G̶ S̶O̶D̶A̶ DIABETES?"

"She is, yes." He chuckled. "And the irony is not lost on me. But my educated guess is that she doesn't really understand the irony. Welcome to the world of parenthood."

Back at home, the evening news did not disappoint. We got a good three minutes of coverage. And there on the screen was Mica, wearing her THE PEOPLE VS B̶I̶G̶ S̶O̶D̶A̶ DIABETES T-shirt, with me to her right and the two mayors behind her, Mayor Lee's hand resting on her shoulder.

That night, as I was putting Mica to bed, I chose the high road. Rather than lecture and pontificate, I took a different tack.

"Sweetie, I got a call from your principal this afternoon. He told me what happened."

She didn't flinch.

"I need you to know that it's not okay for you to do that again. We all make bad choices from time to time, and you made a bad choice today by leaving school by yourself. We still love you, but Mom and I want you to know that we expect it to not happen again."

"But I didn't *do anything*, Daddy. It's not true!" The skin around her eyebrows reddened with shame and anger, an emotional tell unique to her.

"Mica, let's not go there. There were a couple of adults who saw you coming back from the corner store and crossing Valencia Street during recess. And when they checked your backpack, there was a bunch of junk food and drinks in it. Maybe there were a few kids involved, but let's not say it's not true, okay? You'll only make things worse by not telling the truth."

The halos around her eyebrows burned a deeper red.

"Listen, let me ask you something important," I said in a purposefully lighter tone, edging my face closer to hers. "I really wanna know: What flavor of Vitamin Water did you get?"

She looked at me suspiciously, two flames of shame still hovering above her eyebrows. "What?"

"Really, I wanna know. What flavor?"

Hesitating, she answered. "I got . . . berry. Is that okay?"

"*Berry?* You got *berry*-flavored Vitamin Water? You mean the red kind?" She nodded timidly.

"Well, *yuck*," I spewed with an exaggerated quality. "Mica, Mica, Mica. *Grape* Vitamin Water, you know—the purple kind? It's *so* much better. *Way* better. It's all about the grape. You really screwed up, kid. Next time, you *gotta* do the grape."

Her shocked gaze froze on me, and then she burst into laughter and wrapped her precious arms around my neck. We gave each other a big hug, laughed some more, her laughs mixing with her fading tears, and we said good night.

But as I left her room, her puppy eyes on me, I wagged my finger at her and firmly said, "Don't leave school without an adult again, okay?"

I closed her door and strolled across the hallway to my bedroom. Ariella glanced up from her book as if asking me the unspoken question, "How'd the big reckoning go?"

"If you haven't figured it out by now," I proactively announced to her, "you should know that your partner is a parenting *genius*. Who else gets a hug and a smile after scolding one's child for bad behavior? *Moi*, that's who."

She rolled her eyes at me and rewarded me with a smirk.

The next afternoon, my cell phone rang again.

"Dr. Schillinger? Principal Sanchez again. Unfortunately, we caught Mica again. Apparently, she's part of some sort of fourth-grade soda-and-candy ring. We also learned that her nickname is 'Daredevil.' The kids give her their money and make their requests, and then she's the one who dares to do the dirty work."

"*Daredevil?*"

"Sorry. Yes. Anyway, I need to tell you that if this happens a third time, she'll have to suffer some consequences."

"Don't worry. It won't happen again. Thanks for letting me know."

That night, I nominated myself to do the tucking in again, but this time, the ritual would include a consequences conversation. I carefully considered how to approach this repeat transgression. I started in by clearly laying out for her the three rules she broke: 1) going off campus without permission and without an adult; 2) crossing a busy Valencia Street; and 3) buying junk food and soda—which not only was against school rules but also was against our family's rules, especially the sugary drinks. She listened stoically. I followed this up with the fact that being a repeat offender added insult to injury, and that were she to do it again and break the rules a third time, she ran the risk of getting kicked out of her school. And that being kicked out would be hard to wipe clean from her record.

Now tears began to well in her eyes.

I didn't know what to do. By comforting her, I worried, I might unwittingly minimize the gravitas I was trying to convey. At the same time, I recognized that by placing this nine-year-old at the brink of the point of no return, she must have felt like I was threatening her with the prospect of a lifetime sentence. I felt paralyzed by my need to hold her accountable and my concern over the possibility of causing her undue fear.

I fell back on my clinical skills: When faced with uncertainty as to what to say next to a patient in an emotionally charged situation, it is often best to wait for the patient to speak. And if nothing comes forth, to ask an evocative question that can provide a means for a release of some kind, one that often is revealing.

She quietly sobbed but said nothing.

"Sweetie, let's take a step back. *Why* do you feel you have to go buy these things?" I asked, expecting her to pivot to an admission of having succumbed to peer pressure, and anticipating my well-rehearsed retorts about the benefits of resisting such pressures.

My question unleashed a torrent of tears from her. I couldn't help but take her in my arms and rock her as she wailed. I held her this way for five minutes or so, until her crying died down, leaving her only with the strange inhalational spasms that are the sequelae of a long cry.

"Why, sweetie? Tell me *why* you feel you have to go buy these things."

"Do you promise not to be mad at me?" she asked in between her rapid in-breaths.

"Yes, I promise."

"Okay. It's about the Vitamin Water, Daddy. It's just—just . . . that it tastes *so good*. It's *so yummy*. I can't resist it. I *have* to get it. Don't be mad at me, Daddy. And at least it's healthier than sodas 'cause, you know, it has healthy vitamins inside."

"Oh, sweetie, they are *tricking* you into believing it's healthy by calling it Vitamin Water, even though there is nothing at all healthy about it. That's what they do, they act real sneaky and get you to buy something that they've *made sure* you'd love, and buy something that they've *tricked* you to think is good for you. Did you know all that already?"

"No, I didn't, Daddy."

"Well, it's true. And I know you and your friends are way too smart to let them trick you anymore."

MELANIE'S VICTORY AT THE POLLS

In the subsequent week's elections, the SSB tax proposals passed in all three cities, with implementation set for mid-2017 or early 2018. To date, SSB tax initiatives have succeeded in six cities in the US and thirty-three countries across the globe. Evaluations have demonstrated rapid, significant, and sustained reductions in SSB consumption, especially among lower-income groups. Funded by the National Institutes of Health, our research team carried out a study three years after the 2014 Berkeley tax had been implemented. Comparing trends in Berkeley to trends in neighboring and as-of-yet untaxed San Francisco and Oakland, we discovered that the effects of the SSB tax far outstripped the estimates of economists: residents of the city of Berkeley, when compared to residents in the two neighboring untaxed cities, had reduced SSB consumption by an average of 50 percent over three years. A subsequent study we conducted that examined the aggregate effect of SSB taxes across the handful of US cities that have implemented them demonstrated an average effect of a 33 percent reduction in SSB purchases. The size of this effect, particularly if scaled up across California or the nation, would yield very significant health benefits in terms of diabetes cases averted, heart attacks prevented, cavities and gum disease avoided, and health care costs offset. In light of these and other findings, the World Health Organization declared that SSB taxes should be implemented worldwide so as to stem the tide of chronic disease, now the leading cause of death in high-, middle-, and low-income countries.

While promising news for public health, these results—and the accompanying drop in sales of SSBs observed across the US—meant that the industry would wage an aggressive counterattack. On the warning label front, a large team of American Beverage Association (ABA) attorneys appealed the federal court decision related to warning notices in San Francisco, this time arguing that warning notices are *discriminatory* insofar as other sugar-containing products, such as cookies and cupcakes, are not required to post such warnings. The fact that over one-third of added sugar in the US diet comes solely from SSBs should have provided sufficient rationale to single out SSBs; however, the court reversed its decision and ruled in favor of the industry. Their ruling, however, did not accept the industry's argument; rather, it was based on an assessment that the size of the warning notice (20 percent of the billboard) was too large. This left a window for the city to reintroduce a SSB ordinance with a smaller-size warning, which, to its credit, it did in December 2019. Because the city would be forced to pay the ABA's exorbitant legal costs were it to lose this case, as the case wore on the city began to reconsider whether to proceed. Furthermore, the possibility that an appeal by the city would be rejected by what now was a pro-industry Supreme Court could lead to legal precedent that would jeopardize the constitutionality of all consumer-protecting warning notices across multiple industries. The risk to public health were this to transpire was simply too great to continue. The city decided to withdraw the ordinance.

In 2018, through its connections with the Trump administration, the SSB industry shepherded into the revision of the North American Free Trade Agreement a proactive provision banning warning notices on SSBs, potentially prohibiting not only cities, counties, and states but also nations from enacting such warnings.

On the SSB tax front, the industry resurrected an old legal ploy known as *preemption*. Using a strategy of industrial interference resembling Big Tobacco's strategies between 1990 and 2010, the SSB industry started getting industry-friendly regulations and legislation passed at high governmental levels so as to prevent lower-level entities such as cities or counties from regulating, taxing, or otherwise inhibiting the consumption of their products. In a momentum-shifting swing, California—home to four million adults with diabetes, nine million adults with prediabetes, and half a million children with prediabetes—was held hostage to the American Beverage Association's $7-million-funded effort that would have put before voters a referendum to make it nearly impossible for local jurisdictions to impose *any new taxes* on its residents, whether they be taxes to support their fire departments, libraries, schools, or (notably) taxes on SSBs to promote children's health. Fearing that such a broad-sweeping measure would pass and could paralyze cities, the California legislature, together with then-governor Jerry Brown, was forced to choose between two bad options. After only five days of consideration, they opted to surrender, signing a "compromise law" banning any SSB tax in California counties for thirteen years in exchange for the industry dropping the broader referendum. The California legislature passed a law, signed by the governor, that guaranteed that thousands more Californians would needlessly develop diabetes and heart disease.

BRINGING OTHERS INTO THE CENTER OF THE RING

The rapid unfolding of these events made me realize that—much like delivering primary care—advancing public health is a long-term process characterized by many ups and downs. And that reaching one's objectives requires patience, steadfastness, optimism, creativity, partnerships, and a supportive and robust community of stakeholders—one that can stand up to the endless onslaught of the merchants of doubt and purveyors of disease. For too long, public health advocates had mostly been going it alone against the SSB industry, serving as the dominant force at the front lines of the battle. I reflected that, just as succeeding in primary care requires a team, furthering public health requires allies. Based on what I learned from the successes in the AIDS epidemic, those from the most affected communities needed to come forward and bring their voices to the forefront. And they needed to have the platform to do so.

I recalled the power that emanated from the words of my patients in the *San Francisco Chronicle* feature story about diabetes and the SSB tax. And I thought about my daughter: about both her vulnerability to the targeted efforts of the SSB industry, on the one hand, and the familial, economic, and social buffers that protect her from being victimized over the long run, on the other hand. Other children like her—especially the low-income children and children of color in her fourth-grade class, for example—will be the innocent victims of the unhealthy environment in which they are living, an environment shaped and perpetuated by the body politic. Some would even end up like Melanie unless something changed.

What became clear to me was that the children with or at risk of type 2 diabetes represent the secondhand smoke equivalent in the type 2 diabetes epidemic. What we needed was an additional army to combat this enemy, an army populated by individuals who were beyond reproach.

I realized we needed to recruit, inspire, and nurture an Army of Youth and provide them with the platform from which to speak truth to power and inspire others to join a movement.

CHAPTER 22

Melanie Goes Onstage

Only art explains, and that itself cannot be explained. We and art are made for each other, and where that bond fails human life fails.

—Iris Murdoch, *The Black Prince*

IN MY WORK TO CARRY MELANIE'S TORCH BY ATTEMPTING TO SCALE UP diabetes prevention efforts and prevent millions of young people from suffering her fate, I inevitably became aware of my own limitations. My inability to effect diabetes-related policy changes during my five-year term as chief of the Diabetes Prevention and Control Program for the California Department of Public Health had reflected, in part, a failure of communication. My well-crafted presentations to policymakers on the rapidly emerging type 2 diabetes epidemic in California featured compelling bar graphs, convincing prevalence curves, and overwhelming statistics adorned with confidence intervals and P values. Yet my talking points often fell on deaf ears. As I began to understand the limits of *how* I was communicating my message, I gained some traction by pairing scientific content with the stories I had heard from my patients and the events I had witnessed them go through. But even this was not enough. I came to realize that *who* was communicating this message needed to evolve. I needed my patients to speak directly.

While my position as a primary care physician with an ongoing record of caring for communities disproportionately affected by the epidemic, and my career as a public health scientist well versed in the epidemiology, prevention, and management of type 2 diabetes in marginalized patients in public health care settings lent me credibility, they did not appear to be enough to afford me direct influence. However, at times, these credentials provided me the opportunity to be present in the right rooms at the right times—rooms populated by those most affected by the epidemic as well as rooms inhabited by those who make policy decisions. I realized that I had the potential to serve as a credible liaison between marginalized communities whose concerns had yet to be articulated and those in power who needed to hear these voices but had yet to. I recognized that the privileges and station I now enjoyed granted me a platform, a stage from which messengers more effective than I might be able to do what I was unable to do.

A PROFOUND PERFORMANCE

> The theater itself is not revolutionary: it is a rehearsal for the revolution.
>
> —Augusto Boal, *Theater of the Oppressed*

I once was advised by a mentor that staying abreast of advances in medicine, something that requires significant effort, is indispensable to the work of being a great doctor. But that doing so at the exclusion of other things comes at great cost. Because maintaining many interests *outside* of medicine can make one an even better doctor.

"And," she encouraged me, "make sure you mix in with lots of people from outside of medicine. It will pay off in personal and professional ways."

As a seasoned primary care physician, I now have ample experience under my belt to appreciate the benefits of her counsel. Countless times, I found that being in the loop of the everyday goings-on in modern social life, or being familiar with other cultures, or being well versed in a range of disciplines outside of medicine has enabled me to bridge the social distance so often baked into the doctor-patient relationship—enabling me to better facilitate someone's healing or reduce someone's suffering.

I hadn't considered that one day her advice would also serve me in my efforts to promote population health.

Every Sunday morning for twenty years, with the exception of the days I was on duty at the hospital, I played soccer at Rossi Playground in the western section of San Francisco. I looked forward to the two-hour Sunday pickup game both as a means to transition between the joys of a weekend nearly gone and the challenges of the upcoming workweek, as well as a time to socialize with a virtual UN of pickup soccer: amateur players from the US, Ethiopia, France, Germany, UK, Senegal, Israel, Morocco, South Africa, Iraq, Russia, Iran, and others. In their nonsoccer lives, they included a radio announcer, a journalist, a writer, an information technology expert, a programmer, a flamenco musician, a lawyer, an environmentalist, a scientist, a corner store vendor, a photographer, a taxi driver, and an owner of a fine garment store.

But one player—James Kass—was a poet and a performer. He had founded and directed Youth Speaks, a nonprofit whose mission was to empower youths by enabling them to create and perform spoken word poetry. For many years, we had chatted in the gaps in time when errant balls were being chased down or on the sidelines as we took off our cleats and shin guards, learning more about what each of us did in our work lives. On each occasion, we left these conversations with the same conclusion: that one day we had to find a way to work together. To bring together his artistic team and their skills in communicating and reaching young people—especially young people of color—with my medical and public health team and our skills in promoting health literacy. We agreed to many lunches to brainstorm ideas about how to collaborate, but the inertia was too great. For years, no lunch ever transpired, and no collaborations ensued.

Until I heard *her*.

I had been invited to attend a Youth Speaks fundraiser, an annual, formal dinner event. Not one who enjoys attending fundraisers, I begrudgingly accepted the invitation. James made a long pitch to us, hoping to transform us from dinner guests into donors. A few of the young and freshly minted artists were then carted out on to the stage to demo their talent and to highlight the unique ways that Youth Speaks' pedagogy bears fruit. I was not prepared to be blown away.

The lights dimmed, and the curtains rose. On the stage glowed the open face of sixteen-year-old Erica, an African American poet. Adorned with a pink gown that openly celebrated her large body, she proceeded to perform her original poem "Death Recipe." It was a debut experience that to this day makes the hair on my arms stand up in attention. A complex poem about the junk food industry, stress, food addiction, body image, self-destruction, and diabetes.

I can still remember the shocking opening of her poem in which she described her community's death recipe as veiled in the freedom to eat. That they eat like they're still slaves, but now they're just slaves to a modern version of the system.

I knew at that moment that this poem was to become the start of something bigger than any of us in that room could have imagined on that night. She went on, describing some of the ingredients in her daily diet, such as sugar, flour, hydrogenated oils, high-fructose corn syrup, whey powder, Dye Yellow 40, and Dye Red 52. She spoke these lines with an impassioned choreography, pulling back on an imaginary bow and shooting arrows out to the audience as she shouted, "Dye, Dye, Die!"

She continued, calling out the ultra-processed food that surrounds her, drawing attention to the fact that our food is speaking to us. That if the word *dye* is in our food, we should get rid of it.

I fell deeper under her spell as she shifted her focus to describe the negative impacts of junk food on her physical and emotional well-being. How she yearns to incorporate movement into a three-minute poem without running out of breath and how she just wants her smile to be authentic when she puts on her face. Because she isn't happy and is simply tired of hiding behind bulky clothing.

Then she transitioned her piece to call out the ways in which ultra-processed foods have been purposefully designed to lead to cravings and addiction. How she "fiends" for high-fructose corn syrup despite knowing its untoward health consequences. How no matter how hard she tries, she just needs to have her soda and needs to get her sugar high off a cookie.

Finally, she moved on to the diabetes-related consequences, and I held my breath to take it all in. She described how, despite knowing that most of her family has diabetes, she is still addicted to candy. How she sucks on candy as she walks one aunt into her dialysis appointment and accompanies her other aunt who is blind at age thirty-two. How her unhealthy eating behaviors are fixed, despite her grandmother dying of a heart attack at age fifty-one, her little cousin having to inject insulin, and her uncle having an amputated foot.

And then she ended the poem in a suicidal gesture, reciting its last words as she slid her index finger across her throat. For a few seconds after, there was only silence. A deathly silence.

Then Erica took a bow. The room erupted in applause. A standing ovation. All for a poem about type 2 diabetes as a social disease, about the body politic attacking the body of a child.

As the evening came to a close, I sought out James.

She's the one, I needed to tell him. She had shown me the answer for both how and why we could work together.

BRINGING ON THE NOISE:
THE BIGGER PICTURE CAMPAIGN

> The poetics of the oppressed is essentially the poetics of liberation: the spectator no longer delegates power to the characters either to think or to act in his place. The spectator frees himself; he thinks and acts for himself! Theater is action!
>
> —Augusto Boal, *Theater of the Oppressed*

I had a few months left in my term as California's chief of diabetes prevention and control, and we had $30,000 of unspent money left over from our five-year grant from the Centers for Disease Control and Prevention (CDC) that needed to be spent. While what I envisioned for the products of our work with Youth Speaks bordered on the subversive with respect to official department communications, the fact that in a few months I would no longer be the responsible principal investigator of the CDC grant emboldened me to commit these funds to support this novel partnership. A marriage of art and public health, whose goal would be to help young people of color transform themselves from *targets* of metabolic risk to novel *messengers*, active agents of change who could shift the conversation about diabetes toward the bigger picture: its social and environmental drivers.

Our campaign, the Bigger Picture (www.thebiggerpicture.org), was rooted in art as social action. It included a training and curating workshop process to support talented young people of color to develop original spokenword poetry, resources to amplify their work through the co-creation and production of hip-hop music videos that accompanied the poems, and platforms to disseminate their voices. It allowed their stories and their experiences to be in the spotlight, giving youths the chance to call out and confront the structural root causes of type 2 diabetes and their effects. The hope was that creating and disseminating such a campaign would not only enable young people of color to resist the market forces to overconsume SSBs that Melanie faced as a child and young adult but also advance policies to improve the unhealthy social and environmental conditions in which children of color often find themselves trapped.

To help me develop this program on the public health side, I recruited Sarah Fine, a young woman with a youth development background who, as an added bonus, had inherited from her father a revolutionary spirit and strong social justice focus. She was the daughter of the late Dr. Richard (Dick) Fine, perhaps the most influential physician-advocate who ever worked at San Francisco General Hospital. A product of the 1960s, Dick had first established himself in the early 1970s by developing the outpatient care operations at the hospital at a time when the institution, and the city as a whole, offered no follow-up services or care to patients being discharged from the hospital. An informal mentor of mine, Dick was the go-to guy for progressive causes in medicine and public health, a trusted social activist who served as the undercover physician to the Black Panthers in the late '60s; who was appointed by the Indians of All Tribes group to serve as their physician during their nineteen-month occupation of Alcatraz Island; and who, in his role as chief of the medical staff at San Francisco General Hospital, championed the care of patients with AIDS when certain physicians were refusing to provide surgical care to AIDS patients for fear of acquiring the disease at a time when we had little idea what caused the disease or how it was transmitted. Dick both shaped and embodied the contemporary culture of our institution, one that shamelessly embraces social medicine.

On the artistic side, James recruited Hodari Davis and Jamie DeWolf. Hodari is a deeply inspiring poet mentor, a creative genius, and the person most responsible for developing Youth Speaks' unique pedagogical framework. Hodari was to become the poet mentor to partner with me to develop and run the Bigger Picture writing workshops. Jamie, himself a slam poet and product of Youth Speaks, had since become a filmmaker; he was hired to work with the youths to transform their spoken word pieces into deeply compelling three- to five-minute films that could be disseminated on social media.

Hodari, Jamie, and I started with an after-school workshop involving eight youths, all of whom were veterans of Youth Speaks and some of whom were current or former slam poetry event winners. Virtually all of them reported that they had close family members with diabetes and its complications, including many young relatives. The workshop ran for two hours a day over five afternoons. My job was to share my experience as a primary care doctor at a public hospital and to teach the young artists that type 2 diabetes is a consequence not simply of individual lifestyle choices or genetic makeup but of broader, dysfunctional systems that constrain and shape behavior. That there are social forces that reduce costs of obesogenic food, incentivize its marketing to people of color, unequally allocate physical activity opportunities, and perpetuate poverty, food insecurity, and stress—all in ways that disproportionately focus diabetes risk within marginalized communities. The intent of this systems frame was to direct their attention to the structural causes of the epidemic.

I realized my presentation might be hitting home when, as I was presenting the maps of San Francisco that demonstrate the upside-down T in which the overlapping geographic hot spots of poverty, diabetes hospitalization rates, and high consumption of sugar-sweetened beverages are contained (see Chapter 18), a young poet named Aisha—a girl who had barely engaged thus far—stopped the lesson. She stood up and walked over to the large screen at the front of the room.

"Wait a minute," she said, her face blazing in the light from the projector. She pointed to her neighborhood, in the heart of the upside-down T. "I *live* here."

"Yes, I know," said Hodari gently. "It's hard to see this laid out this way."

He turned to the group sitting around the table.

"How many of you also live in one of these hot spot neighborhoods?"

All the poets raised their hands, followed by a general grumbling and some cursing.

Aisha, shielding her eyes from the bright light, blurted out, "What the fuck? *Why are they doing this to us?* Why?"

Turning off the projector, I responded, "That's the question we are asking here and one of the questions your poetry can try to ask or even answer. That's also the sort of righteous anger your words can evoke in others, the injustice that your words can call out."

Aisha stormed back to her seat, shaking her head from side to side. She then packed up her bag and started getting up to leave.

"Where are you going? Are you okay?" asked Hodari.

"I got to get to my job by 6:00. Plus, it's in one of those neighborhoods. And I got to get in costume first."

"What's your job?" I asked.

"My job? I get in a big chicken suit and walk around the mall, giving out Fried Chicken Candy to kids, trying to get their parents to buy some for them. I tell the parents that they can put them in a candy bowl or in their favorite casserole. I'm real good at what I do."

"Wow. There's definitely a Bigger Picture poem or two in that story."

By the end of the weeklong workshop, the youths had written poems that synthesized their new knowledge with their lived experience, reflecting the underlying tenet of Youth Speaks' pedagogy: "Life as primary text." I discovered that their poems tapped into adolescents' deeply held values of social justice, resistance to manipulation, defiance against authority, desire to protect their families and communities, and intrinsic drive to have a voice and sense of agency in effecting change in their world. Here was another example of the power that storytelling and listening can have in the public health sphere. Hearing their drafts, Hodari, James, Sarah, Jamie, and I knew right off the bat that these young people could shift the discourse about type 2 diabetes, whether they were to be performed at high school assemblies, public health and medical conferences, or policy gatherings.

We ran many such workshops. After each workshop, top poems were selected and turned into poetry videos by Jamie and the poet. Each youth poet's vision for how to tell the story was central to production; the videos featured the poets themselves and often their family members, with their own homes and neighborhoods as backdrops. One video poem got picked up by Upworthy, another by the Huffington Post. Soon, we had sufficient, high-quality content and enough talented young artists to reach for health policy platforms that I had access to. The Bigger Picture became the first social media campaign to feature wholly youth-generated artistic content to promote social action in health. The National Academy of Medicine in Washington, DC, as part of its Roundtable on Health Literacy, invited Panamanian American Gabriel Cortez to perform his poem. It was the first time that poetry had been recited at the National Academy of Medicine, an acclaimed, highly influential, and often stuffy scientific body. Gabriel's subversive and transformative poem—about the "Coca-colonization" of Latin Americans and the militaristic targeted marketing of people of color—received a standing ovation from the audience, composed mostly of white men wearing white lab coats.

Perfect Soldiers
by Gabriel Cortez

My grandpa flashes a gold tooth when he smiles,
like I dare you to take something from between my lips.
His tooth shines from the light of the TV screen
when my family watches Telemundo during dinnertime.
While I practice my Spanish, Grandpa unhinges
the English from his throat, at least for a little while.
This is how we both learn to be Panamanian-American,
through television and food.

He tells us of our ancestors.
How they raised maize and yucca from the earth,

hands steeped in indigenous soil.
How as warriors, we drank cacao and water
bitter from the gourd, a medicine sacred to the gods.

Between growing up in Colón, Panama,
and a tour in the U.S. Army,
my grandpa is a proud old soldier
marching through a never ending war.
At 66 we are scared that another stroke
could do what no war ever could
and cut him to the ground.

He drinks
like Aunt Maritza didn't lose
both her legs to diabetes last year.
Like half our neighborhood doesn't look
like the emergency ward of a hospital.
Like he hasn't seen the pictures,
how it is impossible to tell the difference
between a roadside bomb victim
and someone who just forgot to take their insulin.

Grandpa keeps at least two twelve-packs
of soda in the fridge at all times.
Sunny Delight, Tampico, Hi-C,
a jug of Kool-Aid in the back.
Dr. Pepper lines our refrigerator door
like a vest of dynamite, an arsenal of ways
for us to self-destruct.

It is how you learn to drink growing up in a country
where soda is cheaper than clean water.
Where hunger is a canal carved deep into your belly.
Where the only options for work are the docks and the ARMY

because your country is as occupied by Coca-Cola
as it is by the U.S. military.

When you must march to the call of whatever feeds family first,
you drink whatever fits conveniently in your hands.
I understand Grandpa. But don't you know
we are still at war with a country that wants us dead?
How us children of Panama and America learn early
to walk softly and carry a big stick
like a U.S. assault rifle in one hand,
Coca-Cola bottle in the other.

Our country wasn't enough,
they are colonizing our bodies,
our taste buds.
It isn't a coincidence the military
and beverage companies
call us their target audience.
Our black and brown bodies marching
to the center of their crosshairs.

At home, a Coca-Cola commercial
followed by a U.S. ARMY commercial
flickers across my grandfather's tooth
and they both shine like the discharge of a gun.

I learned to drink like Grandpa.
Like Colón, Panama.
Like 14 billion dollars spent
on soft drink advertising last year.

The threat of diabetes is as common in our family
as hard work, obedience, and discipline.
It is as common as Coca-Cola in our refrigerator.

And we drink until the glass is empty
because we ain't never learned how to pull maize from the soil
but we did learn to pull the tab of a Coke can.
Don't it sound like the linchpin of a grenade?
Both explode under pressure,
ain't we just time bombs then?

We march until they cut the legs out from under us.
Ain't we perfect soldiers.

Sixteen-year-old Marje Kilpatrick's poem, having already been viewed on-line by tens of thousands of people, was then presented to hundreds of professionals at an international public health symposium on the relationship between oral health and physical health. Her evocative narrative of being a child in Richmond, California, has been described to me as the most compelling elucidation of the (mostly invisible) social and commercial determinants of health, illuminating how untoward social and environmental conditions shape the health of populations. Especially type 2 diabetes, through the overexposure of added sugar to children of color. And it speaks to the need to end the silence.

Chocolate Smile
by Marje Kilpatrick

In my neighborhood,
We stay quiet
While our sisters stand under streetlights
Letting the shine adorn their skin,
They prance in silver six-inch heels
With clothes that caress their curves,
Coated in chocolate.

In my neighborhood,
We stay quiet

While fiends crave a fix in the form of a fluid,
Swimming beneath a needle,
Letting it corrupt their insides
And run tracks up their arms
And within their damaged veins.

In my neighborhood,
We stay quiet
While our brothers stand on cracked pavement,
Selling broken dreams in the form of a little blue pill.

In my neighborhood
Every mouth is wired shut.
Rape culture
Quiet.
Education system
Quiet.
Police brutality
Quiet.
Institutionalized racism
Quiet.
Type 2 diabetes
Quiet.
Shhh!

They won't tell you about the little girl
Who once held the corner store at her fingertips,
Whose innocence was corrupted with Coke bottles and Ho-ho cupcakes
They won't tell you about that sweet smile,
Feet on pavement,
The way her pink knocker balls used to swing,
Sipping on chocolate milk like remembrance of Mama's nipples.

They won't tell you
How she sucked on Tootsie Pops since she was three years old.

Holding lukewarm bottles of soda
Too scared she'd lose her grip.
Hot Cheeto stains on the collar of her shirt
And the side of her lips,
Stuck in between her teeth
Using the tip of her tongue to savor the last of her dose.

They won't tell you
About that dimple-filled smile,
With big gaps
And big dreams coated in sugar,
The way she hid jawbreakers between her cheek and teeth
Turning her smile three shades of blue,
The ebony of her skin against the rainbow of her smile.

Chocolate like beauty,
Like goddess,
Like ancestry.
Chocolate like Hershey's Kisses building on the back of her neck.

Chocolate like she was raised in the center of the hood,
With hip-hop her late-night lullabies
And staticky cable with her Saturday morning breakfast
Chocolate like every corner near her home
is adorned with a liquor store.

Chocolate like she ain't never heard of Whole Foods,
Just a hole in her only food can fill.
Chocolate like Mama don't have health insurance,
Like a trip to the dentist cost more than Mama's rent.

Chocolate like her teeth becoming one with her skin
This is for the girl who held the corner store at her fingertips,
Whose mouth used to ring of adrenaline-induced laughter,

Her sweet smile now rotting away with her innocence.
Jagged teeth in her mouth has her gums aching.

They won't tell you
How her smile was corrupted by blue slushies and black licorice,
Leaving brown potholes in their wake.
And we still remain quiet
While they drain us of everything sweet
But the color of our skin and the sugar in our hips.

In my neighborhood
Our thighs are heavy,
Our asses thick
Our culture being weighed down
By silence.

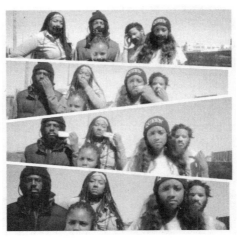

Courtesy of Youth Speaks.

POETRY AND POLICY

Within a few months, the poets and their work were being harnessed to advance progressive diabetes social policy. In the San Francisco Bay Area, stakeholder entities, such as the American Heart Association, the Boys and

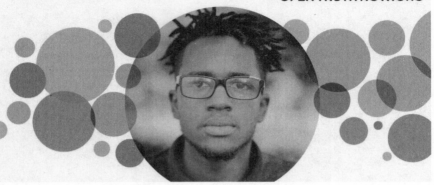

Sugary drinks are making us sick.
OPEN TRUTH NOW.ORG

Courtesy of the Open Truth Campaign, a collaboration among the Shape Up San Francisco Coalition, the Bigger Picture campaign, Alameda County Public Health Department, Sonoma County Department of Health Services, the American Heart Association Greater Bay Area division, and the Clinical & Translational Science Institute at UCSF.

Girls Clubs, and county health departments, adopted the messaging for their prevention efforts. The Open Truth initiative used Bigger Picture messaging to educate the public about the health consequences of sugary drinks, highlighting industry's targeted marketing to youths of color. Riders on the Bay Area Rapid Transit system (BART) could scan the images of the poets posted on the trains and at stops and view their video poems.

A Bigger Picture poet performed at the SSB tax press conference held by the mayors of San Francisco and Oakland. Sixteen-year-old Obasi Davis's poem, "Targets," reveals why:

> *My middle school*
> *On 14th and Adeline,*
> *Wading in a concrete sea of decay,*
> *A central pivot between two liquor stores*
> *That witness more dead bodies than a funeral home*
> *And create more walking cadavers than a zombie apocalypse.*
>
> *Two stationary assassins*
> *Gunning for the preteens caught in the crosshairs*

My classmates and I were all unintentionally killing ourselves
At thirteen.
Targets.
Guzzling down a soda while walking past wheelchaired
amputees and crack addicts
Because we weren't aware of our own bodies collapsing
After the sweet, euphoric sting leapt from our tongue.

Tasty poisons are misleading,
Because we all want to trust gullible taste buds.
But look behind the façade.
Sugary drinks are the leading cause of diabetes.
Sodas kill more colored people than Jim Crow,
Drowning us in corrosive pools of sugar water.

Soda companies reaping the profits of our addiction,
Pushing bottles like weight on corners.
I've seen fiends
From East Oakland to the Mission
Ingesting carbonated poison.
It's no coincidence
That over 40% of Black and Latino youth will get
type 2 Diabetes in their lifetime.

It's strategy.
A minority hunt.
With liquor stores for hit men,
And sugar for bullets
Aim for the sweet spot.

Shortly thereafter, Obasi was selected as the youth poet laureate for the city of Oakland.

Another poet performed his piece outside the federal court where the hearing on sugary beverage warning notices was to be adjudicated. Another performed her poem—an ode to fresh water—at a community event to mark the kickoff of the city's project to install freshwater stations in the soda-engorged neighborhoods bounded by the inverted T on the San Francisco map. Numerous additional performances demonstrated the ways in which the campaign has promoted civic engagement among youths typically considered "disengaged and disenfranchised."

To date, the campaign has produced over thirty videos emphasizing a broad range of public health messages related to the prevention of diabetes through social action. The video poems have been performed for over twenty thousand Bay Area high school students and have been viewed online nearly two million times. At its inception, the Bigger Picture was centered in the San Francisco Bay Area. In 2016, after training sister spoken word organizations, it expanded to seven other California regions hit hard by diabetes, with products featured in a special story in the *New York Times*. This enabled the campaign to extend to such areas as California's Central Valley, home to the fresh fruit and vegetable basket of the country and, paradoxically, the epicenter of California's diabetes epidemic. Eighteen-year-old poet Anthony "Joker" Orozco from Stockton, California, brought attention to this travesty with his poem entitled "Empty Plate," which addresses the legacy of poverty that afflicts migrant families and the fact that farmers who harvest for the fresh produce markets do not earn enough to afford the food themselves:

> *Abuelas y abuelos, tias, tios, primos y carnales*
> *Who picked processed and packed produce*
> *Their pockets couldn't afford to begin with.*
> *Backs breaking, bones aching,*
> *Harvesting healthy fruits and veggies*
> *Acre by acre,*
> *The bounty of California's breadbasket*
> *That almost never blessed the tables of farmero families*

He then calls out the parallel reality of fresh food deserts and the panoply of fast-food outlets endemic to the south side of Stockton, California:

Today it's practically multiple choice,
Being murdered or choosing death by diet.
A decision between
8 spots 3 blocks apart.

THE CROSSROADS

We are all actors: being a citizen is not living in society, it is changing it.

—Augusto Boal, *Theater of the Oppressed*

To date, most public health communication campaigns have focused on changing individuals' health behaviors. They have done little to stem the rising tide of obesity and type 2 diabetes. The Bigger Picture, however, has brought together the arts and public health with the goal of shifting how we view diabetes away from a traditional focus of individual "shame and blame" and toward calling out the social drivers of the disease. The initiative has shown how listening to those most affected by marginalization, and the diseases it generates, can inform public health. The model has shown tremendous promise, potentially worthy of scaling to a national and even international levels. The idea for co-creation in the Bigger Picture emerged from a well-tested health communication approach. In this case, engaging members of a target community in creating messages increased message relevance and motivation and led to the development of novel ways to reframe a health problem and its solutions. Creating new messages (and new messengers) to tell stories that reflect the lived experience of the target population has provided inroads that open up new possibilities for change, and new reasons for our society to make critical decisions to benefit the common good.

Melanie's story and many of the stories I have shared show us what can happen when we, as a society, make the wrong choices. I don't know whether our society ultimately will make the right choices when it comes to public health. But with the voices of these young people telling us the way, I am more hopeful. Poet José Vadi understood that we are at a crossroads and, riffing off Erica's "Death Recipe," he wrote a Bigger Picture poem that encourages us all to rewrite our recipe in a life-affirming way.

The Corner
by José Vadi

We're standing on The Corner
Between Healthy and Heart Attack,
Not sure which way to cross.
On one side, an organic grocery,
On the other, deep-fried death.

Our bodies pull us away from the produce aisle
into Value Meal Heaven,
Ignoring the question of
"Just what part of a chicken
Is a nugget anyway?"

Every bite a last meal telling us
"This is just temporary."
But greener more nutritional options
Are right across the street.

Yet our bodies demand mechanically processed meat,
And water costs more than milk,
When broccoli costs more than beef.
They want a pound of flesh
For every 90 pounds of sugar
We eat in a year.

Our whole block is at this trough,

Thinking we're full
Before being back on The Corner
Starving for the next meal.

They turned our bodies into battlefields.
Turned our cookbooks into combo meals
And told us to "Drive Thru."
My wallet says to super-size it.

We can tell you five different paths
To the deep fryers sizzling past midnight.
Nobody dares to turn off their neon lights.
But their cheap digestible cyanide
Turns my kiss into snakebites

Take an X-ray of my guts and you'll see
the proof's in the puddin'.
When our diets
Make parachute pants out of our jeans

Our ankles become cankles,
Our blood: a stained sewer circulating in our bodies.
Only gangrene amputees will be our legacy,
Corporate sponsored deadly delicacies

How much longer must we lose the battle
Before we start the war against diabetes HERE,
on The Corner
Of Healthy or Heart Attack,
Life or Stroke

Because we don't want to end up on The Corner,
Pricking our thumbs with a lancet
To measure our sugar levels every day

Before we finally decide
Which way to cross . . .

How far do we have to slip
Before we end this edible misery
And rewrite
Our recipe?

Song for My Father

To the Dark Side and Back Again

A BEACON AND A SANCTUARY

The young man lies on the emergency room gurney still wearing work boots caked with dried mud. He stares straight ahead, up to the ceiling, only rarely blinking. The triage nurse elicited no name and found no ID on him. His orange hospital card simply has the pseudonym "Giraffe" embossed on it, with an accompanying medical record number. He looks to me like an undocumented day laborer, one of the many male Mexican immigrants who stand on the corners of Cesar Chavez Street hoping to score a few twenty-dollar bills working dangerous roofing and construction day jobs. His temperature is nearly 105 degrees, but his heart rate is only 64 and his blood pressure and oxygenation are normal. He does not respond to commands and demonstrates no threat response, not even flinching as I feign a strike with my open palm to his innocent face. Both a firm sternal rub and a squeeze of his thigh do elicit vocal pain responses, so he is still with it, if only barely. A differential diagnosis rapidly runs through my mind, scrolling like the opening credits for a film I didn't choose to watch. Hyperthermia or heatstroke? Some sort of infection and evolving sepsis? An AIDS-related illness? Spinal meningitis? Encephalitis? Drug overdose—maybe speed, antidepressants, or antipsychotics?

His chest bears a cross lying atop a backdrop of spotted red skin. Sweat is beading on his forehead, and his shirt is soaked through. I recall the aphoristic warning, "If the patient is sweating profusely, so too should the physician."

I quickly begin the fever workup. I start to draw blood cultures, being especially careful to clean the inner elbows with alcohol to ensure that no skin bacteria contaminate the samples. But the patient keeps squirming, making it impossible for me to safely and effectively get this critical job done. I call one of the experienced ER nurses over to help.

"Do me a favor and firmly hold his arm down. He keeps moving around, and I need to get blood cultures—first from this arm and then from the other."

She does her job well; not a move escapes his arms. I get what I need, and we send the blood-filled bottles off to the lab. We obtain urine cultures, and I start broad-spectrum IV antibiotics and IV fluids. I request a lumbar puncture tray from the nurse. We need to do a spinal tap, and fast, to rule out meningitis. I am also worried about the possibility of a "toxidrome"—a potentially fatal reaction to chemical pesticide agents used in gardening and farming. Do we need to don hazmat suits and decontaminate him first? Another aphorism helps me to remember the classic signs of anticholinergic agent poisonings: "Mad as a Hat, Red as a Beet, Blind as a Bat, Dry as a Bone, and Tacky as a Leisure Suit." Well, mad he is, red he is, blind he may be, dry he is not, and tachycardic he most certainly is not, not with a heart rate of 64. So, no hazmats and no decontamination are needed, I decide.

I grab the arm of a random medical student walking briskly past me and glance at her name tag.

"Listen . . . *Ellen*. I need you to do something really important. Are you up for it?"

"I hope so. Yeah, I think so. I mean, I can try my best," she responds with the ambiguous confidence characteristic of medical students.

"Then your job is to go into that giant waiting room, or to the cafeteria or the parking lot, or onto Cesar Chavez Street if you have to. I really don't care. Just find someone—*anyone*—who knows this guy. Look at him closely so you can describe him. Talk to the triage nurse and get a description of who dropped him off. Then go find them. When you do, take a really good history. Ask them about the circumstances leading up to his getting sick. I want to know *everything*, not just the usual stuff, okay? So, gimme HIV risk factors, travel history, psych history, substance use, occupational hazards or exposures. And try to convince them to come back with you so I can dig deeper. Tell them that their friend really needs them here, and promise them that nothing bad will happen to them if they do come back."

"Okay, I can do that," she says.

"Good. You speak Spanish, right?"

"Medical Spanish, yes."

"What does *that* even mean? We need a fluent Spanish speaker. Grab an interpreter to go with you. Please. *Medical* Spanish," I scoff.

As she rushes off, I work with another nurse—a young one, someone I have never worked with before—over the next twenty minutes, prepping Giraffe for the lumbar puncture. We remove his work boots, peel his clothes off, and position him onto his side, curling his knees up to hug his chest to maximally expose the spaces between the vertebrae of his lumbar spine. I carefully pick my spot, making a midline mark in the divot between the fourth and fifth lumbar vertebrae. I glove and gown up and carefully clean his lumbar area to create a sterile field, applying the rust-colored antiseptic liquid in ever-enlarging concentric circles whose bull's-eye is located at the mark I made.

"Do we have everything we need?" I ask.

"Everything but his informed consent," my nurse shoots back at me.

"Oh, please. Don't start. I know my Nuremberg Code, thank you very much. This guy lacks decision-making capacity. He doesn't even know his mama's name. This lumbar puncture is an emergency procedure. So please glove and gown too so we can get this show on the road. And tell people not to open this curtain until we come out with our liquid gold. Hopefully, crystal-clear liquid gold."

"Okay, but make sure you chart that Nuremberg thing."

"Yeah, will do. Okay, move out from behind me, and please switch over to the other side. I need you to hold him down by his arms so he absolutely doesn't move. If he moves, he can endanger himself and put me and this lumbar puncture at risk. Can't have that happen."

She swings around across the gurney from me and gently holds his arms down. "Okay, señor, I'm just going to hold you and support you while the doctor does his thing. Don't worry."

I withdraw from the kit the long spinal needle still in its sheath and place it on its side and fill a syringe with lidocaine to numb the skin before I insert the long needle. I feel around for the lumbar landmarks one last time to make sure that my X marks the right spot. As I carefully place the short, narrow-gauge lidocaine needle beneath his skin at the target, he lets out a yelp, and his back unexpectedly bucks, dislodging the needle.

"Whoa, cowboy! Relax. Just *relax*. Okay, we *cannot* have that happen again," I inform my nurse. "Especially not when I am putting in the long LP needle."

She looks across at me with an uncertainty that undermines my confidence. I pull off my sterile gloves and walk around to her side.

"Watch me." I grasp both of the patient's wrists, pinning them down to the gurney. I place the weight of my body onto his thighs, using my elbow to pin his knees down.

"This is how it's done. You have to completely immobilize him. You can still talk nice, but you can't let him move. Got it? We don't want to have to use restraints or sedate him."

I return to my side, glove up again, and look over at her across the gurney. She's positioned as I asked but avoids my gaze. Again, as he begins to squirm, she loosens her grip—just as I am about to puncture the skin above his vertebrae to inject the lidocaine.

I take a step back and look at her. She seems shaken.

"Look, I know what I am asking you to do here looks and feels dehumanizing, violent, and even brutal to you. And in some ways, you're right. This is a violent act that we are conducting on him. What probably makes it even harder for you is that perhaps we are forcing ourselves onto a defenseless, undocumented immigrant. Someone who has no voice and whose backstory we don't know. But this is the only way we can express our care and even love for this fellow human being. We don't know who he is. But he is someone's son, someone's brother, maybe someone's lover. So please hold him firmly, but tenderly, so we can help him. Just like you would do for a family member with possible meningitis who desperately needed our help to live."

She gets him back onto his side and into the fetal position and tightly wraps her arms around him. She gives me a nod to go ahead.

This time, she does the job of forcibly restraining him perfectly. The lidocaine goes in with only minimal disruption. The lumbar puncture needle also goes in smoothly and then pops through to the fluid-filled space. I withdraw the needle, leaving behind the narrow metal catheter that extends out perpendicular to his back like a tap sticking out of a maple tree.

The spinal fluid slowly drips out and it indeed is clear, and the opening pressure is normal. While we still need to await the official cell count from the lab, it seems unlikely that meningitis is the cause of this patient's febrile syndrome.

Ellen, the medical student on a mission, rushes back in, breathless. "I found a guy who knows him, who brought him here. In the cafeteria, like you said."

"And?"

"Okay, he refused to come back down, but he told us a lot. The patient's name is Eduardo. He's a distant cousin. He's about twenty-five years old, just arrived in San Francisco two days ago. Walked and hitched rides all the way up from Chiapas over the last month. Crossed the border about seven days ago. Cousin said he seemed fine until this morning, when he got confused and felt hot. No other symptoms. No alcohol since he arrived, not sure about before. He doesn't think the guy uses drugs. No other HIV risk factors that he knows of. Says he's a religious Catholic, but he doesn't know him that well. This Eduardo is a farmer back in Chiapas, but he hasn't worked since he got to the US. No psych history that my guy is aware of, and he didn't see him take any medicines since he got here."

"You're awesome, Ellen. That's a huge help. High five."

Chiapas, I think. *That's malaria country.* Another aphorism hits me: "Fever in a traveler equals malaria, until proven otherwise." This has got to be malaria.

I call the CDC hotline and receive confirmation that Chiapas does have the kind of malaria—an especially virulent brand caused by *Plasmodium falciparum*—that can cause central nervous system disease, altered mental status, and death.

Well then. I am going to try to save this man's life. That's what this whole thing is all about.

I call the lab and ask if the blood I submitted is sufficient to run so-called thick smears to try to detect the malaria parasite. They put me on hold for a bit and then tell me that it is and that they'll run one. But they recommend I send more smears every eight hours at least two more times to increase the chance that they will find it. I love our micro lab. It's the best in the country, hands down.

I admit Eduardo Giraffe to the hospital with the presumptive diagnosis of "*Malaria, possibly cerebral. Rule out sepsis.*"

I go by his room over the next few days. On day three, he is still burning up and remains delirious. He looks about the same as he did before, which isn't good. I grab one of the most basic tools of our trade—the chart hanging from the foot of his bed that displays the trajectory of his vital signs on graph paper—and I analyze his fever curve. A spiky sine wave of ups and downs. The relapsing fever so characteristic of malaria. But why have all the thick smears been negative?

Another set of points on the chart captures my attention. His heart rate has remained in the 60s throughout, irrespective of his temperature. Fever and a fast heart rate should go together like hand in glove. But with him, no ups and downs, just a flat line connecting the dots of slow heart rates. *Only a few infectious diseases do this*, I remind myself. Known as *relative bradycardia*, or *Faget sign*, this dissociation between fever and heart rate have got to provide the answer. I need to go look it up in my infectious disease textbook.

As I am descending the elevator, the hospital chaplain, dressed in black, enters and we exchange nods. The doors close. We are alone, so I ask him, "Chaplain, can you do me a favor? Actually, it's for a patient."

"Yes, of course. That's what I'm here for."

"There's this guy in 5C, bed 12A. An undocumented immigrant. I don't know much about him other than that, apparently, he is super religious. Catholic is what I was told by a cousin. He's out of it, and he's alone. Has some febrile illness that leaves him dazed. We haven't figured it out yet. I'm worried about him. He's hanging in, but it could go either way. I think that maybe a visit from you—"

"Say no more. Do you have a name?"

"Eduardo is all I know."

The doors open at the lobby level.

I walk out, holding the door open for the chaplain. "You coming out?"

He smiles. "No. I'm going back up to the fifth floor."

"Thank you, Chaplain. God bless."

I walk across the sidewalk and enter my redbrick building, one of the original hospital wards built in 1915. I pull open the heavy gilded copper door mottled by green patina, run up the stairs to my third-floor office, and crack open the block-size *Infectious Disease* textbook, Volume 1. I find "Faget Sign" in the index and riffle through the pages to find a table containing a short list of communicable diseases associated with high fever and slow heart rate: *Tularemia, Brucellosis, Yellow Fever, Typhoid Fever*. Tularemia and brucellosis are possible given his history of working on a farm, I think to myself. Tularemia you get from deer ticks and other infected animals, but I think of it presenting more with fever, enlarged lymph nodes and skin ulcers, not delirium. Not my guy. Brucellosis is contracted from undercooked meat or milk from domestic farm animals like pigs and cows. Could be it. I recall it causes undulating fever and muscle pains, but no altered mental status. Probably not my guy either. Severe cases of yellow fever, a mosquito-borne illness, are relatively rare, and such patients should have an enlarged liver and jaundice. My guy's liver tests are pristine, and he certainly is not yellow. That leaves typhoid fever. Common in Central America, usually starts with bloody diarrhea, can last for four weeks . . .

My thoughts are interrupted as my hospital pager goes off: x8172. It's the microbiology lab. Always a moment filled with anticipation. I grab my desktop phone and quickly punch in the four numbers I know so well.

"Dr. Schillinger here, Medical Service, returning your page. You have something for me?"

"Yes, Doctor," replies our Filipina American lab tech. "I have a micro result for you. Patient: Giraffe, medical record number 0177634. His blood cultures are growing out gram-negative rods. *Salmonella typhi*, two out of two sets. I am documenting that you were informed of these results at 2:35 p.m. today."

Typhoid fever. Right. In the second and third weeks of untreated typhoid fever, you can see delirium and an encephalitis-like presentation. The so-called blank typhoidal stare. Classic. The rose spots on his chest. And relative bradycardia. He has it all. The clue to save his life was there the whole time—on his mundane vital signs chart penned by a caring nurse onto graph paper. And then my trusted lab came through to confirm the answer.

Typhoid fever. A scourge of humankind, once a disease of epidemic proportions that wiped out tens of millions of people each year. In the 1880s, Dr. Karl Joseph Eberth, a gray-bearded German pathologist from a Bavarian town north of Munich, discovered that a specific bacterium caused the illness. Initially named *Eberthella typhi*, and eventually renamed *Salmonella typhi*, this microbe still leads to serious illness in over twelve million people a year. A communicable disease transmitted by the fecal-oral route, typhoid fever has become rare in areas of the world with the resources to institute public hygiene measures, including systems for clean drinking water, sanitation, and plumbing. Now, fewer than four hundred cases are reported in the US each year. With a mortality rate as high as 20 percent in the pre-antibiotic era, typhoid fever in the modern era—when correctly diagnosed and treated—has a fatality rate of about 1 percent.

I laugh to myself and feel a warmth spread throughout my body. We *are* going to save this guy's life, albeit from a different disease than the one I first was convinced he had. I feel proud of the field I have chosen for myself, proud of the storied and benevolent profession I have worked so hard to become part of. Proud to be one in a long line of clinicians and researchers who harness science to understand the mechanisms of disease, those who carefully and methodically discover novel pathways to improve our diagnostic skills and who develop innovative ways to treat and cure ailments and plagues. And most of all, I feel proud of *where* I work. All this accumulated knowledge and training, all the skilled and caring people, the technology, the tests, and the equipment—all brought together within this single public institution, organized around its singular mission. A beacon of humanity amid the dysfunctional morass that is US health care, a sanctuary from the brutal realities of our society.

While I recognize this feeling to be a momentary and unusually favorable assessment of the more complicated reality of my hospital, I run with it for now. Because we have just harnessed the best of medicine—past and present—to save a man's life. That is what it's all about.

HEALTH AND HYGIENE

It is almost twenty years later, and thousands of patient encounters are under my belt. I am in Munich, Germany, representing the US in the conduct of a multinational study on diabetes funded by the European Commission.

Deutschland: The land—and its people—that held my young father and his immediate family captive and starving for a year in a concentration camp. A nation that killed all his extended family, including his six uncles, his one aunt, and their families.

Munich: The city where it all started. The birthplace of the National So-cialist movement that culminated in the Nazis' Final Solution to "the Jew-ish problem," a problem defined as the racial defilement of the pure Aryan race by the impure, inferior, and diabolic Semitic race. Fundamentally, it was a problem of biology, of very bad blood. Fixing it was a matter of restor-ing racial hygiene, of tackling it as a medical problem, a genuine and cen-tral concern of public health and of the exciting and new field of genetics. A political movement driven by the founding members of the Nazi Party, a disgruntled set of criminals and hacks. But these individuals were both malevolent and prescient enough to harness a set of warped public health principles and cozy up to the undisputed leaders in German medicine to further the goals of their movement. A movement instigated, catalyzed, propelled, and at times perpetrated by the great and accomplished Ger-man medical and scientific establishment, the envy of the modern world. As is now widely acknowledged, the Final Solution was a culminating public health initiative based on a misguided medical quest for racial improvement and perfection. A medical crusade to "cleanse" German society of popula-tions viewed as biological threats to the nation's health. Its ultimate con-sequence was not a healthier society but a clinically engineered genocide masked as a benevolent campaign designed to rid the German people of Jews, homosexuals, Romani, the mentally disabled, and any others scientif-ically deemed to be subhuman.

Munich is also the city closest to Dachau, one of the many Nazi concen-tration camps in Germany. Yet Dachau stands out among all others for the special role it played in the Holocaust and in the history of modern medicine.

To be a Jew in modern Germany is to be in a state of suspended animation—adrift between the unthinkable horrors of its past and the more sanguine reality of its present. To suffer from a hypervigilance stemming from a brutal history of extreme marginalization and mass murder while simultaneously being coaxed to relax in the context of a welcoming and open society.

This is my first time visiting Germany. I had always avoided it. The trauma of my father's past had been thoroughly communicated to me and had infiltrated my core from a young age. I felt no pull to visit this country, no desire to grace its killing fields with the presence of a son of a survivor. No need to close this loop.

But here I am. I have two days of work and one day free. It is only 7:00 a.m., so a full day awaits me. I decide I will first visit the Olympic Village, home to the dramatic 1972 Summer Olympic Games. Infamous for being the site where eleven Israeli Olympic athletes were taken hostage and then killed by a Palestinian terrorist group, broadcast on television for all to see. While I was only seven years old at the time, the memories are still crystal clear to me. But the village also is a site famous for the swimming pool that Mark Spitz conquered, the pool in which he won seven gold medals. These medals represented one Jewish athlete's affirmative response to Hitler's Berlin Olympic Games of 1936. Finding a place to do my daily swim while traveling is always a challenge. But today, I decide I will spend the first part of my free day in Munich vicariously reliving Spitz's gold-plated victories. I will swim in Spitz's center lane.

I take a cab to the Olympic Village, a modernist compound with structures covered in tarp-like roofs. I pay my entrance fee to the fabled pool, the Munich Schwimmhalle, and confidently enter the men's locker room, labeled *Herren*, or *Gentlemen*.

I am immediately assaulted by the yells and orders of German men.

"*Es ist verboten zu betreten!*"

"*Zieh deine Schuhe aus!*"

I look up to see angry German faces glaring at me, fingers pointing. I am shaken. I recall from my study of the anti-Jewish decrees that *verboten* means "forbidden." I also recall, from my knowledge of how the Nazis efficiently processed the Jews (and their belongings) as they forced them into the death camps, that *Schuhe* means "shoes."

"*Es ist verboten zu betreten! Zieh deine Schuhe aus!*"

Oh . . . now I get it. *No shoes allowed in the locker room.* I show them my open palms to calm them down, and with their eyes still on me, I sit on a bench and remove my shoes. I proceed to the locker number I was provided by the ticket clerk, located at the very end of the locker room. I undress and put on my bathing suit, cap, and goggles and look around to find the entrance to the pool. I see two doors labeled *Dusche*, which must mean "shower." Of course, we have to shower before we swim.

I enter the door closest to me and find myself alone in the shower hall. Eight showerheads loom above me. To be a Jew in Germany standing under eight showerheads is again to be in a state of suspended animation, albeit a more irrational state. If I turn the handle, will warm water come out and rinse off the dirt I have accumulated so I can swim clean with the Germans? Or will Zyklon B gas come out so Deutschland can forever be cleansed of my intrinsic impurity?

Screw this. I need to rinse off. I am going to swim like Spitz. I turn the handle and look up. But nothing happens. I shift left and try the next handle. Nothing. No water. And no gas either.

Then, from the opposite door—the one that I assume leads in from the pool—five naked women enter the shower hall. They freeze as they see me, crossing their arms to cover their breasts and their ankles to hide their pubic regions. A few of them scream, but one giggles.

What is going on? Did I somehow enter the women's shower?

"You must to *push!*" says the giggler, a blonde. "You must *to push*. For the water to come."

I push on the handle and promptly get sprayed by cold water. I step away from the showerhead, dripping. They all laugh at me.

"*Danke!*" I yell to them and race back to the relative safety of the men's locker room.

Thoroughly embarrassed, but newly schooled in the ways of German swimming culture, I enter the correct shower room, with shoes off, and shower. I walk into the pool area, find the exact platform, and dive into Mark

Spitz's center lane. I triumphantly swim my twenty fifty-meter laps. One kilometer. It feels great. Freestyle, breaststroke, backstroke. No butterfly and no relay. I am just a Jewish doctor, after all, not a Jewish Olympian. But when I finish, I raise my two arms toward the roof in victory, just like Mark Spitz once did.

With this, I too have proven that we are a worthy people.

A SUBHUMAN LABORATORY AND TORTURE CHAMBER

Suddenly hit with jet lag, I return to my hotel to take a quick nap. I eat a light lunch and head over to the concierge.

"Excuse me, sir. I would like to visit Dachau this afternoon. Can you tell me how to get there?"

"Certainly, sir," he says to me with a smile. "It's quite efficient, actually."

He reaches under his standing desk and pulls out a Munich subway map, unfolding it before me.

"You simply take the S-Bahn line, or the green S2 line, from here," he cheerfully says, pointing to a green dot labeled MARIENPLATZ, "and ride eight, nine, ten, eleven stops . . . until you reach the stop called DACHAU. It departs every twenty minutes. Get a transfer on your way out of the station, cross the street, and then take a short bus ride to the camp. Very easy!"

He smiles at me again. So content with the efficiency of his city.

"I'm sorry. There must be some confusion. I am looking to visit the *concentration camp* Dachau and its museum. You are telling me to get off at a *subway stop* called Dachau?"

"No confusion at all, sir."

He smiles again. "The concentration camp is at the DACHAU station, as I told you."

"You mean Dachau—the concentration camp—is right in Munich itself?"

It is then that I recall the World War II footage showing the British liberators carting the culpable townspeople of Dachau past the remains of concentration camp victims who had been tortured and killed only a few kilometers from their homes. Footage of German men and women civilians holding kerchiefs over their noses, forced to look at the reeking piles of skeletal, naked corpses stacked one on top of another in deep, open trenches. Forced by the soldiers to take up shovels to dig and cover the bodies to avoid the spread of diseases such as scrub typhus and—perhaps—to punish the townspeople for their complicity in the atrocities.

"Well, Munich has expanded, so yes, Dachau is part of the city," he proudly explains.

"How bizarre. Well, thank you for the directions."

"Anytime, sir. Always at your service. I hope you have a *wonderful* day!"

I pocket the subway map and slowly walk through the lobby toward the hotel exit. I am going to visit one of the most infamous concentration camps. *Have a wonderful day.* Did he really just say that?

The subway station is well marked, making it easy to find my way. The subway car itself, despite being packed with passengers, is prompt and clean and glides along effortlessly. To be a Jew in a German train is also to live in suspended animation—to again be trapped in a bizarre space between past and present. These trains and their railway lines were the means of transport to death on a massive scale. Boxcars stuffed with eighty people, systematically moving millions of starving, thirsty, suffering people across Europe to deliver them to a well-organized network of death camps. And yet here I am, alternately squeezed in between businesspeople rushing home for a quick lunch, sandwiched between young mothers with their strollers and university students with their overstuffed backpacks.

The subway train ascends aboveground for a few minutes.

"*Nächste Halt . . . Dachau! . . . Nächste Halt: Dachau!*" bellows the conductor on the overhead speaker as the train decelerates.

Next stop: Dachau.

A shiver passes through me. Now, a feeling as if I am walking toward my own death. Is this what it could have felt like for them, only much worse? Their fears were anticipatory and authentic; theirs were lived fears. My fear is retrospective, merely a traumatic doppelgänger one generation removed, like a nuclear shadow permanently cast by the atomic blast in Hiroshima.

The train glides to a stop, and the doors open onto a platform that houses a large white-and-blue sign posted on a pole: DACHAU. I warily step out as the train glides away. I am the only one on the platform. I spot the bus stop in front of a kiosk, and I cross the street to wait. The bus soon arrives, and I am shuttled the three kilometers to the camp. This was the same path that, seventy years prior, the soon-to-be camp inmates, fresh off the harrowing five-day train ride, were forced to march. And now, as I descend off the lush bus, I am facing the same entrance to the Dachau complex that they faced, the same gate they were forced to enter.

The wrought iron really does spell out *Arbeit Macht Frei*. I had thought that aphorism had been Auschwitz's unique literary gift to mankind. *Work Shall Set You Free*. So, this too was meant to appear to be a work camp. As I will soon find out, for many it indeed was a work camp. Although the kind of work these inmates were compelled to do represents the most dehumanizing form of forced labor ever devised.

I pass through the gates, slowly walking under the overarching and imposing brick structure. The open space before me is massive in scale. Appearing the size of three or four empty football stadium parking lots, this twenty-acre compound—now largely flattened grounds of dirt and gravel—once accommodated at least thirty-four prisoner barracks. Arranged in perfectly symmetric and geometric patterns that reflect the careful planning that went into the camp's rapid construction, the rectangular barracks each housed over 180 inmates, sleeping in groups of three or four, in fifty or so bunks.

I slowly walk the grounds. Only two prisoner barracks are preserved; they occupy a tiny corner of the expansive compound. Sequentially arranged and evenly spaced concrete gravel beds are all that remain of the other thirty-two barracks. Six abandoned guard towers still loom over the fenced-off borders.

I enter so-called Barrack X, a long, low-roofed brick building topped with a disproportionately tall, rectangular brick chimney. This is the gas chamber and crematorium. I shuffle into the anteroom and see a large doorway with painted letters above the threshold: BRAUSEBAD.

SHOWER-BATH. I pass through this doorway and stand in the middle of a sizable and spotless shower hall. Around me are ventilation ducts. Above me, embedded in recesses along the ceiling, are sixteen round showerheads. False showerheads. Once the doors closed behind the inmates, these showerheads released lethal gas. This floor was repeatedly littered with bodies murdered in the name of public health. I look around the corner, just behind the far wall of the Brausebad, and see the intricate piping network and steering wheel-like valves. Valves that released the lethal gas into the shower room. Separate valves that closed the ventilation ducts. And still other valves to slowly and safely release the expended deadly gas out into the environment. German engineering at its best.

I proceed on and enter the attached crematorium. A well-designed death processing plant made of brick and metal. Metal railways to quickly roll carts with the dead bodies from the so-called bathhouse into the crematorium and deposit them in front of one of the three large brick ovens. Cast-iron doors are flung wide open to welcome the next customer. Metal parallel bars stick out perpendicular to the mouth of each oven, enabling the easy transfer of each corpse first from the cart on the rails and then onto a gurney that would ride on top of the perpendicular bars and smoothly glide the corpse into the coal-burning oven. And then out and away down the rail line, carrying any remains like a conveyor belt of human bones and ash. And then the cart would roll back to the Brausebad to do it all over again. And again, day in and day out. With scientific precision, reliability, and most of all—with German efficiency.

For my last stop, I enter Barrack 5, what I soon discover was the medical experiment barracks. Here, tens of thousands of brutal and unprecedented medical experiments were performed on thousands of inmates, including Jews and "renegade" Catholic priests, most from Poland, many of whom died

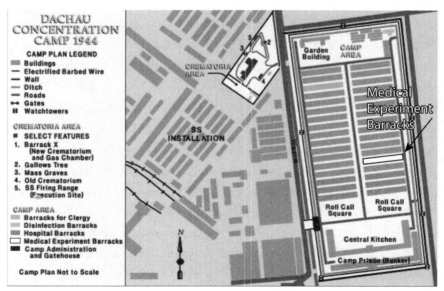

Courtesy of United States Holocaust Memorial Museum, https://encyclopedia.ushmm.org /content/en/map/dachau-concentration-camp-1944.

at the hands of German physician-scientists. Here, men and women were forced to work—not to build armaments, sew military uniforms, harvest food for the men on the front, or mine for coal to fuel the military effort but to give their bodies up to enable "discoveries" in science, to serve as unwilling subjects in medical and surgical experiments. Experiments intended to better understand, for example, if and how German pilots could withstand the profound hypothermia in the North Sea or the rapid changes in altitude they were exposed to in the Northern Atlantic dogfights. Experiments to test methods of making seawater drinkable and studies of blood coagulation to identify methods to stop potentially fatal bleeding. And research intended to inform medical care in the southern sphere of operation, where German infantrymen were dying of malaria.

I slowly walk past a cot with an empty clipboard for a vital signs chart hanging from the foot of the bed. Moving along to the barrack's far wall, I study the medical experimentation exhibit. I see the ruddy, clean-shaven, confidently smiling face of Dr. Sigmund Rascher, posing in his SS uniform. Dr. Rascher was appointed to be Dachau's Sturmbannführer (literally "assault unit leader," an unusual title for a physician) by his close confidant Heinrich Himmler, Hitler's second in command and the grand overseer of the concentration camps—the man most singly responsible for the Holocaust. As Sturmbannführer, Dr. Rascher directed all the medical experiments at Dachau carried out from 1942 to 1945. Beside his photo lies a sample of his written reports addressed and submitted directly to Himmler. Nearly all the clinical research notes composed and filed by the Nazi doctors in Dachau were destroyed by them as the Allies approached, signifying that Rascher and company were well aware that these experiments represented atrocities against humanity and, after the war, could provide tangible evidence of war crimes. But letters such as these, sent up the chain of Nazi hierarchy, were preserved and outlined their clinical research findings in detail.

Beside these letters, under the glass, lies a systematically shot collection of clinical photos displaying the face and upper body of a Jew with a shaved head, wearing striped pajamas. This horrifyingly unforgettable series of photos represents a visual unfolding of different stages in a state-of-the-art "experiment" that exposed the "study participant" to rapidly ascending altitudes, accompanied by rapid decompression. His tormented face icily presents a montage of sequential torture in an objective, clinical fashion. The final photo in the series, one that puts a cherry on top of this medical atrocity, does not show a subsequent iteration of facial distress but instead reveals the back of his shaved head: his sawed-off cranium, exposing the swollen and hemorrhaging brain that resulted from the experiments in rapid ambient pressure change.

Next in line, under the glass case, is a photo of Dr. Klaus Schilling, director of the malaria unit in Dachau from 1936 to 1945. A balded, serious man in a white lab coat, sporting round Kafka-like glasses so fashionable among the German intelligentsia of the day, Dr. Schilling was an international expert in tropical medicine, obsessed with finding a cure for malaria and a vaccine against it. From 1905 to the beginning of World War II, Dr. Schilling, a Munich native, had held the enviable post of director of the tropical medicine division of the Robert Koch Institute. *The* Robert Koch. The father of microbiology and the founder of the field of infectious diseases. It was the great German scientist Dr. Koch who first discovered the causative organisms for

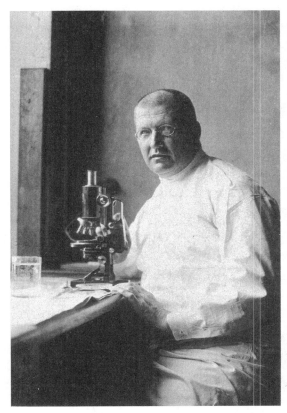

Dr. Klaus Schilling, director of the malaria unit in Dachau concentration camp from 1936 to 1945.

tuberculosis, anthrax, and cholera, among others. It was this same Dr. Koch who developed "Koch's postulates," which form the basis for our modern understanding of communicable diseases. These postulates define the observable criteria required to definitively determine that a specific microbe is responsible for a specific infectious disease.

Dr. Schilling indeed had big shoes to fill. Dachau ultimately provided the perfect setting for him to make his mark. Over many years, he purposely infected over a thousand prisoners with malaria, directly injecting some with serum from other infected patients, and exposing others to mosquitoes chock-full of malaria protozoa. Sometimes he would repeatedly infect them, often on a daily basis, just to see what the human body could tolerate. He purportedly was driven by the need to prevent or cure malaria among German soldiers serving in North Africa. These torturous and often fatal experiments represented unique atrocities not only because of the questions Dr. Schilling was trying to answer and the unscientific methods he employed but also because of the study subjects he selected. While some subjects were the usual Jewish inmates, many were Catholic priests, presumably selected because their blood was believed to be genetically more akin to "pure Aryan blood." Of the many hundreds of priests preferentially sequestered in Dachau, only eighty-two survived.

As I stroll toward the far end of the glass-covered case, shaking my head in disbelief, I am frozen by what I see next. In front of me is a page from one research subject's medical chart, penned on graph paper, adorned with numerous clinical details and notes, and signed by Dr. Schilling himself. As I lean in to view it up close, I recognize that it is an extended vital signs chart, one that displays over time the sinuous fever curve and associated heart rates of a subject who was purposely and repeatedly infected with malaria. The seventy-year-old chart clearly communicates—using the scientific symbols and medical language of our present day, derived from our modern understanding of the clinical signs of disease and health—the illness trajectory of one experimental victim over fourteen days. Relapsing fevers with closely correlated highs and lows in heart rate.

I am shaken and feel as though I will vomit. I step back from the glass case. *I* use these same charts. We rely on these charts to help our patients in our day-to-day work. These charts represent one of the most basic tools of the trade. The same kind of vital signs chart was what helped me get closer to Eduardo's diagnosis and initiate his path to recovery. How could this be? How could all the observational tools, the accumulated medical knowledge, the clinical skills, the tests and the equipment, the trained personnel . . . how could this all have been so perfectly and willingly planned, organized, and harnessed to so systematically *dehumanize?* All of this brought together under the auspices of a society that listened to and was led to believe the virulent messages authored by its scientific, medical, and public health leaders. All of these atrocities executed within this single public facility, organized around a singular, sociopathic mission. For the purpose of furthering science and advancing medical discovery. And all in the name of public health.

THE DOPPELGÄNGER

Back at my hotel that evening, I call my father, Dr. George Schillinger. We three sons always call him by his Hungarian diminutive nickname, Gyuri. He is a retired surgeon who worked in Buffalo, New York, for many years. I want to process with him the role that German medicine—and its individual physicians and public health leaders—played in the Holocaust. He is just finishing up with breakfast. I begin to tell him about my visit to Dachau. He jumps in.

"Deany, I will never, *ever* set foot in that country again. You couldn't kill me to visit a camp. I spent enough time in one. May 1944 to April 1945. Why would I want to go back?"

I gently remind him that I am not calling to convince him to visit Germany or any concentration camp but rather to share with him my visceral reaction to what I saw and experienced. And to hear his thoughts about it—as a survivor and a fellow physician. So I describe to him the malaria chart. Now he listens.

"You know? I don't think I ever told you this story," he begins. Usually this means that I will have to hear one of his Holocaust stories for the umpteenth time and that there is nothing I will be able to do to stop this train once it is rolling.

"A few years before I retire, I had Polish patient, an older man who had urinary retention. Really bad. Could barely pee, and his kidney function had suffer as a result. So, we had to go in there and take out prostate. Not sure what took him so long to come in. But there he was."

He pauses for dramatic effect, as he loves to do.

But this is a new story for me, so I willingly play my role.

"Okay, so what happened next, Gyuri?"

"Well, he was Polish guy from Cheektowaga. A priest. Nice guy. Heavy accent. Indwelling Foley catheter. Anyway, I saw him in my office so I could do pre-op exam and explain him what I needed to do, get him to consent for the procedure. Just bread-and-butter visit."

"But it didn't turn out that way, is that what you're going to tell me?"

"Let me talk! First, he said he told me he'd never consent to the procedure. I told him we'd discuss that later. So, then I had him on table, and I was examining him. You know, basic exam. Just going through motions. As I palpated his suprapubic region and tried to tap out his bladder, I noticed a large diagonal scar running across his left-upper quadrant. So, I said, 'That's strange location for a scar.'"

I interrupt him again. "Wait. Don't tell me."

"Yes. Just listen. So, I asked him if he got into car accident? Or did someone stab him? Or did he have some kind of colon surgery? But he said to me: 'No, Doctor, I am concentration camp survivor. Dachau. They used me for medical experiments.'"

"Jesus H. Christ, Gyuri," I say. "No way. How could you not have told me this story before?"

"Leave me be. How am I supposed to remember what I have told you and what I haven't? Can I continue now?"

"Yes, of course."

"So, I told him I'm survivor too, and we shared a few stories. 'Although I'm not a survivor of medical experiments,' I told him, 'I am a survivor of the world's most destructive public health experiment ever.' So, then I asked him what they did to him. 'Why that scar?' He said, 'I have no idea, Doctor. They did lots of things to me. To all of us, over long period. They never told us what they doing. That was maybe the scariest part. Not knowing what happen or what coming next.'

"After I listened, we shared more horror stories about our mutual experiences at the hands of the Nazis. And then he consented to a procedure that saved his life."

"Incredible, Gyuri. What a story. Did you know that only eighty-two priests survived Dachau? How bizarre that one of the eighty-two ended up being *your* patient. What are the chances?"

We chat some more, and I tell him I love him, and we hang up. My jet lag finally gets the better of me, and I drop off to a dreamless sleep.

Three days later, I am on the runway at Munich airport. Thankfully, it's a direct flight back to San Francisco. As nearly always happens to me, the smell of jet fuel and the gentle motion of the plane as it taxis down the runway before takeoff create a hypnotic effect. I doze into a half sleep, the intermittent and semiconscious slumber of aviation.

Still on the plane, I dream I am back at San Francisco General Hospital, attending on the medical wards. I enter the room of a patient we admitted the afternoon before, an elderly Polish man with *Streptococcus pneumoniae*, known as "the old man's best friend." He'd been quite sick for a week before he finally came in with what turned out to be double pneumonia. He's got four liters of oxygen flowing through tubes into his nostrils. I unbutton my white lab coat, push my rounded spectacles up the bridge of my nose, and inspect the vital signs graph at the foot of the bed.

"Nice to see you awake, Mr. Kuligowski!" I tell him with a smile. "I'm Dr. Klaus Schilling. I'm sure you remember me from a long time ago. But you probably don't remember me from last night. I can tell you: you look better today. You have a classic pneumonia. Both lungs. Fever's still up, but don't worry. It can take two to three days to come down. Your oxygenation still isn't great. The antibiotics will kick in soon, I hope. And then we'll get you outta here and back home. Let me take a listen to you. May I?"

"I *do* remember you," he says. "I asked for you by name."

I laugh, assuming this is his attempt at humor. No one at San Francisco General Hospital's emergency room asks for a doctor by name. I sit him up, part the back of his gown, and direct him to breathe in and out deeply so I can clearly listen to his lung sounds. A whole lot of junk still in there, bilaterally. As expected.

"Okay, you can lie back now. Did you have a bowel movement yet?"

Not waiting for an answer, I pull up his gown and see a large Foley catheter in place and a long diagonal scar over the upper-left quadrant of his abdomen. Had I not seen that yesterday?

"What happened to you here?"

He looks up at me. "I was tortured in World War II. In Dachau. By doctors. I was in your medical experiments."

I forcefully grab his wrist, as if to pin him down, and coldly ask in a whisper, "What did we do to you?"

"Many things. Too many things. Unthinkable things. But what I remember most were the fevers. The high fevers and the nightmares. Scarier than
the torture itself were the nightmares. And the hallucinations. The talk
among the prisoners was that it was malaria. That they were experimenting
on us with malaria."

I tighten my grip on his wrist.

"Right. I remember. We took your spleen out so we could examine it under
the microscope and study how the malaria bug sets up shop and does its
damage."

"Maybe so. I never knew."

"And when you don't have a spleen, you become vulnerable to a number of
infections. Especially those caused by pneumococcus, which happens to be
the exact bug causing the pneumonia you have now."

"So, you're saying I am still suffering from what they did to me?"

"Yes, I guess I am. But tell me, after all you've been through with evil doctors, how did you gather up the courage to seek care, to come to the hospital
and again put yourself in the hands of doctors like me? Is that why it took you
so long to come in the first place?"

"Yes, you are right. I did delay coming. But I knew I could come to *you*. I
knew I could trust you and that you would take care of me. I asked for you by
name, for you specifically. Not for Dr. Schilling, but for you, *Dr. Schillinger*."

I slowly release my grip on his wrist and carefully reposition my hand, now
with my palm resting on the back of his hand. "How did you know that you
could trust me? And do you still believe you can?"

"You are a Jewish doctor, no? And a Jewish scientist?"

"I am, yes, guilty on both counts."

"As a Jew, you have suffered as I have. You have been tortured as I have. You have been experimented on as I have. And as a Jewish doctor and scientist, you recognize more than anyone that the wealth of knowledge and resources and the exceptional privilege provided to you as a physician can either be used for diabolical ends or for divine ends. I know that you will always recognize that conflict, and I trust that your own experience of subjugation will lead you down the right path."

Now I shift my hand to hold his in mine. It is warm. "Thank you for your trust. I hope you are right. You are a Catholic priest, right?"

"I once was, yes."

"Allow me to ask you, Father, as you are a man of faith: How do you reconcile your experiences in Dachau with your belief in the existence of a benevolent and loving God?"

He gently smiles. "My experience, and those of others like me—many not so fortunate as I have been—was not just the experience of a martyr. We have changed the world. We have changed *your* world. Remember, it is because of those experiences, those atrocities, that modern medicine and its research machine developed ethical standards. The outcome of the Nuremberg trials that I am most comforted by is not that the Nazi doctors were convicted of the crimes they committed. Or that some were put to death for their crimes. No. It is because of us that the Nuremberg Code came to be. For the first time, the world created clear rules about what was ethical and legal—and what was not—when conducting human experiments."

I squeeze my eyes tight, trying to remember.

"Yes," I say. "You did accomplish that. The ten points of the Nuremberg Code of 1947. I'm sorry, but I can't remember them all. I'll try:

> "*Voluntary consent of the human subject is essential.*
> "*The experiment should be designed to yield fruitful results for the good of all of society, unprocurable by other methods or means of study.*
> "*The experiment should be so conducted as to avoid all unnecessary physical and mental suffering and injury.*
> "*No experiment should be conducted where there is an a priori reason to believe that death or disabling injury will occur.*

"*Proper preparations should be made and adequate facilities provided to protect the experimental subject against even remote possibilities of injury, disability, or death.*

"*During the course of the experiment the human subject should always be at liberty to bring the experiment to an end if he has reached the physical or mental state where continuation of the experiment seems to him to be impossible.*

"*During the course of the experiment the scientist in charge must be prepared to terminate the experiment at any stage, if he has probable cause to believe, in the exercise of the good faith, superior skill and careful judgment required of him that a continuation of the experiment is likely to result in injury, disability, or death to the experimental subject.*"

"That's very good, Dr. Schillinger. It is good that you remember seven of these points. But I—Father Josef Kuligowski—will be the perennial reminder for those who would hijack the marvels of medicine and the wonders of science to do evil. Any evil. Do not forget that. And—as you continue in your medical work, your scientific work, your public health work—do not ever forget me."

Nine hours later, we begin our descent, with the sun rising over the Sierras. I lift the window shade to see we are approaching the Bay Area from the northeast. We fly over the Richmond–San Rafael Bridge; the skyline of the awakening city sparkles before me, off to the right of the advancing plane. I find Market Street, its diagonal incision crossing the city, and I search south to find my hospital campus in the distance, taking it in with a bird's-eye view. A seemingly unplanned and haphazardly arranged thirteen-acre compound: a collection of old, art deco–style redbrick buildings adorned with green-colored copper roofs surround a brutalist, blocklike, gray, long, concrete building with a rooftop chimney spewing steam from its boiler room, all set off by a singular, contemporary, tall, glass-covered circular structure with a garden rooftop, situated at the compound's westernmost border. Each set of buildings representing a different era in US medicine, each set designed to affirmatively respond to the unique social epidemics of its day. The first set of structures, built in 1915, served as hospital wards whose primary purpose was to quarantine and care for the city's many low-income residents suffering from cholera, typhoid fever, and tuberculosis. It ultimately evolved to spawn an International TB Center of Excellence. The second building, constructed in 1972, marked an important epidemiologic transition in the city and our country. Its primary function was as a trauma center, designed to respond to the unmitigated gun violence occurring in the context of a drug epidemic, but quickly expanded to become the epicenter of the AIDS epidemic and ultimately served as the engine and the model for our nation's response to it. And the third-generation structure, built in 2016 in response to new seismic codes, financed by an $800 million municipal bond measure that passed with an unprecedented 83 percent majority, is the Grand Central Station for the poor person's epidemic of our day: type 2 diabetes, a noncommunicable disease that can lead to kidney failure, amputation, heart attack, or stroke. And onto the backs of those very same individuals and populations left to struggle with these modern-day epidemics piled the opportunistic pandemic of COVID-19.

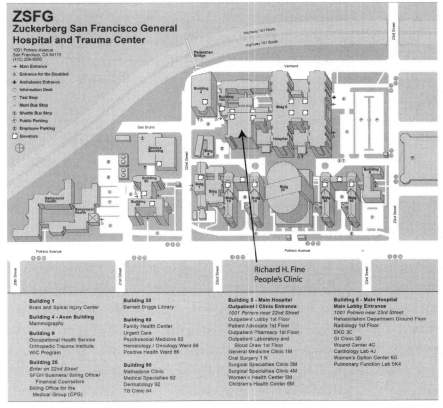

Courtesy of the San Francisco Department of Public Health.

We fly over the campus, toward the airport. I remember Eduardo. And I remember Dachau and Father Kuligowski. As the hospital compound disappears behind me, a warmth again spreads through my body. A pleasant visceral sensation reminds me of how fortunate I am to work at this unique and special place, one in which some bad things but mostly good things have been happening every day for 150 years: sometimes even real miracles, and sometimes small disasters. And some of them involving me. A public institution—with its singular mission—that at least aspires to respond to social ills in a positive way. A sanctuary for so many, helping the most marginalized recover and heal from the brutal realities of our society. And yes—despite its blemishes—perhaps a beacon of humanity casting its light to outshine medicine's darkest past.

Physicians are endowed by society with a degree of power and authority, part of which comes from our unique knowledge of clinical science and our experience in treating and sometimes curing illness. But much of this power comes from the fact that our role is to care for people who are sick, who are truly suffering, and who genuinely and urgently need our help. As such, people often willingly relinquish their own power to us; they ask us to wield our powers to help them become well again.

Physicians most often take this responsibility to heart, and we try to deliver care in a humanistic fashion. However, given the numerous and growing pressures of the job, the diverse and sometimes perverse incentives that drive individual physicians and health systems, and the social and structural inequities that are the engine for disease, this model of humanistic medical care is often undermined. In fact, the delegation of power and authority to physicians, especially when it occurs in the context of a discriminatory society that generates unequal exposures to health hazards and unequal access to health care, can lead to dehumanization in medical care. This risk is amplified in the under-resourced settings that disproportionately care for marginalized patients. And when institutions and their health care staff dehumanize "the other," bad things happen to patients and their communities.

It is my belief and my experience that we can inoculate ourselves against this risk when we bring together the best that science has to offer with the gift that patient narratives offer, positively influencing the culture of medicine and the institutions in which we work. We can only achieve this alchemy by eliciting our patients' stories, by truly listening to these stories, and by acting on them in affirmative ways. Such stories can break down barriers and open up windows into other people's lives in ways that not only assist in diagnosis and treatment but also create deep connections that humanize and improve the experience of illness, suffering, coping, recovery, or death. While the stories I have shared reveal how true this is for the individual patients I have cared for, this also holds true for the many of us who will find ourselves subjected to illness and suffering. This means that we all have a stake in ensuring that health care systems not only provide equitable care but also deliver the kind of care in which each individual's unique story is elicited, valued, and incorporated into their treatment plans.

Apart from making the case for the critical role that places like my own flagship public hospital play in our country, what else do the stories I've told mean for public health? When we aggregate these stories across patients, when we attend to the patterns that comprise what I have called a *narrative epidemiology*, what emerges is a larger, mostly untold story. This story tells of the ill effects of marginalization on health—how unequal exposure to hazardous environments and unhealthy social conditions emerging from this marginalization—and the social policies that have created them—generate unconscionable and consequential inequities, drive health care spending, and drain resources from other worthy causes. These are scientifically proven facts, but when animated by a narrative epidemiology, such lessons become clearer, more relevant, and more meaningful to all of us. Through this process, the alchemy of science and story could generate changes in public policy that would humanize our society, reducing preventable suffering and death.

It is my hope that we more purposefully and consistently elicit and attend to each other's stories, breaking down the walls that divide us and opening up more doors to see into and identify with each other's real lives and experiences. And that we should tell these stories to others inside and outside our circles, creating opportunities for more mutual understanding and empathy. These narrative acts will help us to feel more connected to one another. And in so doing, we will become more generous, more inclusive, and more healing in how we relate to one another as individuals and communities, and in how we craft health and social policy for us all.

Acknowledgments

I HAVE MANY PEOPLE TO THANK FOR THE CONTRIBUTIONS THEY EACH MADE in helping me turn this idea for a book into a reality. I first want to thank Eyal Press, an amazing writer, social critic, and childhood friend from Buffalo, New York (*Go Bills!*), for his unwavering support of my efforts and for his assistance in getting my book the attention it needed. I also am deeply grateful to Joanne Kagle, who granted me the three dimensions of time, space, and place with which to work on my book, trusting only that I might have something important to say. My close friend and an accomplished writer in her own right, Beth Kobliner, gave me her unwavering confidence and encouragement, reassuring me that someone, somewhere, someday, somehow, would absolutely say yes to publishing this book.

Bonnie Nadell of Hill Nadell Literary Agency took on the challenging task of helping me prepare my book proposal and eventually steering it to acceptance. Her clear guidance around message and her straight talk around structure allowed me to transform a series of individual patient vignettes into a more impactful whole. Clive Priddle at PublicAffairs was the first publisher to truly understand what I was trying to do and to embrace it. He also was wise enough to assign the gifted editor Anupama Roy-Chaudhury to take me on as her patient. She helped me diagnose what needed fixing (and surgical cutting!) and provided sage clinical advice to ensure I connected each story to the main themes of the book.

Cannon Thomas, PhD, of CTP Strategies was with me every step of the way—from initial conception to final execution. He has a magical gift of enabling his clients to identify those aspects of their lives and their work that are most meaningful to them, to focus on their skills and their talents, and to help them blend skillful effort with values-based determination to achieve the goals they set out to achieve. I am deeply grateful to him in so many ways.

A number of other friends and writers helped me move through this prolonged process. The wonderful writer and editor Emilia Sowersby graciously offered up her skills to help me get my book proposal into shape, and she served as a gentle sounding board whenever I hit the inevitable speed bump in the editorial process. Jason Thompson validated the challenges inherent to writing a book while working as a clinician and busy academic, and he provided important advice about sticking to my main message when I was veering adrift. I also am thankful for Josh Davis's early encouragement and for his kind introduction to his literary agent, Bonnie Nadell, who then became my agent. I am sure that the nature of his introduction did as much for my cause as did her read of my early manuscript. Longtime friend and writer Ayelet Waldman also gave me the push I needed to finish this book and try to get it published. She also connected me to writer and editor Meredith Maran, who helped me brainstorm how to frame the book in ways that were true to my intentions. Mark Steisel provided me with early editorial feedback and advice that served me well.

I am also thankful to the remarkably talented young poets from Youth Speaks, who were kind enough to allow me to reprint some of their poems. Their amazing video-poems, and other poems from the Bigger Picture campaign, can be viewed at www.thebiggerpicture.org.

I am deeply indebted to my brilliant and truly committed colleagues at San Francisco General Hospital, especially those in the Division of General Internal Medicine and the Center for Vulnerable Populations. There are too many to individually name. I am so grateful for the positive influence they each have had on me, and I am proud of our collective efforts to humanize medicine and public health.

I am most grateful to my primary care patients, all of whom I care for in the Richard H. Fine People's Clinic at San Francisco General Hospital. They have openly shared with me the most intimate details of their lived experiences, communicated the nature of their greatest fears, expressed the depths of their suffering, transmitted both their gratitude and their criticisms, and revealed the wellsprings of strength that sustain them. I hope that this book functions as one means to advocate on their behalf for robust safety net health care systems, for meaningful primary care–based relationships, and for the kinds of positive social and policy changes that will better their living conditions and their health.

My parents, George and Zahava Schillinger, transmitted to me from my earliest days, in different ways, how important communication is to success and even to survival. The inspiring careers of my aunt, Sara Joel, and my late uncle, Dr. Nahum Joel, provided me with invaluable examples of the power of story and of science. Theirs is the core lesson of this book.

Finally, I want to thank my life partner and champion for equal justice, Ariella Hyman. You always have been, and continue to be, my truest inspiration.

Credits

The chapters entitled "The Disability Blues" and "Patagonia Pastorale" were originally published in the *Journal of the American Medical Association* on January 7, 1998, and October 4, 2006, respectively. Permission to reprint these stories was granted by the American Medical Association on October 26, 2023.

The chapter entitled "The Quixotic Pursuit of Quality" was originally published in *Intima: A Journal of Narrative Medicine* in the Fall 2015 issue at theintima.org. Permission to reprint this story was granted by the publisher.

The table and figure used in Chapter 11 was reprinted with permission from *The Medical Management of Vulnerable and Underserved Patients: Principles, Practice and Populations*, 2nd edition, edited by T. King, M. Wheeler, A. Bindman, A. Fernandez, K. Grumbach, D. Schillinger, T. Villela (New York: McGraw-Hill Education, 2016).

A portion of the proceeds from the sale of this book will be donated to the San Francisco General Hospital Foundation, https://sfghf.org/.

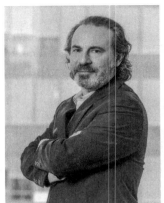

Dean-David Schillinger is a primary care physician, scientist, author, and public health advocate. He is an expert in health communication and has been widely recognized for his work related to improving the health of marginalized populations. He is credited with a number of discoveries in primary care and health communication and is considered a pioneer in the field of health literacy. He is the inaugural recipient of the Andrew B. Bindman Professorship in Primary Care and Health Policy at the University of California San Francisco (UCSF). Dr. Schillinger has served as chief of the UCSF Division of General Internal Medicine at San Francisco General Hospital and chief of the Diabetes Prevention and Control Program for the California Department of Public Health. In 2006, he cofounded the UCSF Center for Vulnerable Populations, a leading research center committed to addressing the social, environmental, and commercial determinants of health through research, education, policy, and practice. He currently directs the UCSF Health Communications Research Program.

PublicAffairs is a publishing house founded in 1997. It is a tribute to the standards, values, and flair of three persons who have served as mentors to countless reporters, writers, editors, and book people of all kinds, including me.

I. F. STONE, proprietor of *I. F. Stone's Weekly*, combined a commitment to the First Amendment with entrepreneurial zeal and reporting skill and became one of the great independent journalists in American history. At the age of eighty, Izzy published *The Trial of Socrates*, which was a national bestseller. He wrote the book after he taught himself ancient Greek.

BENJAMIN C. BRADLEE was for nearly thirty years the charismatic editorial leader of *The Washington Post*. It was Ben who gave the *Post* the range and courage to pursue such historic issues as Watergate. He supported his reporters with a tenacity that made them fearless and it is no accident that so many became authors of influential, best-selling books.

ROBERT L. BERNSTEIN, the chief executive of Random House for more than a quarter century, guided one of the nation's premier publishing houses. Bob was personally responsible for many books of political dissent and argument that challenged tyranny around the globe. He is also the founder and longtime chair of Human Rights Watch, one of the most respected human rights organizations in the world.

.   .   .

For fifty years, the banner of Public Affairs Press was carried by its owner Morris B. Schnapper, who published Gandhi, Nasser, Toynbee, Truman, and about 1,500 other authors. In 1983, Schnapper was described by *The Washington Post* as "a redoubtable gadfly." His legacy will endure in the books to come.

Peter Osnos, *Founder*